Mononeuropathies:

Examination, Diagnosis and Treatment

Mononeuropathies:

Examination, Diagnosis and Treatment

A. Staal
Emeritus Professor of Neurology,
Erasmus University, Rotterdam

J. van Gijn
Professor and Chairman,
University Department of Neurology, Utrecht

F. Spaans
Professor of Clinical Neurophysiology,
University of Maastricht

Drawings by
D. Hasan
Lecturer in Neurology,
Erasmus University, Rotterdam

W. B. SAUNDERS

London • Edinburgh • New York • Philadelphia • Sydney • Toronto

WB SAUNDERS
A Division of Harcourt Brace and Company Limited

ISBN 0-7020-1779-5

British Library Cataloguing in Publication Data
A catalogue record for this book is available from the British Library

Library of Congress Cataloging in Publication Data
A catalog record for this book is available from the Library of Congress

Medical knowledge is constantly changing. As new information becomes available, changes in treatment, procedures, equipment and the use of drugs become necessary. The authors and Publishers have, as far as it is possible, taken care to ensure that the information given in the text is accurate and up to date. However, readers are strongly advised to confirm that the information, especially with regard to drug usage, complies with latest legislation and standards of practice.

The Publishers and authors have made every effort to trace the copyright holders for borrowed material. If they have inadvertently overlooked any, they will be pleased to rectify the matter at the first opportunity.

Commissioning Editor: Miranda Bromage
Project Supervisor: Mark Sanderson
Senior Project Editor: Carol Parr
Design: Sarah Cape

The publisher's policy is to use paper manufactured from sustainable forests

Typeset by Saxon Graphics Ltd, Derby, UK
Printed and bound in Great Britain at the Bath Press, Avon, UK

Contents

Foreword

Neurologists have no monopoly on mononeuropathies. Orthopaedic surgeons, hand surgeons, neurosurgeons, diabetologists, infectious diseases specialists, general physicians, and others are all likely to see, and attempt to treat, surprisingly large numbers of patients with mononeuropathies. Therefore, no one type of specialist sees the 'whole picture'. They, and I, need a monograph like this one, which paints in what we each individually should know about but don't, even though maybe we once did. We may all have the anatomy of the carpal tunnel at our fingertips but not many of us know quite where the the posterior cutaneous nerve of the thigh is to be found, let alone how to examine it neurophysiologically. And, although we all know that unwisely placed injections in the buttock cause a sciatic nerve palsy (despite probably having never seen a case), we need a list to refer to of all the possible causes, however surprising (can credit cards in the back pocket really do such compressive damage?). This monograph supplies us with all the diagnostic information we need, as well as with what there is to know about prognosis and treatment, a rather evidence-free zone in most instances. The information is provided in a user-friendly and well-illustrated way, with clear diagrams and informative case vignettes. But this is just what one would expect from these Dutch authors, who not only write with enthusiasm and knowledge of their subject, but also with the authority of people who actually see patients in real clinical life with all its uncertainties, frustrations and occasional triumphs.

Charles P. Warlow
Edinburgh

Preface

This book reflects our shared interest in mononeuropathies, for some of us a life-long affair. But, is this sufficient reason for giving in to 'the incurable disease of writing', as Juvenal called it, and producing another book on the subject? After all, we have not only admired but endlessly thumbed successive editions of Mumenthaler and Schliack's monograph, and Stewart's more recent concise and authoritative volume. The pretext for putting together our own book is the inclusion of a few special features – none of which is unique on its own, but perhaps are as an ensemble.

First, a mononeuropathy has to be recognized through physical examination before it can be explained and treated. The diagnostic process is simple in execution but complex in conceptual background, because it involves detailed knowledge of muscle function and skin innervation, knowledge that few neurologists have at their fingertips. We ourselves have time and again taken recourse to the pictures in that invaluable British booklet, 'Aids to the Examination of the Peripheral Nervous System'. But, once the deficit has been successfully localized in one or more single nerves, the reader has to turn to another book for instruction about possible causes, prognosis and treatment. In this monograph we have tried to bring the two elements together, in a guide to both the examination and the nosological information. With regard to the examination element, numerous original drawings have been made by Dr Djo Hasan. However, in many cases the design of the 'Aids ...' format could not be improved upon, and we gratefully acknowledge our indebtedness to the consecutive editorial committees of that venerable publication.

A second characteristic is that we have interspersed brief case vignettes throughout the text. We hope the personal flavour of these scenes from clinical life will complement the systematic narrative, by providing some instruction as well as a modicum of diversion. Also, we have included brief sections about electrophysiological investigations. Lastly, several citations refer to publications in languages other than English, but we hope to have resisted successfully the temptation to make the bibliography exhaustive rather than informative.

We are obliged to Fleur Bominaar for expert secretarial support, and to our families for having so graciously endured our preoccupation with this project.

Chapter 1
Introduction

Mononeuropathies are common disorders in the sense that even general practitioners have to deal with them occasionally, although for most family doctors the experience will be limited to the carpal tunnel syndrome and perhaps a drop foot from peroneal nerve compression or a weak hand from ulnar nerve compression at the elbow. Other mononeuropathies should be regarded as the exclusive domain of the neurologist, who is expected to diagnose and treat all varieties, common or rare.

Mononeuropathies give rise to paraesthesia, numbness, weakness and wasting, and sometimes also to pain as a prominent symptom. The causes are manifold, but the great majority are associated with focal compression. Compression of peripheral nerves within narrow passages of normal anatomical structures are called 'entrapment neuropathies'. In the past many arguments have been exchanged about the pathogenesis of nerve compression: mechanical damage to myelin sheaths and axons or ischaemia due to compression of the vasa nervorum. We prefer to remain on the fence in this issue, and tend to agree with what has been said about carpal tunnel syndrome in particular: 'It is as naive to blame the pathophysiology of nerve compression solely on ischaemia as it is to do so just on primary mechanical damage'

(Rosenbaum and Ochoa, 1993). There is no doubt that focal damage to a nerve can lead to segmental demyelination and paranodal myelin swelling (Ochoa *et al.*, 1972); this is later followed by axonal degeneration and further demyelination, or by remyelination if axons have remained intact. On the other hand, chronic endoneurial oedema in entrapped nerves is a likely consequence of haemodynamic derangement (Sunderland, 1978). The electrophysiological correlates of these changes in the structure of nerves are described at the end of this chapter.

Anatomy

Peripheral nerves are made up of fibres from dorsal and ventral roots. On each side of each spinal segment these join together to form spinal nerves, which after only a short distance across the intervertebral foramina again divide into dorsal and ventral rami; the dorsal rami innervate the paraspinal muscles and skin, and the ventral rami of the cervical and lumbosacral spinal nerves combine to form the brachial and lumbosacral plexuses. The individual nerves to the limbs originate from these plexuses. The ventral rami of thoracic origin form the intercostal nerves, except that from the first thoracic nerve, which joins the brachial plexus.

Causes of mononeuropathies

The vast majority of the mononeuropathies are caused by compression or stretching of nerves in narrow but otherwise normal anatomical passages, or by anomalous muscles or fibrous bands (*entrapment neuropathies*). Alternatively, superficial nerves may be compressed by external pressure. Another important category is formed by *iatrogenic damage*. This occurs mostly during surgical procedures, either by direct pressure or stretch (at the site of operation or via retractor blades), or by malpositioning during general anaesthesia. Other causes are local disease processes, including *infectious diseases* such as leprosy, herpes zoster, diphtheria and Lyme disease, *space-occupying lesions* such as cysts, nerve sheath tumours or compartment syndromes, *ischaemic nerve lesions*, and *physical causes* (lightning, burns or frostbite). Autoimmune disorders associated with mononeuropathies may be confined to the peripheral nervous system (neuralgic amyotrophy), or the diseases may be systemic, such as in rheumatoid arthritis, connective tissue disease, polyarteritis nodosa or temporal arteritis. Another category of causes is that of *metabolic and endocrine disorders*: diabetes mellitus, thyroid diseases and acromegaly. Efforts to be complete at this stage are doomed to fail, but this list at least gives the most frequent causes of mononeuropathies.

In patients with systemic disease a mononeuropathy may evolve into a plexopathy, a *multiple mononeuropathy* or a polyneuropathy. Therefore, the mononeuropathies associated with more or less generalized conditions will be dealt with in separate chapters at the end of this book. In contrast, the local causes of mononeuropathy are often more or less specific for the anatomical region and are listed under the heading of the nerve in question.

Epidemiology

Some compression neuropathies are far more frequent than others. The most common entrapment neuropathy is the carpal tunnel syndrome, which occurs most commonly in adult women, with a prevalence rate as high as 9% (de Krom *et al.*, 1992). Other mononeuropathies are equally distributed across the two sexes, except when associated with more or less sex-specific activities (for example, peroneal nerve palsy from paving a road with cobblestones, or compression of the superficial radial nerve by handcuffs), or with gynaecological operations (in which the femoral nerve may be damaged).

No formal studies exist of the frequency of mononeuropathies other than compression of the median nerve at the wrist. In the hospital records of one of us, lesions of the ulnar nerve at the elbow came second, being four times less common than the carpal tunnel syndrome and twice as common as the third most common mononeuropathy, peroneal nerve lesions at the knee. Radial nerve lesions at the upper arm and ulnar nerve lesions at the wrist were much more uncommon; all other mononeuropathies are sufficiently rare that a general practitioner caring for some 2000 patients never will see an example in his or her lifetime.

The history

When should a compression neuropathy be suspected? It is an old dictum in neurology that the cause of a disorder is hidden in the patient's history and that the site of the lesion is detected by examination. This is not always true in compression neuropathies. Often, one can determine the site of the lesion by asking about habits or postures relevant to the nerve in question. Of course, to begin with one should listen patiently to the patient's story, with as few interruptions as possible. The symptoms should be described in plain language, without contamination by medical terms or interpretations by other physicians. One should be wary of physician-patients or allied health professionals who begin by telling that they have a radial nerve palsy. From the outset it has to be made clear what a patient means by terms such as 'numbness', 'weakness', or 'loss of control'. A limb may be called 'numb' or 'dead' when it cannot be moved, or 'lame' when the skin is insensitive to touch. Only after the symptoms have been listed in the patient's words may these be translated into neurological notions. The diagnostic hypotheses that have been formed during the history-taking will often prompt direct questions, aimed at confirming or refuting the initial conjectures. Too penetrating questioning may be misleading, as this may erroneously induce the patient to admit the symptom that is sought. This is one of the most crucial issues in history-taking, and even after many years of experience one may catch oneself committing errors that we teach our residents to avoid. It seems a platitude to say that disorders unknown to the physician are not unearthed, but it is an oft-forgotten truth. One needs to be familiar with a certain pattern of history in order to piece together a comprehensible history, but even with such experience the penny may not always drop. At the end of the history-taking it is often helpful to recapitulate the symptoms in non-medical terms as one has understood them, and to ask the patient if the given summary is a fair one.

Since in mononeuropathies compression is by far the most frequent cause, this possibility should be explored before other, more esoteric conditions. The typical situation in compression neuropathy is that of a healthy person of either sex and any age presenting with recent weakness or numbness in a single limb, for example a foot drop. The patient may be worried about having had a stroke, as many adults are most familiar with that explanation for a sudden loss of function in one arm or leg. However, enquiry into the immediate past will uncover an unusual activity, such as squatting for hours during yesterday's gardening. Further questioning may show that, during that action, the foot 'went to sleep'. Other than with chronic pressure, subacute compression or stretch of a nerve is nearly always painless. If there was no such episode of intensive gardening but the foot drop was noticed on awakening, one should ask about the possibility of an unusually deep sleep, brought about by sleeping pills or heavy drinking. A negative answer does not rule out compression, but a history of intoxication is almost conclusive for the diagnosis. The collective list of activities associated with a particular nerve is formidable; these will be dealt with in the chapters on individual nerves.

An important question in retrieving the cause of a compression neuropathy is about symptoms of the same kind in the patient's own past, or in that of family members. A positive answer to this simple but sometimes neglected question may lead to a probable diagnosis of hereditary neuropathy with liability to pressure palsies (see Chapter 25).

A minority of mononeuropathies are caused by factors other than compression, and the history-taking may uncover these. In many developing countries, leprosy affects millions of people, including people from western countries living there. Neurological manifestations are polyneuritis, mononeuritis multiplex and mononeuritis, in all cases with nerve thickening, especially of cutaneous nerves. Lyme disease (borreliosis) is endemic in some areas, and tends to involve nerve roots rather than peripheral nerves, but the subject of tick bites should be brought up with patients who work in forestry or who have recently spent a holiday in woodland. Herpes zoster also typically involves single roots, and it is associated with characteristic skin lesions; the condition is mentioned here because it may involve the territory of intercostal nerves. Iatrogenic factors will rarely be suppressed in the history. Examples are injections in the buttock (sciatic nerve lesions), intra-arterial puncture in the axilla (damage to median and ulnar nerves), venepuncture (lesions of the median nerve at the elbow), tight cuffs applied for bloodless operations on limbs, X-rays, and overheated, incorrectly placed electrodes during operations. Physical causes outside the medical sphere are a defective microwave apparatus, laser beams, and accidental electrocution. In fact the list of possible causes of mononeuropathy is almost endless.

In summary, the general point we wish to emphasize is that the physician should adopt a detective-like inquisitiveness. Persistent probing for possible circumstances in which symptoms occur should become a compulsive habit, at least before other causes are entertained. It is certainly true that a great many disease conditions can contribute to mononeuropathies even at common sites of entrapment such as the carpal tunnel, from leprosy to acromegaly, but these are far less common than compression by normal anatomical structures. A sound history-taking can never be replaced by laboratory investigations, however extensive. Sometimes it may even be necessary to invoke the help of relatives: it is not exceptional to find that the patient is unaware of certain habits or postures that may have been noticed by other members of the family.

Sensory symptoms

The rate at which a mononeuropathy develops as a result of external compression, stretching or of entrapment in a narrow canal or muscle compartment may be as fast as hours (for example, a radial nerve palsy occurring in an intoxicated sleep) or as slow as days, weeks, months or even years, as occurs in

the carpal tunnel syndrome or in ulnar nerve compression at the elbow. Patients with a pre-existing polyneuropathy, such as in diabetes, alcoholism or hereditary polyneuropathy, are probably particularly vulnerable to compression neuropathies.

Precipitating activities or circumstances are often important clues to the diagnosis. In some cases paraesthesia are continuous, but in carpal tunnel syndrome the symptoms appear especially at night and also during activities such as needlework or driving a car. In the foot, paraesthesia and pain may develop only on standing or walking, which points to Morton's neuroma or tarsal tunnel syndrome, depending on whether the symptoms occur only in the foot or also in the leg. We should like to stress again that paraesthesia are much more specific for a neuropathy than is pain alone, and that these sensations often, although not invariably, remain within the territory of the compressed nerve. Pain is a much less specific symptom, as it may be felt somewhere in the course of the nerve, far outside the area of sensory innervation of the nerve, and sometimes even proximal to the point of compression. Of course the patient does not complain about paraesthesia but about a hand or foot 'going to sleep', 'tingling', 'pins and needles', 'a feeling of electricity', 'a funny feeling' or 'a bad circulation'. These symptoms are mostly experienced in the distal distribution of the nerve, especially in fingertips or toes. An exception is meralgia paraesthetica, where symptoms may be experienced only in the central part of the innervation area of the lateral cutaneous nerve of the thigh.

Sensory deficits are often described as 'numbness' or 'a dead feeling'.

Motor symptoms

Motor symptoms are often not clearly explained by the patient or not even noticed at all, especially when the affected limb is also painful. Conversely, if patients have a painful limb they may complain of severe weakness whereas there is none on examination. And, if weakness does exist, the patient may call it 'numbness'.

Finally, the history-taking should include questions about the general health of the patient, and about professional activities and family structure. The former part of the history may give important clues about predisposing factors for neuropathies such as diabetes, rheumatoid arthritis and hypothyroidism, and the latter may uncover alcoholism or activities that may be hazardous for peripheral nerves. In fact a history-taking is never finished, and repetition of some questions in a second encounter may still produce important information.

The neurological examination

The neurological examination concerns an integrated system relating to the entire body; for this reason it is rarely, if ever, wise to limit the examination to the part of the body where the symptoms are, as a surgeon or dermatologist is used to doing. For example, in case of foot drop one should not forget to examine the facial muscles and the arm on the same side, in order not to miss a hemiparesis, of which foot drop is the most prominent symptom.

The sensory examination

If the history includes numbness of a body part one should ask patients to outline the area themselves. Of course this must be verified by the examiner, preferably with a piece of cotton wool and by pinprick. Needles worn in doctors' lapels have, rightly, gone out of fashion in the era of hepatitis virus and human immunodeficiency virus, and disposable needles tend to draw blood easily; a splinter of an orange stick broken in two will often produce the necessary sensation of sharpness without transmitting microorganisms or messing up the patient's clothing. The area of the sensory deficit is mapped from the centre to the periphery (the patient cannot indicate

negative perceptions, except in conversion disorder). If there is only slight sensory deficit, examination of two-point discrimination may help to delineate this. The examination of vibration sense or position sense is not helpful in cases of suspected pressure neuropathies. It is not uncommon to find no sensory disturbance at all in the area where sensory symptoms (positive or negative) are experienced. The distinction of a presumed peripheral nerve lesion from disorders of cervical and lumbar roots on the basis of a sensory deficit may be difficult, first because the extent of the area may differ according to the examiner or the occasion, and secondly because the territories often overlap. Other symptoms and signs are often decisive.

If an area of the skin is less sensitive one should look for old or recent (surgical) scars, which may point to a neuroma of a cutaneous nerve. Palpating the affected part of the skin with light pressure of the fingertips may also disclose a small tumour, such as a neurofibroma in von Recklinghausen's disease, or a thickened cutaneous nerve in Charcot–Marie–Tooth disease or in leprosy. If paraesthesia are present one should try and find a spot from where these symptoms may be elicited by light tapping, which locates the site of the lesion (Hoffmann–Tinel sign).

If the sensory findings remain vague, or if the patient is not cooperative, it is best to stop this part of the examination. Some patients are apt to report exquisite subtleties of sensation; as a rule this results not only in loss of time but also in implausible hypotheses. It is better to tell the patient from the start that slight differences in perception should be ignored. In general, the longer it takes to do a sensory examination the less reliable the results are.

The motor examination

One should start with inspection of the limbs in search of atrophy, fasciculations, abnormal swellings or abnormal postures such as a dropping hand. This is followed by a systematic examination of muscle strength. The technique for testing individual muscles is discussed in the chapters on the different nerves. Yet we should like to mention the general rule that a muscle is best tested in a position where it is maximally shortened, so that optimal force is produced. For example, the biceps brachii is tested with the patient's arm flexed, and the tibialis anterior with the foot in dorsiflexion. Of course there are exceptions, two to be precise: the quadriceps femoris and the triceps brachii. If either of these two extensor muscles is maximally shortened, that is, if the limb is straightened at the elbow or the knee, it is usually impossible for the examiner to change this position of the limb even in the presence of moderate weakness. The reason for this is a combination of two factors: first, the large force of the extensor muscle in question, especially the quadriceps; and, secondly, the tendency of the knee or elbow joint to 'lock up'. Therefore the triceps brachii and quadriceps femoris muscles should be tested with the limb in flexion, where these muscles are at a mechanical disadvantage (see Figures 7.3 and 16.4).

Strength can best be graded according to the system of the Medical Research Council (MRC), despite considerable interobserver variation, especially when strength is only slightly diminished (grade 4). When a muscle is tested it should be clear to patients what they are being asked to do, if possible by the physician first showing the movement. If words are necessary these should be given in plain language, such as 'pushing away', 'pulling', 'cocking up the feet', etc.; terms such as 'extension' should be avoided. If necessary, patients should repeatedly be encouraged to use all available strength. If there is much pain a single second of full strength is enough. Sometimes, weakness in one muscle makes it impossible to test the strength in another. For example, it is not possible for a patient to separate the

fingers (interossei; ulnar nerve) if there is paralysis of the extensors of the wrist and fingers (radial nerve), unless the fingers are passively supported; even then spurious 'weakness' may lead the unwary to false conclusions about the site of the lesion.

Testing the tendon reflexes is again an objective part of the examination. Unfortunately, in mononeuropathies these are often normal because the nerve in question is not part of the reflex arc. Even if it is, the tendon reflexes may be normal if weakness is only slight.

Examination of the autonomic nervous system

Inspection of the skin may reveal ulceration, a pale colour or a dry and scaly surface in the distribution of a given nerve. Absence of the normal skin dimpling after the hand or foot is held under water for five to ten minutes is fairly typical but not often tested. If the abnormalities of the skin prove to be painless on pinprick the possibility of diabetic polyneuropathy, syringomyelia or leprosy should be considered. In leprosy the skin may also show depigmentation. Complete analgesia occurs only if a peripheral nerve is virtually sectioned, which does not occur in compression neuropathy. All this having been said, in most compression neuropathies the skin looks normal.

Diagnostic pitfalls

Some problems commonly obstruct the road to a rapid diagnosis and adequate therapeutic advice (Table 1.1). In the history-taking, preceding events do not always receive the emphasis they deserve. Few patients will fail to mention a fracture or an operation (mononeuropathy caused by ill-fitting plasters or malpositioning during anaesthesia), but they may remain silent about intoxications, or simply disregard relevant activities such as sitting habits (peroneal nerve), posture while driving (ulnar nerve at the elbow), kneeling in the garden for hours (peroneal nerve), prolonged bed rest (ulnar or peroneal nerve), long cycling tours (ulnar nerve in the palm), or seemingly harmless circumstances such as keeping a bunch of credit cards in one's back pocket (sciatic nerve), or handling screwdrivers, pliers or the mouse of a computer (ulnar nerve in the palm). In order to keep this monograph readable as well as relevant, we have largely omitted references to occupational palsies associated with handicrafts that no longer exist, whereas we have done our best to include most of the modern leisure activities that have replaced manual labour as one of the main causes of mononeuropathies in the industrialized world (for example, damage to the suprascapular nerve by playing baseball).

Of course the distribution of the symptoms is an important element in diagnosing a mononeuropathy. One should, however, take care not to dismiss too rapidly the possibility of compression of a single nerve if the pain and paraesthesia are reported somewhat outside the recognized skin territory of the nerve in question. For example, patients with an otherwise classical carpal tunnel syndrome may report pins and needles in all fingers, including the fourth and fifth (inexplicably, the reverse situation seems to arise much less often with ulnar nerve compression at the elbow, in which paraesthesia tend to be limited to the appropriate area, namely the fifth finger and the ulnar half of the fourth finger). Another pitfall in localizing the lesion is that pain, whether a dull ache or sharp stabs, may be felt far proximal from the entrapment point at the wrist; the best example is again the carpal tunnel syndrome, in which the pain may radiate up the entire arm, to the shoulder or even the neck. The probable explanation is that 'nerve trunk pain' is not, as in the case of paraesthesia, a phenomenon mediated by the sensory fibres within the nerve that innervate a specific area of skin, but presumably by separate nociceptive nerve endings in the nerve trunk (Asbury and Fields, 1984). These intrinsic pain receptors (nervi nervorum) have a poor somatotopic representation in the central nervous system, analogous to headache with involvement of the meninges.

In mononeuropathies there may be paraesthesia without pain, unless the nerve contains only motor fibres. But, if there is only pain without paraesthesia, the diagnosis of nerve entrapment should be seriously doubted. Especially in the absence of neurological signs or even the absence of abnormalities on a nerve conduction study or needle electromyography, nerve entrapment is an improbable cause. In the last decades some (orthopaedic) surgeons have developed a deplorable tendency to advocate operation for pain in the absence of any neurological abnormality whatsoever, on the nebulous assumption that the symptoms should be attributed to compression of a nerve that happens to be in the vicinity of the painful area. As a general rule these are 'pseudo-entrapment syndromes', the actual cause being overused muscles, bands, ligaments, joints, or a somatisation syndrome on the

Table 1.1
Pitfalls in the diagnosis of mononeuropathies

- The patient may not be aware that preceding activities or events are often relevant

- Paraesthesia may radiate outside the standard skin territory of a nerve

- Pain may be felt proximal to the site of entrapment

- It is wrong to diagnose a mononeuropathy if there is pain alone, without paraesthesia or deficits

- Compression of only part of a nerve may falsely suggest a more distal site of compression

- Mononeuropathies should be distinguished from lesions in the central nervous system or elsewhere in the peripheral nervous system

basis of a depressive illness or personality disorder. Of course several of these factors may coexist and interact. Most neurologists will have seen patients after unsuccessful operation on a cervical rib or, even worse, on a first rib, for 'pain in the arm' that clearly resulted from a carpal tunnel syndrome. We also know of a patient who had been subjected to 'decompression' of the radial as well as the median nerve, for a painful frozen shoulder secondary to undiagnosed Parkinson's disease with severe hypokinesia of the arm.

To epitomize: the minimal prerequisite for the diagnosis of compression neuropathy and certainly for surgical treatment is a history of pins and needles more or less conforming to the cutaneous innervation pattern of the nerve (that is, assuming the nerve contains sensory fibres); preferably this should be associated with neurological signs (numbness, weakness, atrophy, or, rarely, fasciculations in weak muscles), and at the very least with neurophysiological evidence of nerve compression. Infrequently, there is involvement of autonomic nerve fibres, or a tendon jerk may be diminished or absent, depending on the nerve in question.

Localizing the lesion to a particular segment of a nerve may be difficult, since nerve fibres may be arranged in separate fascicles far proximal from the actual point of division, while some fascicles are more prone to compression than others. For example, in crutch paralysis resulting from compression of the radial nerve in the axilla, the distal extensor muscles of the wrist and fingers are the most severely affected, a distribution that may erroneously suggest a more distal lesion. An added difficulty is formed by the common variations from 'normal' anatomy and variations in motor and cutaneous innervation, within as well as between nerves. All these problems may be overcome by neurophysiological examination, but it is bad practice to order

neurophysiological studies before a full neurological examination has been performed, if necessary after consultation of an *aide mémoire*. Proper neurophysiological studies can be done only if these are prompted by a proper examination.

Apparently peripheral nerve disorders may in fact originate in the central nervous system, the most common example being a foot drop from an upper motor neuron lesion. It sometimes takes time for an extensor plantar response and hyperreflexia to develop, but an assiduous examination will often uncover associated weakness of knee and hip flexors. Also, any presumed mononeuropathy should be differentiated from a disorder of the anterior horn cells, of nerve roots or of the limb plexus.

Electrophysiological studies

Electrophysiological tests are very helpful in the assessment of the site and the severity of focal peripheral nerve lesions and in the early detection and evaluation of recovery. Moreover, they may disclose subclinical polyneuropathies that underlie the local nerve dysfunction with which the patient presents.

Acute and chronic noxious factors may result in damage to the myelin sheath and to the axon itself, of all fibres within a nerve or a fraction of these. These various lesions can be demonstrated by a combination of motor and sensory nerve conduction studies and needle EMG.

In this introductory chapter the general aspects of electrodiagnosis in mononeuropathies will be discussed. Specific findings will be dealt with in the chapters on the various peripheral nerves.

Motor nerve conduction studies

Most peripheral nerve trunks contain both sensory and motor fibres; hence electrical stimulation activates both types of fibre. To obtain separate information about motor and sensory conduction, it is necessary to choose selective recording sites. For motor conduction studies these are muscles supplied by the nerve under investigation. A convenient aspect is that the evoked compound muscle action potential (CMAP) is much higher (300–1000 times) than the evoked nerve action potential, and therefore is easier to record. The *latency time* between stimulus artifact and CMAP onset includes the conduction time along the unmyelinated axonal endings and the neuromuscular transmission time. Because of this inhomogeneity the motor *conduction velocity* (MCV) of the myelinated motor axons cannot be determined from a single latency measurement. In order to assess the MCV in a given nerve segment the nerve is stimulated at the distal and proximal ends of this segment. The difference in latency times is called the motor *conduction time*, and the MCV is calculated from this value and the distance between the stimulation points (Figure 1.1).

Besides conduction velocities, CMAP amplitudes are an important factor in the assessment of mononeuropathies. For reliable measurements of amplitude and latency it is necessary to use surface electrodes with standard positions over the muscle, the so called belly-tendon montage. Supramaximal stimulation is used to ensure that all A-α motor fibres in the investigated nerve segment are activated, so that all available motor units contribute to the CMAP.

Sensory nerve conduction studies

If a nerve contains only sensory fibres, stimulation and recording can be performed at any attainable site along the nerve. As there is no synapse between the stimulation and recording sites, a single latency measurement is sufficient for the determination of the sensory conduction velocity (SCV) in the relevant nerve segment.

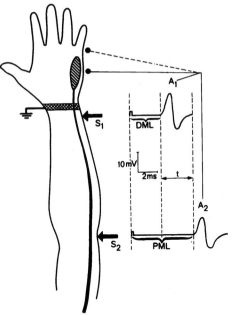

Figure 1.1
**Schematic overview of motor nerve conduction study. The ulnar nerve is supramaximally stimulated at the wrist (S_1) and at the elbow (S_2). DML, distal motor latency, the time between stimulus onset and onset of the CMAP; PML, proximal motor latency; t, conduction time between the two stimulation sites. A_1, amplitude of the CMAP evoked by S_1; A_2, amplitude of the CMAP evoked by S_2.
The distance between both stimulation sites is measured using a centimetre tape.**

Because stimulation of nerve fibres results in an orthodromic as well as in an antidromic volley, propagated with the same velocity, the SCV can be assessed in both directions. For the study of sensory conduction in mixed nerves this means that selective recording of sensory nerve action potentials (SNAPs) can be achieved by stimulation of terminal sensory branches with recording from the nerve trunk, or by stimulation of the mixed nerve and recording from the sensory branches (for example, the digital nerves; see Figure 8.13). Recording with needle electrodes combined with averaging techniques provides information on the range of SCVs in a nerve segment. This is an elaborate and time-consuming technique. In the study of mononeuropathies it usually suffices to get information on the fastest conducting sensory fibres, so that in most examinations surface electrodes are used. In many tests the antidromic technique appears to be the most practical one.

Somatosensory evoked potentials

Stimulation of a peripheral nerve may also be combined with recording of sensory potentials evoked from the central nervous system. These so-called somatosensory evoked potentials (SEPs) can be used as an aid in the study of peripheral nerve lesions. In the case of mononeuropathies their use is mainly restricted to the evaluation of some proximal nerves where no adequate peripheral recording site can be found, for example the lateral cutaneous nerve of the thigh (see pages 99 and 100).

Nerve conduction studies in mononeuropathies

Most mononeuropathies are caused by acute or chronic compression. Nerve compression may lead to local demyelination and subsequently to axonal degeneration. In general, the largest axons are most vulnerable to compression (Aguayo *et al.*, 1971; Ochoa *et al.*, 1972). With respect to nerve conduction studies this is a favourable circumstance, because existing techniques mainly give information about the fastest conducting motor and sensory nerve fibres.

Nerve compression may cause one or several of the following conduction abnormalities:

- Local slowing.
- Local impulse blockade in a portion or in all of the myelinated nerve fibres. In motor conduction studies this results in a lower CMAP with stimulation proximal to the lesion compared with distal stimulation (Figure 1.2).
- Uneven slowing of nerve conduction in the motor axons innervating the

reference muscle. Because of this 'increased temporal dispersion', stimulation proximal to the lesion results in a CMAP with reduced amplitude and increased duration.
- Local slowing and impulse blockade in sensory fibres. Differences in amplitude between SNAPs evoked by distal and proximal stimulation are, however, more difficult to interpret because of the much larger effect of normal temporal dispersion on SNAP characteristics.
- Equally decreased or absent SNAPs with stimulation proximal and distal from a nerve lesion. This finding reflects axonal degeneration. Sensory root lesions proximal to the spinal ganglion cause no degeneration of the peripheral sensory axon, and thereby do not influence the SNAP.

If conduction velocity is measured over a nerve segment that is considerably longer than the demyelinated segment which it contains, the local slowing caused by this focal lesion will be strongly 'diluted'. On the other hand, the shorter the selected nerve segment, the greater the percentage error in the assessment of its length, leading to increasing inaccuracy of the velocity calculation. In order to detect the exact site of a nerve compression, the stimulating electrode may be gradually moved along the nerve to see whether a point can be found where the latency of the CMAP or SNAP suddenly becomes shorter and/or the amplitude suddenly increases. This technique has been called 'inching' (Miller, 1979).

Local slowing of nerve conduction is important for the localization of a nerve lesion, but slowing in itself does not produce symptoms. It is far from rare to find slowing of the median nerve at the wrist or of the ulnar nerve at the elbow without any corresponding symptom. Weakness and sensory loss are due to impulse blockade and/or axonal degeneration. During routine conduction studies demonstration of impulse

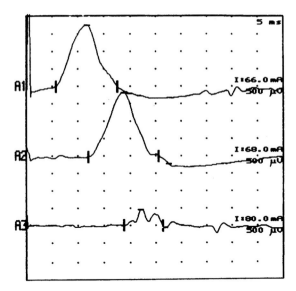

Figure 1.2
CMAPs evoked by supramaximal stimulation of the peroneal nerve at the ankle (A1), below (A2)
and above (A3) the fibula head. The amplitude of the latter is greatly reduced due to impulse
blockade in most motor nerve fibres at the fibula head.
The latency difference between A2 and A3 is 6.8 ms resulting in a strongly reduced MCV of only 13
m/s in the segment of 90 mm between both stimulation sites (43 m/s in the segment distal to the
fibular head).

blockade occurs by using only a few
stimuli. In experimental studies, however,
it has been shown that demyelination may
also lead to impairment of the ability to
transmit long trains of impulses faithfully
(McDonald, 1980). This type of conduction
abnormality is not being studied in the
clinical situation.

Functional loss has a better prognosis if
it is caused by blockade than in the case of
axonal degeneration.

Needle electromyography

The electrical activity in skeletal muscle
can be studied with needle electrodes. In
Europe the concentric needle electrode is
standard, whereas many neurologists in
the USA use a monopolar needle in
combination with a surface reference
electrode. With either approach essentially
the same results are obtained.

The most informative finding is the
occurrence of spontaneous muscle fibre
potentials in the form of fibrillation
potentials, positive sharp waves, or both
(Figure 1.3). This type of activity is usually
caused by degeneration of motor axons,
and is therefore often called 'denervation
activity'. The shorter term 'fibrillations' is
also used to indicate both manifestations
of electrical activity of single muscle fibres.
Following axonal damage it takes two to
three weeks before a change in membrane
properties of the denervated muscle fibres
results in this spontaneous activity.

Fibrillations may disappear as a result
of reinnervation or degeneration of
muscle fibres. In partially denervated
muscles denervated fibres may survive for
many months or even years. This means
that denervation activity should not be
called 'signs of active denervation',
because this term implies a recent or even
progressive disorder.

Loss of motor axons is also reflected in
a reduction of the EMG pattern on
maximal voluntary contraction. Moreover,
partial denervation will be followed by
collateral reinnervation, resulting in

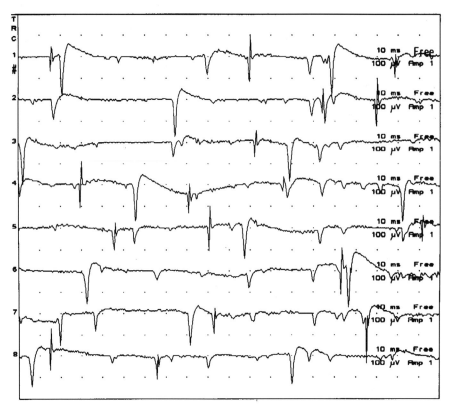

Figure 1.3
Fibrillation potentials and positive sharp waves resulting from degeneration of motor axons. Both types of potential are from denervated muscle fibres. The initial positive (downward) deflection of the positive sharp waves is followed by a protracted negative phase, which probably results from an impeded impulse conduction along the relevant muscle fibres.

enlarged and polyphasic motor unit potentials (MUPs). Recent reinnervation is characterized by polyphasic MUPs with an unstable configuration (Figure 1.4).

Although needle EMG may reveal many other types of activity, the features mentioned above are sufficient for the study of most mononeuropathies.

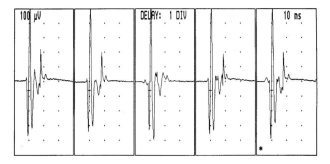

Figure 1.4
Polyphasic MUP resulting from collateral reinnervation in a partial lesion. The MUP shows variation in its configuration during consecutive discharges as a result of unstable neuromuscular transmission in newly formed neuromuscular junctions.

In order to attribute EMG abnormalities to a mononeuropathy, the electromyographer should make sure that they occur exclusively in muscles innervated by the relevant nerve. The site of the lesion is always proximal to the branch to the most proximal muscle in which EMG abnormalities are found. Within a nerve, fascicles may be unevenly damaged, so that EMG abnormalities may still be lacking in muscles receiving their innervation from a point distal to the nerve lesion.

Temperature

Nerve conduction velocities are reduced as the temperature of the limb decreases; a 1 °C change corresponds to a difference in velocity of about 2 m/s. Therefore, all conduction studies should involve measurement of the skin temperature over the investigated nerve segments, and limbs that are too cold should be sufficiently warmed before tests are performed. This may seem less important for the diagnosis of focal nerve lesions where usually comparisons are made between velocities in various nerve segments of a single individual. Without temperature control, however, an underlying polyneuropathy cannot be diagnosed. Moreover, the sensitivity of needle EMG is decreased in cold limbs, because fibrillations are suppressed at lower temperatures (Feinstein *et al.* 1945).

Diagnostic imaging

Computed tomography (CT) or magnetic resonance imaging (MRI) are often useful if local space-occupying lesions are suspected as the cause of nerve compression (Pierallini *et al.*, 1993). Nerves themselves are usually difficult to distinguish, but this has changed with slight modifications of conventional MRI techniques, termed MR neurography (Filler *et al.*, 1996). This technique even visualizes separate nerve fascicles, allowing perineurial, operable lesions (for example, in patients with neurofibromatosis) to be distinguished from infiltrating and unresectable tumours. With nerve deficits after penetrating trauma, MR neurograms allow the distinction between severed nerves needing surgical repair and nerves in which there is still some continuity.

Treatment

Of course, in each mononeuropathy the mode of treatment depends on the specific causes mentioned under the heading of each nerve, but a few general rules should be mentioned. Nerve lesions from external compression generally have a good prognosis for spontaneous recovery. In case of internal entrapment, surgical decompression may be needed. Electrotherapy still enjoys some lingering popularity, but its benefits are unproven (for patients, that is) as well as biologically implausible, and the procedure is unpleasant and time-consuming. Until adequately controlled experiments have established its value, electrotherapy should not be practised, as is true for any medical treatment.

Part one
Mononeuropathies in the arm and trunk

Chapter 2
The dorsal scapular nerve

Anatomy

The dorsal scapular nerve carries fibres from C4 and C5, and innervates the levator scapulae after having pierced the medial scalenus muscle. From there it courses along the medial border of the scapula to the rhomboid muscles (Figure 2.1). The levator scapulae elevates and the rhomboid muscles adduct the medial border of the shoulder blade.

Examination

There are several ways to test the rhomboid muscles. The most simple method is indicated in Figure 2.2.

Causes

Not infrequently, the rhomboid muscles are involved in neuralgic amyotrophy (see Chapter 24). To our knowledge there are no descriptions of isolated entrapment or other compressive lesions of the dorsal scapular nerve.

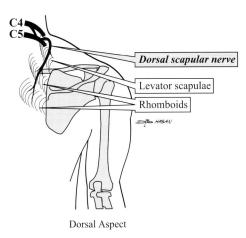

C4
C5

Dorsal scapular nerve

Levator scapulae

Rhomboids

Dorsal Aspect

Figure 2.1
Muscles innervated by the dorsal scapular nerve.

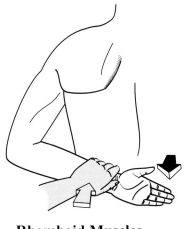

Rhomboid Muscles

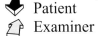 Patient

Examiner

Figure 2.2
The examiner stands behind the patient, who pushes the hand of the examiner backward against resistance.

Chapter 3
The long thoracic nerve

Anatomy

The long thoracic nerve (Figure 3.1) arises from the motor roots of C5, C6 and frequently also from C7. It is the motor nerve of the serratus anterior muscle. Mostly it courses downward through and in front of the medial scalenus muscle, and further descends dorsal to the brachial plexus, along the medial axillary wall where it gives off its branches to the different digitations of the serratus anterior muscle.

History

Dysfunction of the long thoracic nerve manifests itself in difficulty with elevating the upper arm (for example, combing one's hair or shaving). The weakness may be accompanied by a dull ache in the shoulder, mainly caused by strain on muscles and ligaments as the serratus anterior muscle no longer tightens the scapula against the rib cage.

Examination

The serratus anterior muscle is tested by standing behind the patient and asking him or her to push against a wall with both arms almost but not completely extended at the elbow (Figure 3.2), or to elevate the arms to a forward position.

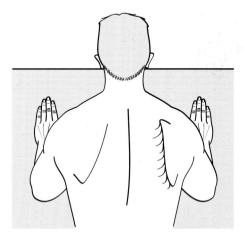

Serratus Anterior Muscle

Figure 3.2
The patient is pushing against a wall with a slightly flexed elbow. Even moderate weakness of the serratus anterior muscle will be evident by winging of the (right) scapula.

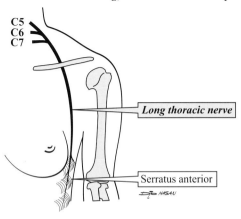

C5
C6
C7

Long thoracic nerve

Serratus anterior

Ventral Aspect

Figure 3.1
Muscles innervated by the long thoracic nerve.

The long thoracic nerve

Even moderate weakness of the serratus anterior muscle will then be evident by winging of the scapula; this may be visible also in the resting position. If weakness is so severe that the patient cannot lift the extended arm forward, the examiner should do this instead and then ask the patient to push the fist forward, against the other hand of the examiner; during this manoeuvre winging of the scapula will then be seen. With paralysis of the serratus anterior muscle, abduction of the arm may be also restricted. The limitation of movement may then be noticed as early as during the handshake at the beginning of the consultation, a movement for which of course elevation as well as some abduction of the arm is necessary. When the examiner takes over the function of the paralysed serratus anterior by pressing the scapula against the chest wall, elevation of the arm again becomes more or less possible.

Electrophysiological studies

Usually the investigation is limited to needle EMG, but motor latencies to the serratus anterior muscle can be measured on stimulation at Erb's point (Alfonsi *et al.*, 1986). The serratus anterior muscle is best studied with a needle electrode introduced between the anterior and middle axillary lines, at the level of the fifth or sixth rib. In order to avoid puncture of the intercostal muscles or even the pleura, the examiner places his index finger and middle finger in the intercostal spaces on either side of the rib. The needle is introduced between these fingers at an acute angle until it touches the rib, and is then slightly withdrawn. The muscle can also be approached at the inner side of the inferior angle of the winging scapula.

Differential diagnosis

Lesions of the roots C6 or C7 may cause weakness of the serratus anterior muscle

(Makin *et al.*, 1986), but in combination with weakness of extensors of the arm, wrist or fingers. In myopathy more muscles of the shoulder and upper arm are involved and the motor deficit is usually bilateral. Disruption of the serratus anterior muscle itself may occur in rheumatoid arthritis (Meythaler *et al.*, 1986) or, at the level of the insertion, by fractures of the scapula (Hayes and Zehr, 1981).

Weakness of the trapezius muscle may somewhat resemble weakness of the serratus anterior muscle, because this may also cause winging of the scapula (upper part), especially on abduction of the arm.

Causes

Involvement of the long thoracic nerve is often seen in neuralgic amyotrophy, but rarely as an isolated lesion (Petrera and Trojaborg, 1984). If such cases are also painless, the diagnosis can be made only by exclusion. Rarely, it may be the sole manifestation in inherited brachial plexus neuropathy (Phillips, 1986).

All sorts of trauma may damage the nerve (Petrera and Trojaborg, 1984): a blow to the shoulder or the lateral chest wall, carrying heavy loads on the back ('rucksack paralysis'), or muscular exertion such as pushing loads above the head, or falling on outstretched arms. A variety of athletic activities has been associated with lesions to the long thoracic nerve (Schultz and Leonard, 1992; Packer *et al.*, 1993), including playing volleyball (Distefano, 1989), professional ballet (White and Witten, 1993) and archery (Shimizu *et al.*, 1990). Sometimes the 'trauma' is so unobtrusive that one suspects a combination of mechanical factors with neuralgic amyotrophy:

> A 48-year-old psychiatrist, after having played the saxophone for about an hour, noticed some weakness of the

right arm on lifting the instrument, which had been fastened by a string around his neck. A few days before, he had played for much longer, during the rehearsals. Yet, in retrospect, for some days he had had an undefined, strange sensation in the right upper arm. For the next three weeks some mild weakness remained, especially on abduction of the arm; when he looked at his body in the mirror it seemed that the contour of the right shoulder had changed. Pain had never occurred, other than a mild ache in the shoulder that he had first felt three days after the onset of weakness; it was never severe enough to interfere with his work or with sleep. On examination, three weeks after onset, the abnormal contour of the right shoulder the patient had noticed proved not to be caused by atrophy, but by winging of the medial border of the scapula on abduction of the arm. The same phenomenon occurred when the patient elevated the arms forward, or when he pushed the extended arms against the wall. Power was normal in all other arm muscles, and there was no sensory deficit. Another three weeks later all symptoms and signs had disappeared.

Many surgical procedures of the chest wall may cause lesions of the long thoracic nerve (Martin, 1989; Kauppila and Vastamäki, 1996); this complication has been specifically reported after thoracostomy for pneumothorax (Fosse and Fjeld, 1991), transaxillary breast augmentation (Laban and Kon, 1990), axillary node dissection for breast carcinoma or malignant melanoma (Duncan *et al.*, 1983), and operations for the relief of so-called thoracic outlet

syndrome, such as scalenotomy and resection of a first rib or cervical rib (Kauppila and Vastamäki, 1996). If the nerve has not been transected the prognosis is usually good. Other iatrogenic lesions have occurred after radiation therapy for breast cancer (Pugliese *et al.*, 1987), or with chiropractic manipulation (Oware *et al.*, 1995).

Borrelia infection is an extremely uncommon cause of long thoracic nerve involvement (Monteyne *et al.*, 1994). A single report speculated that a cervical rib may cause compression of the long thoracic nerve, and that surgical removal led to recovery (del Sasso *et al.*, 1988); it is difficult to dispel the suspicion that the anomaly may have been coincidental in a patient who in fact went through an episode of neuralgic amyotrophy (see Chapter 25). Scepticism should be fuelled even more by the knowledge that such operations may actually cause lesions of the nerve (Kauppila and Vastamäki, 1996) or of the brachial plexus.

Treatment

Spontaneous recovery is the rule in the vast majority of patients with neuralgic amyotrophy, even after complete loss of function. The same applies to traumatic injury, at least if the deficit is partial. At least two years should have elapsed before surgery is considered. The only surgical approach consists of operative stabilization of the scapula, for which different methods exist (Mumenthaler and Schliack, 1993). However, shoulder function remains impaired even after the operation; also, after several years the fixation may give way. In view of these disadvantages it is doubtful whether the procedure should be undertaken at all.

Chapter 4
The suprascapular nerve

Anatomy

The suprascapular nerve arises from the upper trunk of the brachial plexus and carries fibres from C5 and C6. It runs under the trapezius muscle and at the upper border of the scapula, from where it courses beneath the transverse superior scapular ligament to innervate the supra- and infraspinatus muscles (Figure 4.1). Fibres to the infraspinatus muscle run separately through the spinoglenoid notch, which is covered by the transverse inferior scapular ligament. The nerve does not contain skin afferents.

Entrapment sites are at the suprascapular notch and at the spinoglenoid notch (see Figure 4.1); compression results in weakness of both spinatus muscles or of the infraspinatus muscle only, respectively.

Lesions of the suprascapular nerve

History

Injury may be associated with vigorous exercise, especially with sports such as baseball, volleyball or lawn tennis (see below). A modern variety of a pressure palsy of the suprascapular nerve in which the history is also essential is prolonged cradling of a mobile telephone between an ear and the shoulder (Hopkins, 1996).

Suprascapular nerve entrapment is mostly associated with pain at the superior margin of the scapula, radiating towards the shoulder. However, this condition may also occur in a painless fashion. In either case there is difficulty with movements of the shoulder.

Examination

Inspection of the supra- and infraspinate muscles from above and behind may reveal atrophy, but in a frail, elderly patient it may be difficult to decide whether the atrophy is pathological or merely caused by ageing, unless there is clear asymmetry. The deltoid muscle should be intact as it is innervated by the axillary nerve. The strength of both spinatus muscles is tested as shown in Figures 4.2 and 4.3. There should be no restriction of passive shoulder movements (see below).

Differential diagnosis

Non-neurogenic disorders of the shoulder region include the rotator cuff syndrome and tendinitis of the supraspinatus muscle. As with other peripheral nerves, one should be extremely cautious in diagnosing a nerve entrapment syndrome on the basis of pain only, in the absence of neurological deficits. In particular, soft tissue injuries in the shoulder region,

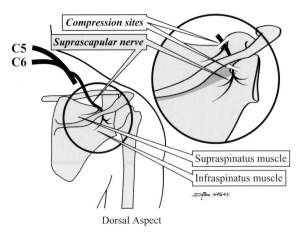

Figure 4.1
Muscles innervated by the suprascapular nerve.

whatever the cause ('frozen shoulder'), are much more common than nerve entrapment. The shoulder pain further inhibits the mobility of the shoulder joint, a vicious circle that may well result in atrophy of the muscles around the shoulder: particularly the supraspinatus but often the deltoid muscle as well, which is strong proof against a neuropathy of the suprascapular nerve. In brief, with a stiff and painful shoulder one should be extremely cautious in diagnosing a nerve entrapment. On the other hand, a suprascapular nerve lesion

may itself be the cause of a frozen shoulder, but this occurs in only a small minority of cases. An increase of the pain by moving the arm across the chest is mentioned by Dawson *et al.* (1990) as a sign of suprascapular nerve entrapment, but this certainly also occurs with other painful disorders of the shoulder joint.

Radiculopathy of C5 or C6 rarely, if ever, leads to isolated weakness of the supra- or

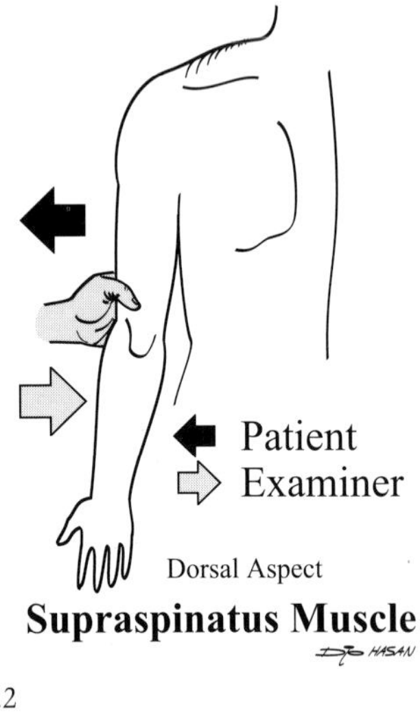

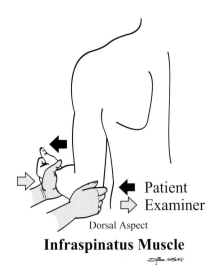

Figure 4.2
The upper arm is abducted against resistance.

Figure 4.3
The upper arm is externally rotated against resistance. The examiner's right hand prevents abduction of the upper arm.

infraspinatus muscles. The pain mostly radiates into the arm with these root disorders, and the biceps jerk is usually diminished.

Neuralgic amyotrophy may be confined to one or both of the spinatus muscles, in which case the mononeuropathy is probably caused by an autoimmune disorder rather than by entrapment. Neuralgic amyotrophy is dealt with in Chapter 24.

Electrophysiological studies

Motor conduction in the suprascapular nerve can be investigated by stimulation of the brachial plexus and recording from the spinatus muscles (Aiello *et al.* 1982; Post and Mayer, 1987). Both muscles are readily accessible by needle EMG, by which method the severity of the nerve lesion may be assessed as well. Needle EMG is, of course, also helpful in distinguishing lesions of the nerve from lesions of the brachial plexus or cervical roots.

Causes

Suprascapular neuropathy is mostly precipitated by trauma, such as a blow on the shoulder or heavy lifting (Kómár, 1976; Rengachary *et al.*, 1979; Lang *et al.*, 1988; Callahan *et al.*, 1991; Arboleya and Garcia, 1993; Vastamäki and Göransson, 1993), or activities involving forceful and extreme movements of the shoulder such as baseball, volleyball, tennis, boxing, fencing, pitching or professional ballet (Kómár, 1976; Aiello *et al.*, 1982; Ringel and Treihaft, 1988; Kukowski, 1993; Vastamäki and Göransson, 1993; Jackson *et al.*, 1995; Antoniadis *et al.*, 1996), or it can be idiopathic (Rengachary *et al.*, 1979; Callahan *et al.*, 1991). In idiopathic cases with acute onset the cause is likely to be an autoimmune, inflammatory disorder, whereas in cases of subacute onset there may be entrapment by the transverse superior or inferior scapular ligament.

Much less common causes are iatrogenic injury (Shaffer, 1994) or a local mass, such as a ganglion cyst, sarcoma, chondrosarcoma, metastasis, or haematoma associated with fracture; these masses can be identified by MRI (Fritz *et al.*, 1992).

Treatment

After a blunt trauma without fracture of the scapula, watchful waiting seems to be the wisest course to follow. With chronic symptoms in sportsmen the first measure should be a change of the provoking activities, at least if this proves acceptable to the patient (Kukowski, 1993). If rest does not result in improvement or if the cause is in doubt, further exploration by MRI scanning and, ultimately, operation seems warranted. Injections with hydrocortisone have been recommended (Kómár, 1976), but as muscle atrophy had occurred in only 21 of the 124 patients in this series most patients probably suffered from soft tissue lesions rather than nerve entrapment.

The usual surgical approach consists of decompressing the nerve by resection of the transverse suprascapular ligament, and if necessary also widening the spinoglenoid notch (Laulund *et al.*, 1984; Hadley *et al.*, 1986; Post and Mayer, 1987; Antoniadis *et al.*, 1996). With isolated weakness and atrophy of the infraspinatus muscle the site of compression may still be relatively proximal, with selective entrapment by the transverse superior suprascapular ligament of the fascicle containing fibres to the infraspinatus muscle. Alternatively, the site of compression may be more distal, and surgery should consist of enlargement of the spinoglenoid notch, with excision of a hypertrophied transverse inferior scapular ligament (Kiss and Kómár, 1990; Henlin *et al.*, 1992). In one-third to two-thirds of operated patients the pain disappears immediately, and most of the remainder recover in the next few months

(Rengachary *et al.*, 1979; Callahan *et al.*, 1991; Vastamäki and Göransson, 1993). A minority may be left with residual pain, weakness, or both; the operation failed in 15% of the 66 patients in one large series (Vastamäki and Göransson, 1993), and some of these may represent neuralgic amyotrophy in which the usual recovery failed to occur. For patients with recurrent symptoms a second decompressive operation may be indicated (Callahan *et al.*, 1991).

Chapter 5
The axillary nerve

Anatomy

The axillary nerve originates from the posterior fascicle of the brachial plexus and carries fibres from C5 and C6 (Figure 5.1). It passes just below the shoulder joint and encircles the humerus from behind until it is under the deltoid muscle, which it innervates together with the teres minor muscle. In this trajectory, at the posterior aspect of the shoulder the nerve passes through the so-called quadrilateral space, defined by the teres minor muscle above, the teres major muscle below, the long head of the triceps medially and the neck of the humerus laterally. The sensory branch, the *upper lateral cutaneous nerve of the upper arm*, innervates only a small area of skin, overlying the deltoid muscle (Figure 5.2).

Lesions of the axillary nerve

Examination

Atrophy of the deltoid muscle is easily recognized, especially when the patient is seated and inspected from behind and above. Due to the decrease in muscle bulk the acromion and the head of the humerus become visible. The power of the anterior and middle parts of the deltoid muscle should be tested with the patient keeping the arm abducted in a horizontal position, against resistance (Figure 5.3). The first 30° of abduction of the upper arm from the trunk are effected by the supraspinate muscle, not by the deltoid muscle. The posterior part of the deltoid muscle is tested by retracting the abducted arm against resistance (Figure 5.4). The teres minor muscle cannot be tested separately, as this muscle works jointly with the infraspinatus muscle (suprascapular nerve) in the outward rotation of the upper arm (see page 24).

Electrophysiological studies

Motor conduction in the axillary nerve can be investigated by stimulation at Erb's point and recording from the deltoid

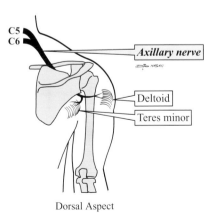

C5
C6

Axillary nerve

Deltoid

Teres minor

Dorsal Aspect

Figure 5.1
Muscles innervated by the axillary nerve.

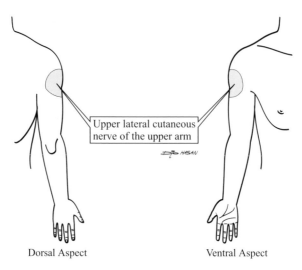

Upper lateral cutaneous nerve of the upper arm

Dorsal Aspect   Ventral Aspect

Figure 5.2
Approximate skin area innervated by the axillary nerve.

muscle (Berry and Bril, 1982; de Laat *et al*, 1994). Needle EMG abnormalities exclusively in the deltoid muscle, and perhaps also in the teres minor muscle (which is difficult to localize), support the diagnosis of an isolated axillary nerve lesion.

Causes

Most lesions of the axillary nerve are the result of acute trauma. It is commonly damaged in subcapital fractures of the humerus (Blom and Dahlback, 1970; de Laat *et al.*, 1994), or by blunt trauma of the shoulder without fracture (Berry and Bril, 1982). An axillary nerve lesion may also result from antero-inferior dislocation of the shoulder joint, for instance by a blow at the tip of the shoulder, for example during soccer or other contact sports (Liveson, 1984a; de Laat *et al.*, 1994) or as a complication of reposition with this type of dislocation. After luxation of the shoulder it is not possible to test the

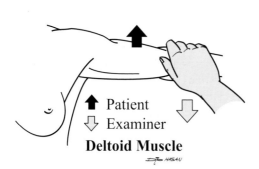

↑ Patient
⇩ Examiner
Deltoid Muscle

Figure 5.3
The horizontally raised upper arm is abducted against resistance.

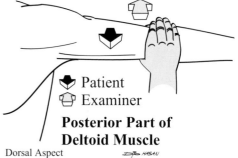

⬇ Patient
⬆ Examiner
Posterior Part of Deltoid Muscle

Dorsal Aspect

Figure 5.4
The horizontally raised upper arm is retracted against resistance.

strength of the deltoid muscle; therefore, it is important to examine the sensory area of the axillary nerve for hypalgesia before repositioning is performed, and it may be wise to explain this to the patient in order to forestall claims for compensation. Unfortunately, sensation may be entirely normal with deltoid paralysis, as the sensory branch follows a short and separate route. Iatrogenic injuries include intramuscular injections in the deltoid muscle (Johnson, 1984) and faulty positioning on the operating table, with the upper arm elevated to 90° for 4.5 hours (Aita, 1984). Birth injury may damage the axillary nerve in isolation, or as part of a lesion of the brachial plexus. Finally, young volleyball players may suffer axillary nerve lesions in the absence of acute trauma (Paladini *et al.*, 1996).

There is some debate about the existence of a so-called *quadrilateral space syndrome*, in which the axillary nerve and the posterior circumflex artery are supposed to be compressed by fibrous bands or overstretched by extreme movements (Cahill and Palmer, 1983). Baseball pitchers are said to be especially at risk (Redler *et al.*, 1986). Diagnostic criteria other than weakness of the deltoid muscle are said to be tenderness over the quadrilateral space and paraesthesia over the lateral shoulder as well as over the posterior aspect of the upper arm (Francel *et al.*, 1991; Linker *et al.*, 1993). We would like to object that it is difficult confidently to diagnose weakness of the deltoid muscle in a patient with a painful shoulder. Some go as far as to diagnose quadrilateral space syndrome in patients without motor deficits but with selective atrophy of the teres minor muscle on MRI scanning (Linker *et al.*, 1993). Others adduce

arteriography as an argument, because the posterior circumflex artery of the humerus may be compressed when the arm is abducted and rotated externally (McKowen and Voorhies, 1987). We remain sceptical, not only of the observation of a compressed artery (such a phenomenon may well be observed in controls), but also of the entire concept of the 'quadrilateral space syndrome'. After all, the axillary nerve is often involved in neuralgic amyotrophy (see Chapter 24), and in about 10% of patients the axillary nerve is affected in isolation (Tsairis *et al.*, 1972).

Treatment

If paralysis of the deltoid muscle after trauma does not show signs of recovery after about four months, nerve grafting may be considered (Petrucci *et al.*, 1982). Partial lesions tend to recover spontaneously (de Laat *et al.*, 1994). In neuralgic amyotrophy recovery may take many months and exploration is, of course, not indicated. Surgical decompression has been advocated in patients thought to suffer from the so-called quadrilateral space syndrome, with reasonable results (Cahill and Palmer, 1983), but the critical reader cannot but wonder whether these uncontrolled results do not merely represent the natural history of an autoimmune inflammatory response, namely neuralgic amyotrophy.

As long as the deltoid muscle is weak, mobility of the shoulder joint should be ensured by active or, if necessary, passive exercises; especially in older patients there is the danger of permanent disability because a frozen shoulder syndrome has developed by the time the nerve injury has healed.

Chapter 6
The musculocutaneous nerve

Anatomy

The musculocutaneous nerve (Figure 6.1) arises from the lateral cord of the brachial plexus and carries fibres from the roots C5, C6 and C7. After a short course through the axilla the musculocutaneous nerve pierces the coracobrachialis muscle while giving off branches to it. From there on it runs between the biceps and the brachialis muscles. Branches are given off to the coracobrachialis muscle, to both parts of the biceps muscle and to the brachial muscle.

The *lateral cutaneous nerve of the forearm* is the sensory continuation of the musculocutaneous nerve. It pierces the fascia lateral to the tendon of the biceps muscle, just above the elbow, and innervates the skin of the radial part of the volar side of the forearm as far as the wrist (Figure 6.2).

History

Isolated lesions of the musculocutaneous nerve are extremely rare, be they of the motor or sensory part alone, or both. The clinical features follow the simple anatomical arrangement (Bassett and Nunley, 1982), although abnormalities of sensation are often less marked than might be expected (Mumenthaler and Schliack, 1993). There may be pain in the elbow and the forearm, and paraesthesia along the radial side of the forearm, but pain may also be entirely absent.

Examination

If motor signs are present, the most important one is weakness of the biceps and brachialis muscles; this is evident from flexion of the elbow against resistance, with the hand in full supination (Figure 6.3). Exceptionally, the coracobrachial muscle is involved, in which case one finds some weakness on elevation of the arm.

Electrophysiological studies

Techniques are available for measuring conduction in both motor and sensory

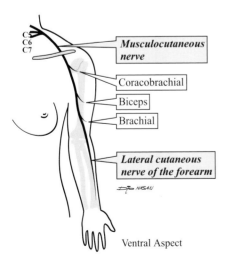

Figure 6.1
Muscles innervated by the musculocutaneous nerve.

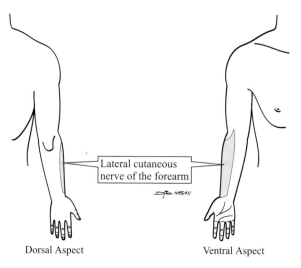

Figure 6.2
Approximate skin area supplied by the musculocutaneous nerve.

fibres belonging to the musculocutaneous nerve (Trojaborg, 1976; Spindler and Felsenthal, 1978; Izzo *et al.*, 1985). Sensory conduction in the lateral cutaneous nerve of the forearm can easily be measured using an antidromic technique (Spindler and Felsenthal, 1978). The demonstration of a sensory nerve action potential can be helpful in distinguishing between radicular and more peripheral lesions (see Chapter 1).

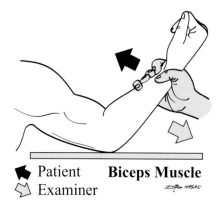

Figure 6.3
The supported and supinated forearm is flexed against resistance.

Differential diagnosis

With an isolated musculocutaneous nerve palsy there is no diagnostic alternative, unless one is misled by a ruptured biceps tendon. In that situation one finds on contraction of the biceps muscle a hardening mass under the insertion of the pectoralis major muscle, and there is no sensory loss. In a C6 root lesion wrist extension is also affected, at least towards the radial side (extensor carpi radialis muscle). Second, the muscle belly of the brachioradialis muscle will not be visible on flexion of the elbow (which it will be in case of musculocutaneous nerve lesions, as it is innervated by the radial nerve). Third, supination will be weak not only with the elbow in flexion (biceps muscle) but also with the forearm extended (supinator muscle, innervated by the radial nerve). Finally, lesions of the C6 root are associated with sensory loss in the hand.

Causes

Penetrating injuries of the upper arm (by knife or gunshot) may be associated with isolated lesions of the musculocutaneous nerve. Other traumatic causes are dislocation of the shoulder (Jerosch *et al.*, 1989; Corner *et al.*, 1990), a closed fracture of the clavicle (Bartosh *et al.*, 1992), and operations of the shoulder for habitual luxation (Zeuke and Heidrich, 1974) or for instability of the clavicle (Caspi *et al.*, 1987), and axillary node dissection for malignant melanoma (Karakousis *et al.*, 1990). Strenuous exercise of the arms can lead to entrapment of the musculocutaneous nerve (Mastaglia *et al.*, 1986), particularly weight-lifting (Braddom and Wolfe, 1978) or performing 500 push-ups (Pecina and Bojanic, 1993). The nerve may be involved in neuralgic amyotrophy, even in isolation (Tsairis *et al.*, 1972). Very uncommon causes are opportunistic infection by the bacterium *Capnocytophaga canimorsus*, probably of the *vasa nervorum* (Banerjee *et al.*, 1993), or paralysis after sleep (Both *et al.*, 1983).

The *lateral cutaneous nerve of the forearm* may be damaged by blows on the forearm or elbow (Young *et al.*, 1990), a heavy weight pressing on the volar side of the elbow (Hale, 1976; Sander *et al.*, 1997), or a forearm splint or surgery in the antecubital fossa, including venipuncture (Yuan and Cohen, 1985; Chang and Oh, 1988).

A 51-year-old professor of neurology, fit enough to have recently run a mountain marathon, underwent elective resection of a carcinoma of the sigmoid colon, Duke grade B. Postoperative analgesia was maintained with intravenous morphine. One intravenous line had been inserted on the dorsum of his left hand and the other on the dorsum of his left lower forearm. Immediately after surgery the patient was not aware of very much apart from the pain from the surgical wound, but the next morning he realized that his left forearm felt vaguely numb. A day or two after surgery it became clear to the gradually more alert professor that the numbness of the left forearm, to both pain and light touch, was precisely in the distribution of the lateral cutaneous nerve of the forearm. Because the intravenous drips were both well away from the nerve and none of the drugs infused was likely to have caused any nerve damage, presumably the nerve had been compressed or stretched in some way while the arm was abducted during surgery. The symptoms and signs gradually resolved in about four weeks.

Excessive exercise with elbow extension and arm pronation may cause entrapment of the lateral cutaneous nerve of the forearm (Felsenthal *et al.*, 1984), and the sensory nerve may also be involved in idiopathic inflammatory plexopathy (that is, 'neuralgic amyotrophy' without weakness).

Treatment

Surgical treatment should be considered only in case of direct penetrating trauma with severe axonal damage or even complete interruption of nerve continuity. In all other situations an expectant attitude should prevail.

Chapter 7
The radial nerve

Anatomy

The radial nerve (Figure 7.1) forms together with the axillary nerve the continuation of the posterior cord of the brachial plexus; it carries fibres from the roots C5–Th1. At the lower margin of the axilla branches are given off to the different parts of the triceps muscle. The radial nerve then passes downwards between the medial and lateral heads of the triceps muscle and winds around the back of the humerus, in the spiral groove. It is at this site that the nerve is most often damaged by compression (Sturzenegger and Rutz, 1991). At the distal third of the upper arm the radial nerve pierces the strong intermuscular septum between the

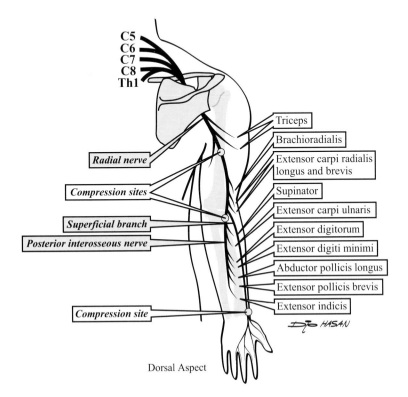

C5
C6
C7
C8
Th1

Triceps

Brachioradialis

Extensor carpi radialis longus and brevis

Supinator

Extensor carpi ulnaris

Extensor digitorum

Extensor digiti minimi

Abductor pollicis longus

Extensor pollicis brevis

Extensor indicis

Radial nerve

Compression sites

Superficial branch

Posterior interosseous nerve

Compression site

Dorsal Aspect

Figure 7.1
Muscles innervated by the radial nerve.

lateral head of the triceps and the brachialis muscle. Far proximal to the supinator muscle branches are given off to the brachioradialis muscle and to the extensor carpi radialis longus and brevis. At some point, varying between 3 cm above and a similar distance below the humero-radial joint, the radial nerve divides into a deep motor branch, which continues as the *posterior interosseous nerve*, and a superficial sensory branch, the *superficial branch of the radial nerve*. The motor nerve passes through and innervates the supinator muscle and then runs dorsal to the interosseous membrane of the forearm to supply the extensor carpi ulnaris, all extensor muscles of the fingers and thumb, as well as the abductor pollicis longus muscle.

The sensory innervation corresponds in its entirety to a strip of skin laterally at the extensor side of the arm, from halfway up the upper arm to the dorsum of the thumb (Figure 7.2). The corresponding sensory nerves, the *posterior cutaneous nerve of the upper arm* and the *posterior cutaneous nerve of the forearm* leave the radial nerve during its course in the spiral groove, having left the parent nerve at the level of the axilla, or coursing as an independent funicular system within the nerve. The *lower lateral cutaneous nerve of the upper arm* arises before the radial nerve passes through the intermuscular septum. It supplies the skin of the lateral and posterior surface of the distal third of the upper arm as well as a small portion of the back of the forearm. In the spiral groove the motor and sensory fibres are easily exposed to pressure, but the sensory nerves are often spared in midhumeral compression of the radial nerve. The *superficial terminal branch of the radial nerve* originates near the elbow and courses superficially on the radial side of the forearm, over the styloid process and towards the dorsum of the thumb. At the level of the styloid process, just proximal to the wrist joint, the nerve lies exposed and can be easily compressed from outside. This nerve supplies the radial part of the dorsum of the hand and ends in *five dorsal digital nerves*, of which two supply the dorsum of the thumb (except the nail area), two the dorsum of the index finger (up to the middle phalanx), and one the first phalanx of the middle finger (Laroy *et al.*, 1998) (see Figure 7.2).

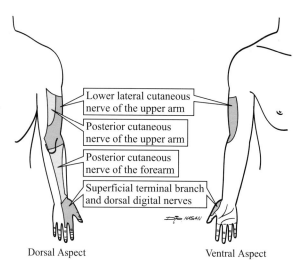

Dorsal Aspect   Ventral Aspect

Figure 7.2
Approximate skin areas innervated by the radial nerve.

Lesions of the radial nerve at the axilla

Clinical features

History Isolated radial nerve lesions at this level are rare. Regardless of the cause (see below) the history is mostly short. The patient notes weakness in stretching the elbow, the wrist, all fingers and the thumb. Pain is not an important feature.

Examination There is weakness of the triceps (Figure 7.3) and of all other muscles necessary for stretching the wrist, fingers and thumb. For a more detailed description of the distal motor deficits, see below. There is only a slightly decreased sensation of the back of the humerus and forearm, and often also of the web between index finger and thumb and of the radial side of the dorsum of the hand.

Causes of radial nerve lesions in the axilla

Apart from all other sorts of trauma, long crutches may be the cause of isolated radial nerve palsy, but usually the median and ulnar nerves are involved as well. Weakness of the muscles innervated by the radial nerve, however, usually dominates the clinical picture. Pressure palsies of both radial nerves at a site proximal to the spiral groove, probably at the posterior axilla, have been reported in a 26-year-old Turkish porter, who used to carry four or five crates with a total weight of 70 kg on his back by keeping both arms outstretched behind his trunk and the forearms in maximal supination, the hands supporting the lowest crate (Kirchof *et al.*, 1962). Full recovery occurred after several weeks.

Lesions of the radial nerve in the upper arm

Clinical features

History Usually, lesions at this level have a more or less sudden onset. There is an inability to extend the wrist, the fingers and the thumb.

Examination As a rule, radial nerve compression at the upper arm spares the triceps muscle and also sensation in the upper arm, since the lesion is usually located distal to the branches to the triceps and to the branching of the proximal sensory nerves. But all the other muscles innervated by the radial nerve will be involved. The brachioradialis may seem to be less weak than the extensors of the wrist and fingers, because of the action of the intact biceps and brachial muscles. The brachioradialis is tested by flexion of the elbow against resistance with the thumb pointing towards the ceiling (Figure 7.4). The supinator, which mostly is only slightly weak, is tested by keeping the forearm turned outward against resistance, with the elbow fully extended; if the elbow is kept flexed, the biceps muscle can also contribute to the supination movement (Figure 7.5).

On inspection the diagnosis can hardly be missed, because of the classical picture of dropping hand and dropping fingers. The extensors of the wrist and of the metacarpophalangeal joints are weak.

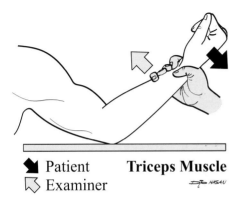

■ Patient   **Triceps Muscle**
◺ Examiner

Figure 7.3
The supported arm is extended against resistance.

The radial nerve

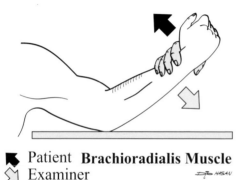

Patient **Brachioradialis Muscle**
Examiner

Figure 7.4
Midway between pronation and supination, the forearm is flexed against resistance.

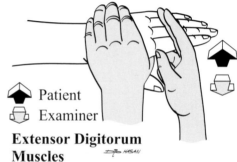

Patient
Examiner

Extensor Digitorum Muscles

Figure 7.6
The fingers are extended in the metacarpophalangeal joints against resistance, while the patient's wrist is held by the examiner.

Testing the strength of the extensor digitorum is shown in Figure 7.6. The abductor pollicis longus is also involved. Weakness of this muscle is not easily distinguished from that of the abductor pollicis brevis, which is innervated by the median nerve. A problem is that both muscles are tested together by the same manoeuvre, and in order to separate their action one has to rely on tightening of the muscles and tendons. To see and feel this,

the abduction movement should be tested in a plane at right angles to the palm (Figure 7.7). Care should be taken that the thumb does not deviate to the radial side (in the plane of the palm rather than perpendicular), because in that case the extensors rather than abductors of the thumb are tested (Figures 7.8 and 7.9). Extension of the wrist is performed jointly by the extensor carpi radialis and the extensor carpi ulnaris, but to some extent either muscle can be tested separately (Figures 7.10 and 7.11).

The posterior cutaneous nerve of the forearm courses with the motor fibres

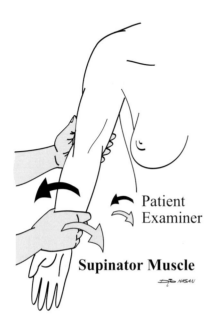

Patient
Examiner

Supinator Muscle

Figure 7.5
The extended forearm is supinated against resistance.

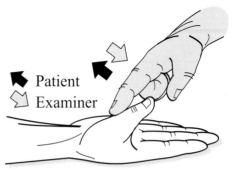

Patient
Examiner

**Abductor Pollicis Longus Muscle
Abductor Pollicis Brevis Muscle**

Figure 7.7
The dorsum of the patient's hand rests on a flat surface, while the thumb is raised to the ceiling against resistance at the metacarpophalangeal joint.

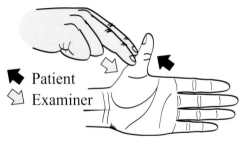

Extensor Pollicis Brevis Muscle

Figure 7.8
The thumb is extended (in the same plane as the palm) against resistance, in the metacarpophalangeal joint.

through the spiral groove, but in radial nerve compression at the upper arm it often escapes damage. Thus normal sensation in the web between the thumb and the index finger can be misleading in localizing the lesion; the history and, especially, the extent of the motor deficits should lead to the correct conclusion.

Electrophysiological studies

Electrophysiological studies may be useful for the determination of the site

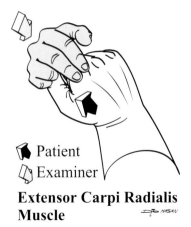

Extensor Carpi Radialis Muscle

Figure 7.10
The hand is extended and abducted at the wrist against resistance.

and the severity of the lesion. Fibrillation potentials, as signs of axonal degeneration, may be found in all or some of those muscles supplied by the radial nerve that are distal to the nerve lesion. The main trunk of the radial nerve and its final motor and sensory branches

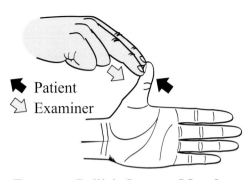

Extensor Pollicis Longus Muscle

Figure 7.9
The thumb is extended (in the same plane as the palm) against resistance, at the interphalangeal joint.

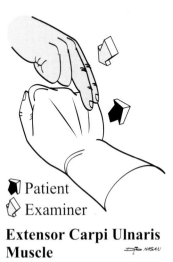

Extensor Carpi Ulnaris Muscle

Figure 7.11
The hand is extended and adducted at the wrist against resistance.

can be stimulated at several sites, so that conduction can be studied in all segments of interest (Trojaborg and Sindrup, 1969). With compression halfway down the upper arm the branches to the triceps are spared, so that no EMG abnormalities will be found in this muscle; conduction studies usually reveal local slowing and signs of conduction block. Trojaborg (1970) found considerable abnormalities of motor and sensory conduction, which returned to normal within 6–8 weeks; these findings are in agreement with the good prognosis in most cases.

Discussion of electrophysiological studies of radial neuropathies in the forearm has been integrated in the relevant section.

Causes of radial nerve lesions in the upper arm

Supracondylar fractures of the humerus and external compression of the nerve are the main causes of radial nerve damage in the arm. Compression usually occurs during an intoxicated sleep, whereas under normal circumstances people are briefly awakened by tingling or pain and then change their position. The classical example is alcohol-induced sleep with the arms folded over the back of a chair or otherwise resting on a hard ridge, a condition labelled in different languages as 'Saturday night palsy', *'paralysie des ivrognes'* or *'Parkbanklähmung'*. Improper positioning during general anaesthesia may have the same effect, as may prolonged application of a tourniquet. Unless there is a history of drugs or alcohol one rarely encounters radial nerve paralysis, although sometimes the quantities of intoxicant imbibed are small and the circumstances prosaic:

> A 25-year old lawyer had driven a friend to the airport, on a warm day. Before parting they had a single glass of beer. On coming back to his car he felt a bit sleepy, and he decided to take a nap in one of the back seats. In doing so he took off his jacket and folded his arms across the front seats, which were made of uncovered steel tubing, the car being a Citroën 2CV. On waking up he could not extend the wrist and fingers of the left arm. Examination, one day later, showed a complete radial nerve palsy below the level of the triceps, without sensory involvement. The deficit resolved in six weeks.

If a radial nerve palsy occurs after normal sleep an additional factor should be assumed, such as a hereditary liability to pressure palsies (see Chapter 25), or an underlying lipoma (Bieber *et al.*, 1986; Fernandez *et al.*, 1987). Shooting practice in a kneeling position with the left upper arm resting on the left knee caused acute wrist drop and numbness at the back of the thumb in ten Taiwanese recruits, after three hours of uninterrupted exercise. Complete recovery ensued in the course of 9–12 weeks, except in one patient who had continued practising for another three hours despite having developed weakness of wrist extension (Shyu *et al.*, 1993). Radial nerve palsy directly after heavy physical effort has been convincingly documented, involving extension at the elbow against strong resistance (Lotem *et al.*, 1971), or the 'windmill' pitching motion of competitive softball (Sinson *et al.*, 1994). The onset may be delayed (Streib, 1992).

> A 39-year-old woman had spent many hours removing paint from a staircase, her right hand moving the scraper while she continuously held a heater in her left hand. At the end of that same day she felt an ache in her left arm (she could not exactly recollect in which part). The next day she experienced weakness of the left hand,

specifically in extending the fingers and the wrist. About a week later she also noticed a numb area at the back of the left thumb. Examination, three weeks after the onset, showed paralysis of all muscles innervated by the radial nerve, except the triceps muscle. The sensory loss corresponded with the territory of the superficial branch of the radial nerve. EMG studies repeatedly demonstrated abundant signs of denervation, exclusively in muscles supplied by the radial nerve. Spontaneous recovery did not start until six months later, and was virtually complete after another period of six months.

Sometimes factors other than exercise are involved, such as diabetic neuropathy in a patient who suffered an acute radial nerve palsy after the prolonged use of a walker (Ball *et al.*, 1989). The structure causing compression of the nerve in cases of overexertion has been identified as the lateral head of the triceps (Mitsunaga and Nakano, 1988), but also as a fibrous arch at the lower part of the humeral groove (Lussiez *et al.*, 1993). Surgical decompression has been advocated (Mitsunaga and Nakano, 1988), but spontaneous recovery is common (Lussiez *et al.*, 1993), although it may take several months.

Radial nerve lesions at the level of the arm have also been reported in patients with severe immobility from Parkinson's disease, leading to compression injury (Little and Furlan, 1985; Preston and Grimes, 1985). Sometimes anatomical factors are identified that may contribute to entrapment, such as an abnormal branching pattern at the level of the spiral groove (Reisecker *et al.*, 1987).

Radial nerve injury at the level of the arm may also occur in newborns, and not only in association with prolonged labour or forceps extraction. Ross *et al.* (1983) reported two cases with complete radial nerve palsy with both skin necrosis and subcutaneous lesions just above the elbow. The site of the lesion, according to clinical and neurophysiological examination, was distal to the innervation of the brachioradialis muscle in one patient and proximal to the triceps muscle in the other; the deficits recovered after six weeks and four months, respectively. In a premature infant, repeated measurement of blood pressure involving the use of a plastic cuff was followed by wrist drop and absence of finger extension on day 20 (Töllner *et al.*, 1980); the deficit fully disappeared, recovery starting three weeks after the onset of weakness.

Callous bone formation following fracture of the shaft of the humerus sometimes causes delayed compression (Edwards and Kurth, 1992), as does myositis ossificans (Fitzsimmons *et al.*, 1993). Recovery must then be helped by surgical intervention. Related situations in which operation may be needed are delayed radial nerve injuries caused by blunt trauma, with soft tissue swelling resulting in solitary paralysis of the triceps muscle (Mizuno *et al.*, 1992), or penetrating missile wounds causing a traumatic aneurysm of the radial artery (Rahimizadeh, 1992). The need for surgical exploration is exceptional since, in general, acute radial palsies with supracondylar fracture of the humerus, such as those occurring after sleep, carry a good prognosis without any intervention (Packer *et al.*, 1972): normal function gradually returns after days or weeks. With severe peripheral nerve damage there is always a point of no return, and recovery may fail to occur after a very long coma in an unfavourable position, for example in drug addicts after an overdose. Neurophysiological studies are indicated if the prognosis remains in doubt clinically.

A most unusual entrapment involving the posterior cutaneous nerve of the arm has been described in an amateur drummer, who had recently increased his musical activities (Makin and Brown,

1985). He experienced a painful burning sensation at the lower posterior aspect of the right upper arm. These symptoms occurred only when he played the cymbals and drew his right arm in hyperabduction across his chest, followed by vigorous extension. Examination showed decreased sensation in the area of the posterior cutaneous nerve of the upper arm. The authors supposed this nerve was intermittently stretched or compressed by the long head of the triceps muscle distal to its origin from the axillary portion of the radial nerve.

A tumour of the nerve should be suspected if the deficits in the distribution of the radial nerve are slowly progressive, and if there is no obvious other cause (Stöhr and Reill, 1980). Space-occupying lesions compressing the radial nerve may also arise from surrounding structures, such as lipomas (Bieber *et al.*, 1986; Fernandez *et al.*, 1987), or fibrous myopathy caused by injection of pentazocine (Kim, 1987).

Management of radial nerve lesions in the upper arm

Especially with slowly progressive radial nerve palsy surgical exploration should be considered, sometimes even after a first, negative operation. Stöhr and Reill (1980) described a 52-year-old printer with slowly progressive dysfunction of the right radial nerve, developing over many months, with pain at the lateral side of the elbow. His work, manually printing music scores, with his right hand in maximal pronation and slight extension, may have been a contributing factor. Only a second operation showed concentric thickening of the epineurium; after resection and interfascicular neurolysis a partial recovery occurred.

Whether early exploration should be performed after closed fractures of the humerus with immediate and complete radial nerve palsy is a problem that has raised acrimonious discussions. It is

easier to reach consensus about partial radial nerve lesions following humeral fractures: these should certainly be left alone. Packer *et al.* (1972), advocates of early exploration, reviewed 31 patients with radial nerve palsy after a closed fracture of the humerus, in 29 of whom the deficit was complete. In 24 patients the paralysis had occurred immediately after the injury, while in the other five it had occurred after closed manipulation. All fractures were displaced, 18 were comminutive, six were oblique and one was segmental. Eighteen patients were operated upon within two weeks after the injury, with complete recovery in 89%. Although the gross pathological findings during operation were rather impressive, we think these do not in themselves justify early surgical intervention, because recovery is the rule even in radial nerve palsies occurring immediately after a fracture of the humerus (Mumenthaler and Schliack, 1993). Besides, Packer *et al.*'s study dates from 1972, and nowadays MRI or even CT studies give much more information than do plain radiographs.

Only in complex fractures immediately followed by radial nerve palsy does early exploration seem a reasonable proposition. The same may apply to radial neuropathy developing after closed reposition of the fracture, but if nerve conduction studies show that the deficit is mainly caused by conduction block a policy of patiently waiting for spontaneous recovery is justified.

Some postulate that in closed trauma resulting in radial neuropathy surgery should be performed if signs of recovery fail to occur for two months after the injury (Privat *et al.*, 1978). Yet spontaneous recovery may occur after an even longer interval.

An 18-year-old girl had suffered multiple elbow fractures which healed with functionally severe sequelae, including severe restriction of pronation and supination movements. A reconstructive operation several years later resulted in a complete radial nerve palsy immediately after the operation. It involved all muscles innervated by the radial nerve distal to the triceps muscle. Electrophysiological investigation was compatible with severe axonal damage (no motor response could be elicited distal to the site of injury). Re-exploration was considered, but three months after the operation an impressive spontaneous recovery of the radial nerve function occurred. Only extension of the thumb remained weak.

Lesions of the radial nerve in the forearm (supinator syndrome, posterior interosseous nerve syndrome)

At the point where the motor branch of the radial nerve, the deep radial nerve or the posterior interosseous nerve pierces the supinator muscle it may be caught by compression, the symptoms most often being slowly progressive (Benini and Di Martino, 1976; Spaans, 1987; Dawson *et al.*, 1990).

Clinical features

History In the beginning there is often only difficulty in stretching the little finger, it getting curled up with tasks such as getting something out of a trouser pocket. This problem slowly progresses to a total inability to extend the metacarpophalangeal joint. Later, similar weakness starts in the other fingers, one after the other. The thumb is usually affected last, but this sequence may also be reversed (Bronisch, 1971). As a consequence, many movements of the hand are bungled up, for example typing or playing the piano; writing remains fairly normal. Grip remains powerful, provided the fingers are passively placed

around an object. Often there is little or no pain, but there are exceptions. Occasionally the supinator syndrome may occur bilaterally (Penkert and Schwandt, 1979).

Examination There is a total inability to extend the fingers and thumb in the metacarpophalangeal joints. The main features of the supinator syndrome can therefore be briefly characterized as 'dropping fingers without dropping hand'. Some extension of the index finger remains possible, in the interphalangeal joints, by contraction of the lumbrical muscles (innervated by the median nerve). There may be some weakness of the supinator muscle. The brachioradial muscle retains normal power; if it is involved the lesion must be sought at a more proximal site, usually above the elbow. There is severe weakness or even paralysis of the extensor carpi ulnaris, but extension of the wrist remains possible since the extensor carpi radialis muscles function normally. The first sign that the extensor carpi ulnaris is weak appears when the patient is asked to make a fist, from a distinct radial deviation of the extended hand. The dissociation between the two extensor muscles of the wrist is explained by the branch to the extensor carpi radialis leaving the main stem of the radial nerve proximal to entry in the supinator muscle. It therefore escapes being involved in the supinator syndrome, other than with radial nerve lesions above the elbow, in which there is a dropping hand as well as dropping fingers. The interossei may seem also weak with a radial nerve lesion (at any level above the wrist), but this is only because fingers cannot be spread apart if not first put in an extended position. The difference becomes obvious when the fingers are supported on a flat surface: in the case of a radial nerve lesion the action of the interossei is possible and the fingers can be spread apart at least to some extent, whereas with a lesion of the upper motor neurone or a combined lesion of the radial and ulnar nerves there is still severe weakness when the patient is asked to separate the fingers against resistance.

EMG studies in the supinator syndrome may show fibrillation potentials in the muscles receiving their innervation from the posterior interosseous nerve after its passage through the supinator muscle, and also in the supinator muscle itself (Carfi and Dong, 1985). An important criterion is the presence of EMG abnormalities in the extensor carpi ulnaris but not in the extensor carpi radialis longus and brevis. Local slowing of motor nerve conduction may be lacking. Sensory radial nerve conduction is normal because the superficial branch of the radial nerve does not pass through the supinator muscle. A separate compression of the superficial branch in the proximal forearm may occur between the tendons of the brachioradialis and the extensor carpi radialis (Spindler and Dellon, 1990).

Differential diagnosis

Other conditions that may resemble a lesion of the posterior interosseous nerve are listed in Table 7.1. Three of these merit some special discussion: upper motor neurone lesions, a C7 radicular syndrome, and spinal muscular atrophy.

Central (upper motor neurone) weakness
Dropping hand and dropping fingers may occur in central lesions, but without sparing of the radial wrist extensors. In addition, with upper motor neurone lesions other muscles tend to be involved as well: not only the triceps, innervated by the radial nerve but affected only by lesions in the axilla, but also the interossei (to be distinguished from pseudo-paresis of intrinsic hand muscles with radial nerve lesions; see preceding section). Furthermore, when in case of central weakness the patient makes a fist or grips an object with the whole hand, one often observes an involuntary extension of the wrist, which is impossible with involvement of the radial nerve. Finally, one has to look for other central signs, the most important being hyperreflexia and increased tone of the arm in question, and extensor plantar reflexes.

A 61-year-old general practitioner found that he could not squeeze normally, at a funeral reception where he had to shake many hands. Two days before he had played an exhausting match of tennis. In the next few days he found that the right hand was increasingly weak with a number of other activities: shaving, turning a key in the lock, holding a mug of coffee, or flushing plugs from the ears of his patients. There was no numbness, and only a vague ache at the inner side of the forearm. He had always been in good health, apart from 'lone' atrial fibrillation (no other risk factors). A neurologist in his home town had diagnosed a stroke, despite a normal CT scan of the brain; he was rather devastated by this diagnosis. Examination showed moderate weakness of the finger extensors, and of wrist extension on the ulnar but not on the radial side; there were no other signs. In the subsequent six weeks the power gradually returned to normal.

Table 7.1
Conditions that may resemble lesions of the posterior interosseous nerve

---

- Upper motor neurone lesions
- C7 radicular syndrome
- Spinal muscular atrophy
- Neuralgic amyotrophy (see Chapter 24)
- Diseases of extensor tendons
- Compartment syndrome of the deep extensor muscles of the forearm (Hardegger and Segmuller, 1982)

C7 radicular syndrome In this syndrome the weakness predominates in the extensors of the fingers, whereas the wrist extensors are mostly spared (the main contribution coming from the C6 root). The triceps muscle is almost invariably involved, with a decrease of the triceps jerk, which, again, can be attributed to the radial nerve only if the lesion is in the axilla. In addition, the history almost invariably starts with pain, mainly in the neck and the extensor side of the upper arm, and with pins and needles in the index and middle finger.

Spinal muscular atrophy This not infrequently begins with partial deficits, often most prominent in the extensors of the wrist. One should look for weakness of muscles of the hand and forearm outside the distribution of the radial nerve.

The 'resistant tennis elbow'

There is a widespread tendency among orthopaedic or even general surgeons to extend the notion of compression of the posterior interosseous nerve to a syndrome characterized by pain only, without motor deficits. This condition was called the 'resistant tennis elbow' by Roles and Maudsley (1972), who advocated surgical decompression of the nerve. Pain and tenderness in the course of the nerve are considered the primary clinical features, the maximum tenderness being attributed to 'the radial tunnel', located slightly more distally than the lateral epicondyle, which is the tender spot in the classical tennis elbow. The authors stated that in some of the 38 patients they described conduction studies were done, and that these showed 'significant delay' in motor latencies measured from the spiral groove to the median portion of the extensor digitorum communis. In other studies information about the EMG findings was also deficient (Lister *et al.*, 1979; Werner, 1979; Ritts *et al.*, 1987). In contrast, two separate studies of 10 and 17 patients thought to be suffering from such an entrapment failed to find objective clinical or neurophysiological abnormalities (van Rossum *et al.*, 1978;

Verhaar and Spaans, 1991). There seem to be no good arguments so far to believe in the existence of a painful posterior interosseous nerve syndrome without evidence of nerve dysfunction, in this case in the form of weakness alone. Unfortunately, the decompressive operation has gained some popularity among orthopaedic surgeons, although not universally (Wadsworth, 1987). To date there have been no sound observations to support the conclusion that pain in the region of the upper forearm without motor deficits should be attributed to nerve compression. A more probable explanation is strain injury of muscles, tendons or fibrous tissues. This is supported by the good results obtained by operative release of the lateral part of the common extensor aponeurosis from the lateral epicondyle, in 62 patients who had suffered from a 'tennis elbow' for six months or longer (Verhaar *et al.*, 1993).

Causes of posterior interosseous nerve lesions

Entrapments of the posterior interosseous nerve just below the elbow are often attributed to local anatomical variations, such as a tendinous structure of the medial half of the so-called arcade of Frohse (Cravens and Kline, 1990), or by a tight passageway through the supinator muscle, or by entrapment of the nerve by the fibrous origin of the extensor carpi radialis brevis and supinator muscles (Goldman *et al.*, 1969). Other causes are listed in Table 7.2. Sometimes the cause is unclear, as in the case reported by Kruse (1958), in which the deficit was preceded by pain in the elbow, one day before; spontaneous recovery ensued after nine months. One might speculate that the posterior interosseous nerve can be affected by a self-limiting inflammatory process, presumably an autoimmune reaction, analogous to the more common variants in the brachial plexus ('neuralgic amyotrophy'); after all, in this condition cranial nerves can be affected as well

Table 7.2
Causes of posterior interosseous nerve lesions

- Entrapment between 'normal' anatomical structures, at the level of the supinator muscle
- Congenital hemihypertrophy of supinator muscle (Dumitru *et al.*, 1988)
- Accessory brachioradialis muscle (Spinner and Spinner, 1996a)
- Lipoma (Hustead *et al.* 1958; Capener, 1966; Löser and Schafer, 1972; Mariette *et al.*, 1987; Lidor *et al.*, 1992)
- Intramuscular myxoma (Valer *et al.*, 1993)
- Cysts (Bowen and Stone, 1966)
- Rheumatoid arthritis of the elbow joint (Millender *et al.*, 1973; Ishikawa and Hirohata, 1990; Fernandez and Tiku, 1994)
- Traumatic aneurysm of the posterior interosseous artery (Dharapak and Nimberg, 1974)
- Ganglia (Ogino *et al.*, 1991)
- Dislocations of the elbow, fracture of the ulna with dislocation of the radial head, or Monteggia's fracture (Morris, 1974)
- Arteriovenous fistulas for haemodialysis (Sawin and Loftus, 1995)
- Metal contraptions with open radial fractures of the radial head (Dawson *et al.*, 1990)
- Elbow arthroscopy (Papilion *et al.*, 1988)

(Billings and Grahame, 1975; Sanders *et al.*, 1988).

CT scanning, MRI and ultrasound studies may visualize processes that compress the nerve before surgical exploration. However, a definite cause may remain obscure even after exploration, although the surgeon can convince himself to have found, and corrected, an anatomical variation. Such a variation, which seemed to explain the paralysis, was described long ago (Woltmann and Learmonth, 1934): the dorsal interosseous nerve instead of passing through the supinator muscle passed between this muscle and the aponeurosis of the common extensor. However, excision of the aponeurosis had not resulted in improvement after one year. This old case history nicely illustrates the uncertain relevance of 'abnormalities' found during explorations. The same aetiological uncertainty exists with regard to certain occupations in which continuous pro- and supination of the forearm is often blamed (Penkert and

Schwandt, 1979). Preferably neurologists should be present during surgical exploration and should meticulously evaluate the subsequent clinical course.

Management of posterior interosseous nerve lesions

Despite the qualifications stipulated above, trying to free a nerve thought to be compressed is, in general, sound practice and will often lead to recovery. After having convincingly established the site of compression nothing is lost by having a look. Bronisch (1971) has extensively described an ear, nose and throat surgeon in whom full recovery was reached after a second decompression in which the posterior interosseous nerve was liberated from a supinator muscle which over great length was altered into tendinous tissue. At the first operation only the upper tendinous ridge of the supinator muscle had been incised, without clinical improvement. Recovery began soon after the second operation.

Lesions of the radial nerve at the wrist

At the wrist the superficial radial nerve lies in such a superficial position that it seems exceptionally prone to damage, by all sorts of pressure.

Clinical features

Symptoms consist of a shooting pain at the radial side of the wrist, together with unpleasant and painful paraesthesia radiating into the thumb and index finger, each time the radial side of the wrist is touched, or accidentally knocked. Compared with the pain the zone of diminished or absent sensation at the radial side of the hand is only a minor discomfort. Conduction studies of the superficial radial nerve can easily be performed with surface electrodes in the segment between the forearm and the wrist or between the thumb and the wrist (MacKenzie and DeLisa, 1981; Chang and Oh, 1990).

Causes and management of radial nerve lesions at the wrist

Tight wrist bands (Bierman, 1959) and, especially, handcuffs are common factors. Appel (1991) mentioned that as a neurologist in the New York City prison system he had seen 80 patients with handcuff neuropathy, out of approximately 7500 subjects seen over a period of 11 years. Stone and Laureno (1991) described five intoxicated patients who were forcibly handcuffed for a short time; the superficial terminal branch of the radial nerve was affected in eight hands. In some the symptoms of this 'handcuff neuropathy' remained for as long as four months or even three years. Since malingering can be suspected in prisoners, sensory nerve conduction may offer valuable objective evidence. According to these authors the most widely used metallic models employ a ratcheted arm that is advanced with pressure to tighten the handcuffs. Officially, overtightening should be prevented by double-locking with a small key; however, this is difficult in struggling prisoners. A more humane handcuff with automatic double-locks is now available. A more respectable source of pressure on the superficial radial nerve is a meeting badge of the type used at scientific conferences; the badge has a clip that may compress the radial side of the wrist when the arms are crossed (Preston and Shapiro, 1997).

Direct injury is, not unexpectedly, another cause of lesions of the superficial radial nerve. In a series of 51 patients with compression of the radial sensory nerve, injury was the cause in more than 80% (Dellon and Mackinnon, 1986). Lindscheid reported 17 patients with symptoms from direct injury to this branch, with follow up between 4.5 and 15 years (Lindscheid, 1965). Often there was continuous and burning pain in the thumb and

unpleasant numbness or inordinate tenderness around the wrist. Touching the skin area in question was most unpleasant. Results from nerve repair and excision of neuromas had good results in two patients in whom the nerve itself had not been severed. In eight patients the injuries were accidental, and eight others suffered injuries to the nerve from surgical procedures such as for stenosing tenosynovitis (de Quervain's disease) or open reductions of fractures of both bones in the forearm; in one patient a tight watch band was to blame. Transposition of a flexor tendon towards the thumb may also result in compression of the superficial branch of the radial nerve (Spinner and Spinner, 1996b). Longitudinal scars at the radial aspect of the wrist should probably be avoided (Lindscheid, 1965). Some patients may become completely disabled, not tolerating the slightest touch to the skin of the innervated zone, and showing the peculiarities of true causalgia (Dawson *et al.*, 1990).

Surgical causes of lesions of the superficial radial nerve other than fractures are shunt operations for haemodialysis, compression by a perivascular tissue reaction to an indwelling catheter, or even infiltration of the arm with silicone gel, following rupture of a subpectoral breast prosthesis (Sanger *et al.*, 1992).

In a minority of patients entrapment of the radial sensory nerve can be attributed only to repeated movements (pronation/supination of the forearm, or movements of the wrist from the radial to the ulnar side, with the arm in pronation and the wrist in flexion), a position which may cause the nerve to be pinched between the tendons of the extensor carpi radialis longus and of the brachioradialis (Dellon and Mackinnon, 1986). Stenosing tenosynovitis (de Quervain's disease) may contribute to entrapment of the superficial radial nerve; in one series of 50 patients this was the underlying condition in as much as 50% (Lanzetta and Foucher, 1993). The list of possible causes of compression or chronic trauma of this nerve is almost endless, but sometimes the cause remains unclear. Transposition of the nerve to a less exposed position may bring lasting relief.

A 40-year-old and lean female horse breeder had for several months had the typical symptoms of painful paraesthesia over the back of the hand and thumb, with numbness. No neurography was performed. On exploration, exactly at the point from where the unpleasant symptoms could be evoked, the nerve tissue showed a red discoloration over a length of about 1 cm. The nerve was normal on palpation so a tumour seemed highly unlikely. Transposition of the nerve to a less exposed site led to complete recovery in about three weeks. Five years later there had been no recurrence. Chronic microtrauma could have been a cause in her profession, but this was repeatedly denied.

Compressive lesions of the dorsal digital nerves

Compressive lesions of the dorsal digital nerves seem to be rare. Professional and daily use of scissors has been reported as a cause of a dorsal digital neuropathy of the thumb, as has a palmar ganglion (Margles, 1994). Wartenberg (1932) mentioned this syndrome under the name of 'cheiralgia paraesthetica'.

Chapter 8
The median nerve

Anatomy

The median nerve (Figure 8.1) carries fibres from C5–Th1 and emerges from the axilla together with the radial and ulnar nerves as well as the axillary artery and its vein, through the inelastic axillary sheath. In the upper arm no branches are given off; the nerve courses through the bicipital sulcus to the elbow, at the medial side of the brachial artery. At the level of the elbow the median nerve runs through the antecubital fossa, medial to the biceps tendon and under the bicipital aponeurosis. Here branches are given off to the pronator teres, flexor carpi radialis, palmaris longus and flexor digitorum superficialis muscles. In the proximal

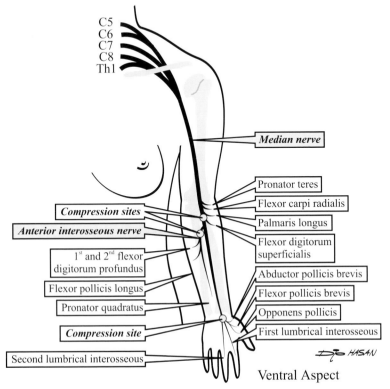

C5
C6
C7
C8
Th1

Median nerve

Pronator teres
Flexor carpi radialis
Palmaris longus
Flexor digitorum superficialis
Abductor pollicis brevis
Flexor pollicis brevis
Opponens pollicis
First lumbrical interosseous

Compression sites
Anterior interosseous nerve
1ˢᵗ and 2ⁿᵈ flexor digitorum profundus
Flexor pollicis longus
Pronator quadratus
Compression site
Second lumbrical interosseous

HASAN

Ventral Aspect

Figure 8.1
Muscles innervated by the median nerve.

portion of the forearm it has a much deeper position, between the two heads of the pronator teres. Distal to this muscle the *anterior interosseous nerve* originates, a purely motor branch innervating the flexor digitorum profundus I and II, flexor pollicis longus and pronator quadratus muscles. This branch lies anterior to the interosseous membrane that joins radius and ulna, and passes further down between the flexor pollicis longus and the flexor digitorum profundus. Just proximal to the wrist the median nerve takes a more superficial course before entering the carpal tunnel. Within or distal to the carpal tunnel is the origin of the *recurrent motor branch to the thenar*, which supplies the abductor pollicis brevis, opponens pollicis and flexor pollicis brevis muscles. The most distal ramifications of motor nerve fibres are to the superficial head of the flexor pollicis brevis and to the first and second lumbricals. It is not rare, however, to find the flexor pollicis brevis entirely innervated by the ulnar nerve, and in other cases it has double innervation by the median and ulnar nerves (Highet, 1943; Rowntree, 1949).

The motor innervation distal to the flexor retinaculum may be quite different from the standard description given above. The median nerve may innervate the hypothenar muscles via an anomalous branch, arising from its course in the carpal tunnel (Seradge and Seradge, 1990), and even an 'all median hand' has been reported (Marinacci, 1964). Conversely, the deep motor branch of the ulnar nerve may communicate with the median nerve in the hand (Riche-Cannieu anastomosis) (Harness and Sekeles, 1971). Another and more common variant is that fibres from the median nerve in the forearm cross to the ulnar nerve, an anomaly called the Martin–Gruber anastomosis, which is found in 15–30% of normal subjects (Amoiridis, 1992; Leibovic and Hastings, 1992), and almost invariably (8/8) in subjects with Down's syndrome (Srinivasan and Rhodes, 1981). Most often

(60%) the anastomosis consists of fibres of the anterior interosseous nerve coursing with the ulnar nerve to innervate 'median muscles', but in 35% the anastomosing fibres from the median nerve innervate 'ulnar muscles', such as the adductor pollicis and first dorsal interosseous muscles (Leibovic and Hastings, 1992). In extremely rare cases an anastomotic branch from the radial nerve may innervate the abductor pollicis brevis muscle, and even the musculocutaneous nerve may give off fibres to muscles that are normally innervated by the median nerve (Rosenbaum and Ochoa, 1993).

The area of sensory innervation by the median nerve is confined to the hand and fingers (Figure 8.2). The *palmar cutaneous branch* leaves the main trunk of the median nerve a few centimetres proximal to the wrist, and courses over the transverse carpal ligament to the thenar eminence. It innervates the proximal half of the radial side of the palm, and also the thenar eminence. There is extensive overlapping with the innervation areas of the digital branches of the median nerve (see below), the lateral cutaneous nerve of the forearm (musculocutaneous nerve), the medial cutaneous nerve of the forearm (brachial plexus), and in the palm with the territories of the superficial radial nerve and the ulnar nerve.

The *digital nerves* (see Figure 8.2) innervate the volar side of the skin of the thumb, index finger, middle finger and the radial half of the ring finger, as well as the adjoining portion of the palm. At the dorsal surface the median nerve innervates almost the entire middle finger, and the middle and terminal phalanges of the index finger and ring finger (radial half). The sensory supply areas show considerable overlap, but the sensory innervation of the hand is less variable than motor innervation. A unique observation is that of a little finger that was innervated entirely by an anomalous branch of the median nerve (Saeed and Davies, 1995).

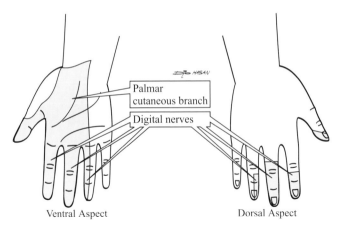

Figure 8.2
Approximate skin area innervated by the median nerve.

Examination

The different muscles in the forearm and hand innervated by the median nerve are tested as shown in Figures 8.3 to 8.12.

Median nerve lesions in the axilla

Apart from trauma associated with accidents or assault, subacute and severe damage to the median nerve in the axilla may be iatrogenic, following repositioning of shoulder luxation, or axillary arteriography producing inflammatory fibrosis, a false aneurysm, or both. In an early series of 62 percutaneous catheterizations via the axillary approach there was injury to the median and ulnar nerves in three patients, leading to severe disability of the hand (Staal *et al.*, 1966; Staal and van Voorthuisen, 1969). Simultaneous lesions to these two nerves in the axilla is not surprising, since both nerves pass

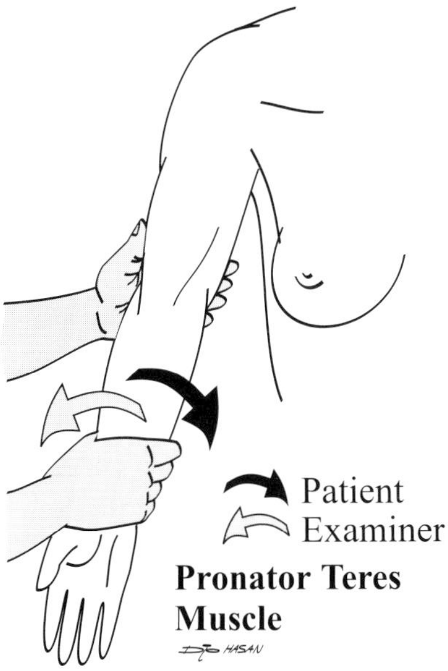

Pronator Teres Muscle

Figure 8.3
The extended forearm is pronated against resistance.

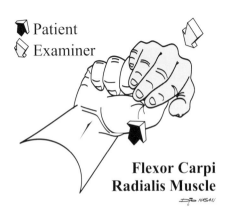

Flexor Carpi Radialis Muscle

Figure 8.4
The hand is flexed and abducted at the wrist against resistance.

The median nerve

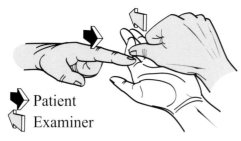

Patient
Examiner

Superficial Flexor Digitorum Muscle

Figure 8.5
The index finger is flexed at the proximal interphalangeal joint against resistance, while the proximal phalanx is fixed by the left index finger of the examiner.

together with the axillary artery and its vein through the non-elastic axillary sheath. With the passing of years this complication has not disappeared (Kennedy *et al.*, 1997). Fortunately, nowadays axillary arteriography has been almost completely replaced by the femoral route. Lipomas may cause compression of almost any nerve at any level; for the median nerve this has been

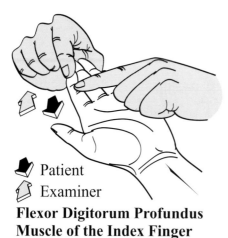

Patient
Examiner

Flexor Digitorum Profundus Muscle of the Index Finger

Figure 8.6
The distal phalanx of the index finger is flexed against resistance, while the middle phalanx is fixed by the left index finger of the examiner.

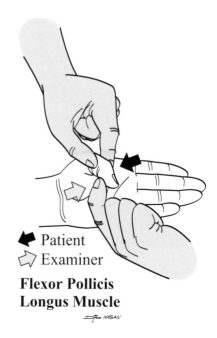

Patient
Examiner

Flexor Pollicis Longus Muscle

Figure 8.7
The distal phalanx of the thumb is flexed against resistance, while the proximal phalanx of the thumb is fixed by the left hand of the examiner.

reported also in the infraclavicular fossa (Weinzweig and Browne, 1988).

Median nerve lesions in the upper arm

Possible causes of median nerve compression in the upper arm include

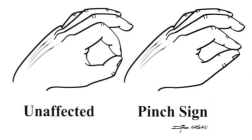

Unaffected   **Pinch Sign**

Figure 8.8
Pinch sign due to paralysis of flexor digitorum profundus of the index finger and of the flexor pollicis longus.

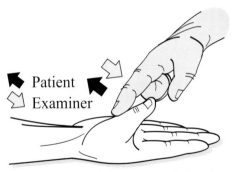

► Patient
▷ Examiner

Abductor Pollicis Longus Muscle
Abductor Pollicis Brevis Muscle

Figure 8.9
The dorsum of the patient's hand rests on a flat surface, while the thumb is raised to the ceiling against resistance at the metacarpophalangeal joint.

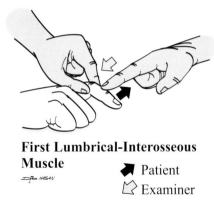

First Lumbrical-Interosseous Muscle

► Patient
▷ Examiner

Figure 8.11
The index finger is extended at the proximal interphalangeal joint against resistance, while the metacarpophalangeal joint is hyperextended and fixed by the left hand of the examiner.

tourniquet paralysis (Bolton and McFarlane, 1978), a nerve tumour (Rosenbaum and Ochoa, 1993), soft tissue tumours such as non-Hodgkin lymphoma (Desta *et al.*, 1994), or closed reduction after supracondylar fractures of the humerus (Thorleifsson *et al.*, 1988).

Sometimes the cause remains unknown in cases with sudden onset followed by spontaneous improvement (nerve infarction?).

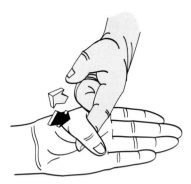

Opponens Pollicis Muscle
► Patient
▷ Examiner

Figure 8.10
The thumb is pointed to the base of the little finger against resistance.

A 49-year-old housewife, while reading the newspaper, noticed a numb sensation in the radial three fingers of the left hand, and difficulty in lifting a glass, all this without any pain. In the preceding days she had heavily indulged in playing golf. On examination there was weakness (MRC grade 4) of pronation, and of the flexor carpi radialis, flexor digitorum superficialis, flexor digitorum profundus I and II, flexor pollicis longus, and abductor pollicis brevis. Skin sensation was diminished at the palmar side of the radial three fingers and at the adjacent palm. Nerve conduction studies, three days after the first symptoms, showed a partial conduction block of the median nerve halfway down the upper arm; two weeks later there were signs of denervation in the affected muscles. The erythrocyte sedimentation rate (ESR) and blood glucose were normal, as was an MRI scan of the left axilla and arm. Three weeks after the onset she experienced a spontaneous burning sensation as well as hyperaesthesia in the numb area as well as a dull ache in the entire arm. This heralded the beginning of spontaneous improvement of the weakness; after about three months all symptoms and signs had disappeared.

Sleep paralysis of the median nerve in the upper arm, from pressure of a partner's head, is a rare event (*'paralysie des amoureux'* or, more conventionally, 'honeymoon palsy').

Median nerve lesions at the level of the elbow

Lesions of the median nerve at the elbow are much more uncommon than those at the wrist. There are two entrapment points in this region, very near to each other: between the two heads of the pronator teres muscle and somewhat more distally, near the origin of the pure motor branch of the median nerve (anterior interosseous nerve), by a fibrous band between the deep head of the pronator muscle and the flexor digitorum superficialis. Neurological signs in both conditions may overlap.

Some orthopaedic surgeons (Johnson, R.K. *et al.*, 1979; Hartz *et al.*, 1981) believe

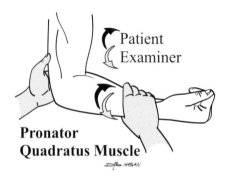

Figure 8.12
The forearm is pronated against resistance, while the elbow is flexed.

in the existence of an entirely subjective pronator teres syndrome, consisting only of pain in the forearm. Apart from the local tenderness of the ventral forearm there may be a vaguely localized numbness in the thumb and index finger. We have strong reservations about diagnosing a pronator teres syndrome in such circumstances, without evidence of median nerve dysfunction such as weakness, sensory change or reproduction of specific paraesthesia by provocative tests (Rosenbaum and Ochoa, 1993), let alone for operating on such patients. In the following sections we shall only deal with conditions associated with objective neurological findings.

The pronator teres syndrome

This syndrome is the least rare form of entrapment of the median nerve near the elbow. There may be some pain along the flexor side of the proximal forearm and paraesthesia in the median nerve distribution in the hand, but definitely nothing like the intense pins and needles experienced in the carpal tunnel syndrome. Pressure on the pronator teres muscle may produce radiating pain or, more convincingly, paraesthesia. It should again be emphasized that the diagnosis remains uncertain without weakness in one or more hand muscles innervated by the median nerve, characteristic sensory loss, or typical EMG findings.

Sensory loss may occur in the entire median nerve area in the hand but, as a rule, it is restricted to the ulnar side of the thumb and to the radial side of the index finger. Because there may be damage to some fascicles of the median nerve with sparing of others (Spaans, 1987), it is difficult to localize exactly the site of entrapment and distinguish the pronator syndrome from the anterior interosseous syndrome if there is no sensory deficit. In a series of seven patients with pronator syndrome associated with heavy manual work, all but one had sensory impairment but no excruciating pain (Morris and Peters, 1976); weakness of the abductor pollicis brevis and flexor pollicis longus was present in all, of the opponens pollicis muscle in five patients, and the flexor digitorum profundus of the index finger in one patient. Five patients recovered and were able to resume their normal activities after corticosteroid injections in the region of the pronator teres muscle, but this treatment was uncontrolled. The use of an electrical screwdriver was the solution in another patient.

A pronator teres syndrome is best confirmed by demonstrating needle EMG abnormalities in the forearm and hand muscles innervated by the median nerve. These may also occur in the pronator teres muscle itself (Hartz *et al.*, 1981; Gross and Jones, 1992), which means that needle EMG does not allow differentiation from more proximal lesions of the median nerve. Abnormal nerve conduction studies are found in a minority of cases. In the absence of electrophysiological abnormalities the diagnosis of pronator teres syndrome should not be made lightly.

The anterior interosseous syndrome

Here we are on firmer ground, but entrapment of the anterior interosseous nerve is rare, amounting to less than 1% of all median nerve afflictions (Rosenbaum and Ochoa, 1993). Pain may be present, but is not a leading symptom and mostly the presenting symptom is subacute weakness in the hand. Marked weakness or even paralysis of the flexor pollicis longus and the flexor digitorum profundus of the index finger (flexion of the terminal phalanx) is the hallmark of the condition; sometimes there is less severe weakness of the pronator quadratus. Typically, the patient is unable to form a small circle by pinching the end phalanx of the thumb and index finger together, the so-called 'pinch sign' (see

Figure 8.8). In addition, the 'straight thumb sign' is seen when the patient attempts to make a grasping movement with the affected hand (Cherington, 1977). The pronator quadratus should be tested with the elbow in flexion (see Figure 8.12). Sensory impairment does not occur, since the anterior interosseous nerve is purely motor.

The abnormally extended posture when the patient attempts to pinch the thumb and index finger together is so typical that other sites of entrapment are practically ruled out, provided there is no sensory loss or weakness in other muscles innervated by the median nerve (apart from the pronator quadratus).

A 50-year-old administrator had for several days had a spontaneous and dull pain in his right forearm, radiating to the index finger and thumb; moreover, the right hand was weak. On examination there was weakness of the flexor pollicis longus and the flexor digitorum profundus of the index finger, but in addition the opponens muscle was weak and sensation was impaired at the radial side of the index finger and the ulnar side of the thumb, indicating involvement not only of the anterior interosseous nerve but also of the main trunk of the median nerve. Surgical exploration, one month later, revealed a fibrous band compressing both nerves. Recovery started two weeks after the operation and was complete after three months.

If the weakness is preceded or accompanied by acute and severe pain in the arm, neuralgic amyotrophy must be considered (see Chapter 24), especially if the pain is in the shoulder or the upper arm (Smith and Herbst, 1974; Goulding and Schady, 1993); the latter authors reported six patients, all of whom spontaneously recovered within 9–24 months. In some of these cases the site of the inflammatory lesion is not the anterior interosseous nerve itself but rather the corresponding fascicle in the brachial plexus, as evidenced by subsequent development of weakness in the shoulder girdle, for example of the serratus anterior muscle (Rennels and Ochoa, 1980).

An anterior interosseous neuropathy is best confirmed by demonstrating abnormalities on needle EMG exclusively in the three muscles supplied by this nerve. As this neuropathy can be a manifestation of neuralgic amyotrophy, arm and shoulder muscles should be examined as well (Wertsch, 1992). A few studies have reported increased motor latencies to the flexor digitorum profundus muscle (Krause and Reuther, 1979) or to the pronator quadratus (Farber and Bryan, 1968; Nakano *et al.*, 1977; Rosenberg, 1990), but in most cases no slowing in conduction of the anterior interosseous nerve has been found. Motor and sensory conduction in the main trunk of the median nerve are always normal in this disorder.

Causes of median nerve lesions at the level of the elbow

A variety of specific causes may be associated with pronator syndrome or the anterior interosseous syndrome (Table 8.1). In the absence of trauma or obvious source of compression the cause is presumed to be 'overuse' of the pronator muscle (Gross and Jones, 1992), although anatomical variations such as fibrous bands probably contribute to the development of the lesion, given its rarity despite heavy manual work being ubiquitous.

Management of median nerve lesions at the elbow

If the history implicates blunt trauma, external pressure, or unusual hyperactivity of the arm, it seems wise to wait for spontaneous regression. However, if the deficits remain the same or even worsen

Table 8.1
Causes of median nerve lesions at the level of the elbow (at the pronator muscle or at the origin of the anterior interosseous nerve)

- 'Overuse' of pronator muscle, probably in combination with one of the anatomical factors mentioned below (Gross and Jones, 1992)
- External pressure, with carrying heavy objects (Gardner Thorpe, 1974)
- Persistence of median artery in the forearm (Jones and Ming, 1988)
- Pressure from the anterior interosseous artery (Franzini *et al.*, 1995)
- Compression by a fibrous band from the supracondylar process to the medial epicondyle of the humerus, or Struthers' ligament (al Qattan and Husband, 1991; al Naib, 1994; Murali *et al.*, 1995)
- Compression by a fibrous band at the humeral head of the pronator muscle (Tulwa *et al.*, 1994)
- Intra-articular fracture of the humerus (Burczak, 1994)
- After closed reduction of a dislocated elbow (Boe and Holst Nielsen, 1987)
- Synovial bursa from partial rupture of distal biceps brachii tendon (Foxworthy and Kinninmonth, 1992)
- Haematoma or false aneurysm after puncture of the brachial artery (Macon and Futrell, 1973; Yip *et al.*, 1997)
- Intravenous injections into the forearm (Blankenship, 1991), venepuncture (Berry and Wallis, 1977), or intravenous catheterization (Finelli, 1977)
- Vascular shunts for haemodialysis (Zamora *et al.* 1986)
- External pressure during general anaesthesia (Gardner Thorpe, 1974)
- Application of a tight band in the treatment of lateral epicondylitis ('tennis elbow') (Enzenauer and Nordstrom, 1991)

over a period of about two months, MRI and surgical exploration are usually warranted (Schantz and Riegels Nielsen, 1992). Often this also reveals the exact site of compression as well as its cause.

Median nerve lesions at the wrist: the carpal tunnel syndrome

Spontaneous compression of the median nerve at the wrist within the carpal tunnel is by and far the most frequently occurring mononeuropathy. It was first recognized in 1913 by Marie and Foix, but it took a few more decades, until the influential publications of Brain (Brain *et al.*, 1947; Kremer *et al.*, 1953), before it dawned on the neurological community that the old syndrome 'brachialgia paraesthetica nocturna' should be attributed to compression of the median nerve at the wrist. It is mainly seen in women. The explanation for the gender difference may be, at least partly, that the cross-sectional area in the carpal tunnel is less in women than in men, as demonstrated by computed tomography (Dekel *et al.*, 1980). MRI allows the true volume of the carpal tunnel (bony canal minus soft tissues) to be determined, but so far studies have not distinguished between the sexes (Richman *et al.*, 1987; Skie *et al.*, 1990).

Epidemiology

The prevalence of carpal tunnel syndrome has been studied in the Netherlands among the population of the town of Maastricht and its neighbouring villages (de Krom *et al.*, 1992). In a random sample of 715 inhabitants, stratified for age and sex and with a response rate of 70%, the authors found a prevalence rate of 9.2% of all adult women, 5.8% of which were newly detected; the remaining 3.4% had been previously diagnosed. The authors' criteria for the diagnosis were a history of being woken up at least twice a week by unpleasant 'pins and needles' in one or both hands, together with neurophysiological confirmation (prolonged distal latencies of the median nerve). The proportion of 5.8% newly detected cases may actually be an underestimation, because 14 of the 51 women who reported nocturnal paraesthesia declined to undergo neurophysiological testing (which confirmed carpal tunnel syndrome in 23 of the 37 others). The age of the subjects interviewed ranged between 25 and 74 years, above age 35 years the prevalence was more or less similar in all age groups, contrary to the often repeated notion that carpal tunnel syndrome is typically an affliction of middle-aged women. As expected the overall prevalence rate for men was vastly lower, amounting to only 0.6% (95% CI 0.02–3.4%). The most powerful risk factors for carpal tunnel syndrome in women, as identified in a case-control study, were small body length and activities involving wrist flexion (de Krom *et al.*, 1990a).

The incidence (rate of newly occurring cases) of carpal tunnel syndrome in patients identified from the files of the Epidemiology Program Project of the Mayo Clinics was 125 per 100 000 person-years (age-adjusted incidence, for the period 1976–1980), of whom 79% were women (Stevens *et al.*, 1988). These data confirm that idiopathic carpal tunnel syndrome is a remarkably frequent disorder, mostly seen in adult women, but not only in middle age. There are a few case reports of carpal tunnel syndrome in children, nearly always secondary to other conditions such as infection or vaccination, Klippel–Trenaunay syndrome (Poilvache *et al.*, 1989), haemophilia (Case, 1967), or a variety of congenital limb deformities (Rosenbaum and Ochoa, 1993). In view of the high frequency it is astonishing that general practitioners and other physicians still so often fail to diagnose carpal tunnel syndrome as the cause of tingling in the fingers or pain in the arm.

Anatomy

The point of entrapment of the median nerve in carpal tunnel syndrome lies under the flexor retinaculum or transverse carpal ligament, which extends from the most distal part of the wrist up to two-thirds of the distance along the medial border of the thenar eminence (see Figure 8.1). This inelastic ligament forms the roof of the carpal tunnel, a narrow channel through which the median nerve (motor, sensory and autonomous nerve fibres) passes together with nine flexor tendons. The ulnar nerve passes over the flexor retinaculum and so escapes compression at this level. The floor of the carpal tunnel consists of carpal bones and their connective tissue components. The space in the carpal tunnel decreases even further on flexion of the wrist (Yoshioka *et al.*, 1993; Howe *et al.*, 1994). In the case of surgical treatment it is important to know that in about one-quarter of subjects the recurrent thenar motor branch does not leave the median nerve distal to the flexor retinaculum, but pierces the ligament about 6 mm proximal to its distal border (Poisel, 1974).

The *motor function* of the median nerve at the level of the wrist concerns mainly the abductor pollicis brevis (see Figure 8.9) and opponens pollicis (see Figure 8.10) muscles. The superficial head of the flexor pollicis brevis and the first and the second lumbricals are also innervated by fibres branching from the median nerve distal to the flexor retinaculum, but these muscles are difficult to test separately. Moreover, the flexor pollicis brevis may receive its innervation partly or entirely from the ulnar nerve. Several other variations in the standard pattern of branching exist; these have been described in the section on the anatomy of the median nerve. Only neurophysiological studies can discover these anatomical variations.

The *sensory innervation* from the median nerve distal to the carpal tunnel includes the palmar surface of the first three and a half fingers. On the dorsal side the skin area of the median nerve includes almost the entire middle finger, and the middle and distal phalanges of the index finger and of the ring finger on the radial side (Laroy *et al.*, 1998) (see Figure 8.2). The palmar cutaneous branch, innervating the proximal part of the palm and the thenar eminence, leaves the median nerve about 5 cm proximal to the wrist, and so it is not involved in carpal tunnel syndrome. However, there may be overlapping innervation from the digital branches of the median nerve, from the lateral cutaneous nerve of the forearm, or from

the ulnar nerve (Rosenbaum and Ochoa, 1993).

History

The symptoms of carpal tunnel syndrome are rather uniform in nature but vary widely in severity, and there may be spontaneous remissions, even almost complete. In the beginning there is an intermittent sensation of pins and needles (the hands are 'sleeping') on the side of the palm, in some or all of the fingers innervated by the median nerve. A considerable proportion of patients report that tingling is experienced in the entire ring finger and even in the little finger; if they remain adamant, the physician may be led to the erroneous conclusion that the ulnar nerve is involved. Apart from this, but often only later in the disease, there may be burning pain, numbness and, early in the morning, a sensation of swelling of the hand, often causing rings to be taken off. The paraesthesia are typically most troublesome at night; the patient wakes up with them. Shaking or rubbing the hands ('letting the blood circulate') gives quick relief, but after a brief nap the history repeats itself, leading to broken nights. Some regard the flicking movements, of the hand(s) in response to the question 'What do you actually do with your hand(s) when symptoms are at their worst' as a better predictor of carpal tunnel syndrome than some provocation tests (Pryse-Phillips, 1984), but this was not confirmed in a later study (de Krom *et al.*, 1990b). Early in the morning the hand may be clumsy with fine finger movements, and it feels swollen and weak. The same symptoms may occur during the daytime, especially while knitting, sewing, wringing, driving a car or during other manual work, which is not necessarily heavy. Needlework becomes impossible. The symptoms may not disappear on holidays. The subjective weakness of grip, which is a common complaint, cannot be confirmed by examination. The 'pins and needles' become increasingly painful and may eventually be accompanied by numbness at the tips of the thumb, index and middle finger. Rarely, there are autonomic phenomena such as red discoloration of the palm of the hand; we have never seen cyanosis. Furthermore, the pain, but not the paraesthesia, may radiate through the forearm, and even the upper arm may be involved as far as the shoulder or even the neck. One may occasionally meet a patient who seeks help because of pain in the shoulder and who, only after persistent questioning, admits to paraesthesia in the fingers.

Because carpal tunnel syndrome is so common it is practical to consider every woman with complaints of the hand and arm as having a reasonable chance of suffering from carpal tunnel syndrome, until the opposite has been proved. The *a priori* possibility of carpal tunnel syndrome increases even further if symptoms are bilateral, because carpal tunnel syndrome often affects both hands, although one hand is always more seriously involved than the other. The dominant hand may be most affected, but there are many exceptions to this rule.

Nowadays it is rare to meet patients performing special handicrafts that demand wrist movements in endless repetition, as was usual in a number of professions until World War II (see section on causes). Overdiagnosis is to be avoided, particularly in males.

Examination

Sensation. In many patients with carpal tunnel syndrome the neurological examination is negative but it is not unusual to find slight numbness on the palmar side of one or more fingertips or more proximally, but only within the distribution of the median nerve. Perception may be diminished for pinprick, touch or both.

Motor findings. Patients may have severe sensory symptoms for more than a decade, without any weakness or atrophy. Only in a small minority does one find weakness of the thenar muscles, with or without atrophy. In these exceptional cases atrophy of the thenar muscle is partial or total, depending on whether the flexor pollicis brevis is innervated by the ulnar or the median nerve (Highet, 1943; Rowntree, 1949). Muscle wasting and weakness is then usually limited to the outer half of the thenar muscle, corresponding to the abductor pollicis brevis and opponens muscles. Weakness of the opponens pollicis muscle can often be diagnosed by inspection only, when the patient is asked to place the thumb at the base of the little finger. To test the strength of the opponens pollicis the examiner should exert counterpressure just distal to the metacarpophalangeal joint of the thumb (see Figure 8.10). Some manual workers, male or female, have such strongly developed thenar muscles that these mechanically interfere with placing the thumb at the base of the little finger, while weakness may be difficult to detect unless the contralateral side is unaffected. The abductor pollicis brevis is the most important muscle for the diagnosis of carpal tunnel syndrome, since it is the thenar muscle that is the least likely to be innervated by the ulnar nerve (Rowntree, 1949). Its strength is assessed by asking the patient to keep the dorsum of the hand on a flat surface and then to move the extended thumb in the direction of the ceiling (i.e. in a plane perpendicular to the palm) (see Figure 8.9). Patients with muscle wasting are less often troubled by paraesthesia and pain than are those without wasting (Fullerton, 1963).

Autonomic changes. Trophic skin lesions may include small ulcers on the fingertips (Rosenbaum and Ochoa, 1993), but these are very rare indeed. Sometimes there is a reddish discoloration of the palm and the palmar side of the fingers, whereas we have never seen cyanosis. Raynaud's phenomenon is not seen in idiopathic carpal tunnel syndrome, unless the two conditions co-exist.

Provocation of symptoms. In most cases with proven carpal tunnel syndrome the manoeuvre of forceful hyperflexion of the wrist by the examiner leads within a minute to unpleasant paraesthesia that are recognized by the patient as being similar to the symptoms for which medical help was sought. The sensations often occur in all five fingers, one after the other, in other words also outside the distribution of the median nerve. De Krom *et al.* (1990b) dismissed all provocation tests as useless, but in their study these manoeuvres consisted only of asking the patient to flex the wrist by placing the dorsum of their hands against each other (Phalen, 1970), or to press the palms of their hands against each other (hyperextension). In our experience, admittedly not backed up by a systematic study, forceful hyperflexion of the wrist by the examiner is a sensitive and specific test for detecting carpal tunnel syndrome. Others claim similarly good results for direct compression of the carpal tunnel (Del Pino *et al.*, 1997). Inflating a blood-pressure cuff around the upper arm adds the effects of ischaemia to those of conduction block by chronic pressure, and this test may also provoke the characteristic tingling sensations within less than one minute (Gilliatt and Wilson, 1953), but Gellman *et al.* (1986) found this test positive in 40% of controls, against 71% of patients with carpal tunnel syndrome. Hyperextension of the wrist by the examiner, together with percussion of the median nerve at the wrist (Hoffmann–Tinel sign), may also provoke symptoms, but false-negative or false-positive results with this test are common (de Krom *et al.*, 1990b).

Given a typical history, with or without positive results of the forced hyperflexion test, objective signs are absent in the

majority of patients. Therefore accurate investigation of sensory conduction of the median nerve at the wrist is of crucial importance to support the clinical diagnosis of carpal tunnel syndrome. Nevertheless, we should confess that we have seen three patients with a classical history and positive hyperflexion test but normal sensory conduction velocities, in whom surgical decompression of the median nerve resulted in dramatic and long-lasting relief.

Electrophysiological studies

An early electrophysiological sign of nerve compression is local slowing of impulse conduction, resulting from damage to the myelin sheaths (Figure 8.13). Therefore nerve conduction studies are essential in the diagnosis of the carpal tunnel syndrome. A large variety of nerve conduction tests has been advocated

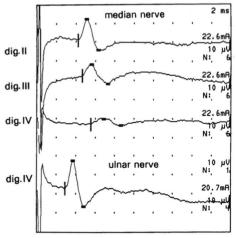

Figure 8.13
Sensory nerve conduction study in a case of carpal tunnel syndrome. Stimulation of the median nerve and ulnar nerve at the wrist and recording with ring electrodes from digits II, III and IV (antidromic method). The distances between the stimulating cathode and proximal recording electrodes were equal (150 mm). From digit II to digit IV median SNAPs are increasingly delayed and reduced in amplitude. This is a common finding in carpal tunnel syndrome. The latency of the ulnar digit IV SNAP serves as an intraindividual control value. Calibration: 2 ms and 10 μV.

(Jablecki *et al.*, 1993). The most sensitive tests are those that use sensory conduction in other nerve segments in the same hand for comparison. As a standard procedure we measure the antidromic sensory conduction times over the ulnar and median nerves in the segments between the wrist and the ring finger, over equal distances (Brenninkmeyer, 1979). Differences in distal sensory latency between the median and ulnar nerve of more than 0.4 ms are abnormal (Jackson and Clifford, 1989; Charles *et al.*, 1990). Median nerve entrapment in the carpal tunnel appears to affect the fibres to the ring finger more than those to the other fingers (Spaans, 1984; Uncini *et al.*, 1989; Uncini *et al.*, 1993; Charles *et al.*, 1990). To detect the exact site of compression the so-called 'inching' technique may be applied, in which multiple stimulation sites along the distal sensory segment of the median nerve are used (Kimura, 1979).

Comparison of responses from median nerve stimulation at the wrist and the palm can be used not only to localize the lesion at the wrist, but also to discriminate between conduction block and axonal degeneration in sensory and motor fibers, which might be useful in predicting outcome (Di Guglielmo *et al.*, 1997).

As a routine test for distal motor conduction in the median nerve the absolute latency to the abductor pollicis brevis is often used. A much more sensitive test is comparison between distal motor latencies to the ulnar-innervated interosseous and the median-innervated lumbrical muscle in the second interosseous space, using equal conduction distances for both nerves (Preston and Logigian, 1992).

Long-standing nerve compression may lead to axonal degeneration and, thereby, to needle EMG abnormalities in the abductor pollicis brevis. Signs of reinnervation (polyphasic muscle action potentials) may occur without signs of denervation (fibrillations). These are mostly mild but chronic cases in which the process of denervation is apparently counterbalanced by an almost equal degree of reinnervation. In typical carpal tunnel syndrome with modest but unequivocal conduction abnormalities there is usually no need for needle EMG.

Diagnostic imaging

Imaging techniques are not required as a standard technique in the diagnosis of carpal tunnel syndrome, if only because the sensitivity and specificity of these methods are incompletely known. Radiological investigations are required only if specific structural lesions are suspected. Routine *wrist radiography* is not cost-effective (Bindra *et al.*, 1997). *Computed tomography* may help to clarify the anatomical relationships in the region of the carpal tunnel (Pierallini *et al.*, 1993), but *magnetic resonance imaging* provides anatomical details not only of the bony structures bordering the carpal tunnel but also of the soft tissue structures, even with three-dimensional reconstructions (magnetic resonance neurography) (Howe *et al.*, 1994). This allows identification not only of congenital stenosis of the carpal tunnel as a cause of compression of the median nerve (Horch *et al.*, 1997), but also of specific abnormalities such as thickening of the synovium of the flexor tendons (Healy *et al.*, 1990; Buchberger *et al.*, 1993), an intracanalicular ganglion, swelling of the median nerve (Middleton *et al.*, 1987), a neuroma (Murphy *et al.*, 1993), or a nerve tumour. *Ultrasonography* has also been found to be a useful technique for demonstrating compression of the median nerve in the carpal tunnel (Buchberger *et al.*, 1993).

Differential diagnosis of the carpal tunnel syndrome

Because carpal tunnel syndrome is so common and the symptoms are so characteristic it rarely occurs that some other condition is mistaken for carpal tunnel syndrome; errors occur relatively more often the other way around. Only *median nerve compression slightly more distal* in the palm, for instance caused by a lipoma, should be borne in mind (De Smet *et al.*, 1994), especially since abnormalities of sensory conduction may be practically the same as in compression at the wrist. Surgical exploration may bring the solution. More *proximal compression of the median nerve* in the forearm may lead to pain in the forearm radiating to the radial three fingers and to the palm of the hand, but the cardinal sign in that case is weakness of flexor muscles of the distal phalanges (flexor digitorum profundus) of the index finger and the thumb. Moreover, in this condition sensory conduction in the median nerve at level of the wrist usually remains normal. *Compression of digital nerves* (see below) leads to much more local symptoms, and again sensory conduction at the wrist is normal. Rare anatomical variants may pose difficulties, such as a bifid median nerve of which the longest portion had a normal course but the other portion passed through a hole in the flexor digitorum sublimis of the middle finger, at its musculotendinous junction in the forearm, causing pain and dysaesthesiae on movements of the middle finger (Fernandez Garcia *et al.*, 1994). *Thenar hypoplasia*, whether unilateral (Danner, 1983) or bilateral (Witt and Oberlander, 1981), may not become symptomatic until later in life (Cavanagh *et al.*, 1979), and the history as well as small muscle compound potentials without signs of denervation and normal conduction velocity at the carpal tunnel should distinguish it from carpal tunnel syndrome. Paraesthesia in the thumb or in the index and middle finger may occur with *lesions of the sixth or seventh cervical root*, respectively, most commonly as a result of a lateral disc prolapse at the C5–C6 or C6–C7 level; again conduction velocities at the wrist are normal in these conditions. The presence of a *cervical rib* or

abnormally long transverse process of C7 in a patient with pain and paraesthesia in the arm and hand is almost certainly coincidental, at least in patients with otherwise typical carpal tunnel syndrome. In true cases of thoracic outlet syndrome there may be thenar wasting, but the pain and sensory deficit are on the ulnar side of the forearm (T1 territory); the sensory conduction velocity of the median nerve is completely normal, but the ulnar nerve sensory action potentials have a decreased amplitude or are even absent (Gilliatt *et al.*, 1978). As a matter of fact, ordering radiographs of the cervical spine after having diagnosed definite carpal tunnel syndrome is unnecessary, as not only cervical ribs but also cervical arthrosis is bound to be coincidental, whatever the degree of degenerative changes. Paradoxically, most diseases that may give rise to diagnostic problems are not neurological in nature: tenosynovitis, stiffness of joints, rheumatic hands or Dupuytren's contracture may confuse the picture and delay the diagnosis of carpal tunnel syndrome. Raynaud's disease may co-exist with carpal tunnel syndrome more often than expected by chance (Pal *et al.*, 1996).

Causes of the carpal tunnel syndrome

Most cases of carpal tunnel syndrome are idiopathic, although obesity is a risk factor (Stallings *et al.*, 1997). There is a long list of specific conditions leading to typical symptoms (Table 8.2). Sometimes the disease in question may already be known to exist (for example, trauma or leprosy), but if carpal tunnel syndrome is the first manifestation of a systemic condition such as hypothyroidism the diagnosis is more difficult. Standard investigations in patients with clinical features of carpal tunnel syndrome should, apart from neurophysiological tests, include erythrocyte sedimentation rate (ESR), blood glucose, and thyroid function tests if the history or physical examination provides clues of thyroid disease.

Table 8.2
Causes of median nerve lesions at the level of the carpal tunnel

---

Idiopathic, with or without occupational factors

Pregnancy (Tobin, 1967; Ekman *et al.*, 1987; Wand, 1990)

Congenital anomalies
- Stenosis of the carpal canal (Dekel *et al.*, 1980; Bleecker *et al.*, 1985)
- Léri's pleonostosis (Watson-Jones, 1949)
- Madelung's wrist deformity (Radford and Matthewson, 1987; Luchetti *et al.*, 1988)
- Anomalous muscle in carpal canal (Schuhl, 1991; Rosenbaum and Ochoa, 1993)
- Ulnar nerve in carpal tunnel (Galzio *et al.*, 1987)
- Enlarged ulnar artery (Hankey, 1988), or large superficial palmar branch of radial artery (Widder and Shons, 1988)

Metabolic disorders
- Diabetes mellitus (Dieck and Kelsey, 1985)
- Acromegaly (Pickett *et al.*, 1975; Luboshitzky and Barzilai, 1980)
- Hypothyroidism (Cremer *et al.*, 1969; Golding, 1970)
- Hyperthyroidism (Beard *et al.*, 1985)
- Amyloidosis (Kyle and Greipp, 1983; Ochoa and Hedley-White, 1995)
- Mucopolysaccharidosis, in children (Haddad *et al.*, 1997)

Connective tissue disorders
- Rheumatoid arthritis (Crow, 1960; Moran *et al.*, 1986)
- Polymyalgia rheumatica (O'Duffy *et al.*, 1980; Richards, 1980; Herrera *et al.*, 1997)
- Mixed connective tissue disease (Vincent and Van, 1980; Winkelmann *et al.*, 1982)
- Sarcoidosis (Bleton *et al.*, 1991)
- Sjögren's syndrome (Binder *et al.*, 1988; Andonopoulos *et al.*, 1990)
- Gout (Moore and Weiland, 1985; Jacoulet, 1994; Tsai *et al.*, 1996)
- Systemic lupus erythematosus (Omdal *et al.*, 1988)
- Chondrocalcinosis (Goodwin and Arbel, 1985; Jones *et al.*, 1987)

Space-occupying lesions in the carpal tunnel
- Haematoma, spontaneous (Copeland *et al.*, 1989; Naess and Blom, 1991), or under anticoagulant therapy (Black *et al.*, 1997)
- Neurofibroma (Strickland and Steichen, 1977); neurofibromatosis (Brooks and Pascal, 1984)
- Chondrosarcoma (Steffens and Koob, 1988)
- Myeloma (Currie and Henson, 1971)
- Metastasis (Witthaut *et al.*, 1994)
- Lipoma (Brand and Gelberman, 1988; Babins and Lubahn, 1994)
- Lipofibroma (Patel *et al.*, 1979; Dap *et al.*, 1992)
- Ganglion (Kerrigan *et al.*, 1988; Nakamichi and Tachibana, 1996)
- Osteoid osteoma (Herndon *et al.* 1974)

Infections
- Septic arthritis (Gerardi *et al.*, 1989)
- Gonococcal tenosynovitis (DeHertogh *et al.*, 1988)
- Tuberculosis (Bush and Schneider, 1984; Gouet *et al.*, 1984)
- Leprosy (Selby, 1974)
- Lyme disease (Halperin *et al.*, 1989)
- Rubella arthritis (Blennow *et al.*, 1982); immunization with live rubella virus (Tingle *et al.*, 1985)
- Rare microorganisms: *Mycobacterium fortuitum* (Randall *et al.* 1982), *Mycobacterium malmoense* (Prince *et al.*, 1988), *Sporothrix schenckii* (Stratton *et al.*, 1981), *Histoplasma capsulatum* (Randall *et al.*, 1982), or parvovirus B19 (Samii *et al.*, 1996)

Hereditary neuropathies
- Hereditary liability to pressure palsies (see Chapter 25)
- Hereditary motor and sensory neuropathy (Charcot–Marie–Tooth disease)
- Familial carpal tunnel syndrome (McDonnell *et al.*, 1987)
- Hereditary neuropathic amyloidosis type II (Mahloudji *et al.*, 1969)

Trauma
- Distal fracture of the radius: immediate (Chapman *et al.*, 1982), or delayed (Altissimi *et al.*, 1986; Kwasny *et al.*, 1994)
- Soft tissue trauma or burns (Adamson *et al.*, 1971)
- Handcuffs (Stone and Laureno, 1991)
- Cycling (Braithwaite, 1992)
- Rock climbing (Heuck *et al.*, 1992)

Table 8.2 (continued)
Causes of median nerve lesions at the level of the carpal tunnel

Miscellaneous causes
- Benign joint hypermobility (March *et al.* 1988)
- mucopolysaccharidoses and mucolipidoses (MacDougal *et al.*, 1977; Norman Taylor *et al.*, 1995)
- Arteriovenous fistula (Chopra *et al.* 1979); aneurysm (Toranto, 1989)
- Arteriovenous shunt for haemodialysis (Harding and Le, 1977; Knezevic and Mastaglia, 1984; Seifert *et al.*, 1987)
- Danazol treatment, for endometriosis (Schmitz *et al.*, 1991)
- Interleukin-2 treatment, for cancer (Puduvalli *et al.*, 1996)
- Insect sting (Lazaro, 1972; Barker *et al.*, 1986)
- Snake bite (Schweitzer and Lewis, 1981)

A 75-year-old woman experienced fairly typical symptoms of carpal tunnel syndrome in her right hand, except that the pain was unusually severe, was present also at rest, and involved the arm as well. There were no neurological deficits, but the sensory conduction velocity of the right median nerve was markedly decreased over the wrist. While she was on the waiting list for surgery new symptoms developed: severe pain in both shoulders, headache, malaise and, finally, a depressive illness. The ESR was raised to 40 mm, whereas the year before it had been 5 mm. A diagnosis of polymyalgia rheumatica was now made, and treatment with oral prednisone 50 mg/day was begun. Within two days all general and focal symptoms had disappeared. After ten months, the dose of prednisone could be gradually tapered to 2.5 mg every other day without any recurrence of symptoms.

The most frequent causes are trauma, especially extension trauma of the wrist, fractures of the distal forearm, rheumatoid arthritis, shunts for haemodialysis and hypothyroidism. Most other causes are much more uncommon, but together they form a formidable list. It should be recognized that systemic 'causes' may contribute to carpal tunnel syndrome but do not exclude the possibility that local treatment is effective.

A 40-year-old man was known for 15 years to have Charcot–Marie–Tooth disease (HMSN type I). For about three months he had severe paraesthesia in all fingers of the right hand. He showed clinical and neurophysiological features of a demyelinating polyneuropathy, but the sensory conduction velocity of the right median nerve over the wrist was disproportionally low, and also much lower than on an earlier occasion. The diagnosis was carpal tunnel syndrome, in addition to the hereditary neuropathy. After surgical division of the transverse carpal ligament the symptoms were dramatically relieved.

A few conditions listed in Table 8.2 deserve separate comment. Many women develop symptoms of carpal tunnel syndrome during pregnancy, most commonly in the third trimester. Usually the symptoms disappear within 4–6 weeks after delivery, or slightly later if breast-feeding (Wand, 1990). Some women, however, do not recover or show recurrent symptoms of carpal tunnel syndrome at a later stage (Stahl *et al.*, 1996).

Occupational 'causes' of carpal tunnel syndrome represent a variable mixture of more or less strenuous hand movements or use of vibration tools and an idiopathic predisposition, in which a narrow carpal canal is probably an important factor.

Many manual workers, including women, will never experience carpal tunnel syndrome. On the other hand, even a certain posture may lead to symptoms of carpal tunnel syndrome, such as that of the statue 'Le Penseur' by Rodin. Wiederholt reports a patient who experienced intermittent symptoms of carpal tunnel syndrome (and ulnar compression) as a result of habitually leaning with his chin on the dorsum of his flexed right hand, with the elbow resting on his knee (Wiederholt, 1992). This report again serves to emphasize the importance of a careful history-taking, and also illustrates that thinking may hurt peripheral nerves. The prevalence of occupational neuropathies has decreased impressively in the last fifty years, at least in the Western world, because many handicrafts have disappeared or were replaced by machines. Yet some manual occupations still predispose to nerve entrapment in the carpal tunnel, for example shoe hemmers (Fortuna *et al.*, 1989), carpet weavers (Senveli *et al.*, 1987), or carpet floorers who use their wrists as hammers (dell'Omo *et al.*, 1995). Bleecker *et al.* (1985) used CT scanning to study the size of the carpal canal as a risk factor for carpal tunnel syndrome in 14 male electricians, all employees of a single shop. The ages ranged between 20 and 60 years. All were daily engaged with light- or medium-weight tools (pliers, screwdrivers, hammers, power tools and cable cutters). Seven workers with symptomatic carpal tunnel syndrome and three with 'subclinical' carpal tunnel syndrome (prolonged distal motor latency) had, on average, a significantly smaller cross-sectional area of the carpal tunnel than the four unaffected workers. Several other occupations that involve repetitive wrist motions have a much higher frequency of carpal tunnel syndrome than the general population (Silverstein *et al.*, 1987).

In particular musicians perform endlessly repetitive movements and thus may suffer nerve damage from whatever instrument they play. Lederman (1989) described 229 instrumentalists with playing-related symptoms. Nine musicians had carpal tunnel syndrome, this being bilateral in four. Two other musicogenic median neuropathies included an anterior interosseous nerve syndrome with ipsilateral focal dystonia and a pronator teres syndrome. From our own experience we should like to add that beginner musicians in particular may have symptoms in one or both arms without objective findings, either clinically or neurophysiologically. Probably, muscles, tendons and especially the mind are all taxed by the duty to study longer and to perform better. 'Thoracic outlet syndrome without neurological signs' (Lederman, 1989) is hardly a convincing diagnosis. Rest and guidance are often the best therapy, depending on the talent of the musician. A change in playing technique or even of profession may be necessary, depending on whether the brunt of the stress bears on body or mind (Lockwood, 1989).

Patients with paraplegia from spinal cord disease who have regained an independent life are at special risk of developing a carpal tunnel syndrome, as they tend to overuse their hands in propelling a wheelchair or carrying their body weight during transfers (Aljure *et al.*, 1985). A man or woman with paraplegia and tingling hands is much more likely to have carpal tunnel syndrome than post-traumatic syringomyelia or another form of progressive spinal cord disease.

Carpal tunnel syndrome with an acute onset is strongly suggestive of haemorrhage.

A 69-year-old right-handed man had been busy hammering a hole in a stone. A few hours later he experienced an excruciating pain in the palm and thumb, radiating to the other fingers. He was on oral anticoagulants after an operation for an aortic aneurysm. On examination, the same day, there was loss of superficial sensation at the palm of the right hand, and also of the volar surface of the thumb and the three adjoining fingers. Nerve conduction at the wrist was blocked for motor and sensory fibres in the median as well as in the ulnar nerve. After the coagulation defect had been reversed, operative decompression was performed the next day. A haematoma under pressure was evacuated. Immediately afterwards all symptoms had disappeared.

Treatment of carpal tunnel syndrome

A change of professional or other habits that provoke symptoms is not always sufficient. The choice between conservative and surgical treatment has to be made without the backup of clinical trials and much depends on the personality of the patient and the physician. Splinting of the wrist in 30° of extension may give immediate but only temporary relief. In addition, it is a cumbersome method during the daytime and splinting should preferably be advised only overnight. We are not impressed by the results of medical therapy such as pyridoxine (Smith *et al.*, 1984) or diuretics. Injection of steroids into the carpal tunnel may be helpful initially but in most patients the symptoms recur (Crow, 1960; Gelberman *et al.*, 1980; Ozdogan and Yazici, 1984; Irwin *et al.*, 1996), and complications are by no means rare (Gottlieb and Riskin, 1980; McConnell and Bush, 1990; Tavares and Giddins, 1996). Similarly, a short course of low-dose oral prednisone (20 mg/day for one week and 10 mg/day in the second week) gave rapid relief but after eight weeks the effect had waned in most patients (Herskovitz *et al.*, 1995). Laser light neurolysis has been recommended on the basis of a single study, without controls or long-term follow-up (Weintraub, 1997).

Since none of the conservative measures provides permanent relief, patients with long-standing (six months or a year) symptoms should be treated by surgery, preferably under local or regional anaesthesia, done by an experienced surgeon (hand surgeon or neurosurgeon). Even in cases with weakness and muscle atrophy the recovery after surgery may be excellent (Phalen, 1966; Rietz and Onne, 1967). Apart from the duration of symptoms, surgical intervention is indicated in all patients with weakness, sensory loss or both. Some advocate serial nerve conduction studies to determine if and when surgery is indicated (van Rossum *et al.*, 1980), but this will often be impractical. Pregnant women with severe symptoms, and especially those with weakness, are also candidates for surgery, under local analgesia, since otherwise the expectant mother may not be able to properly handle the baby after delivery.

Surgical treatment involves complete sectioning of the transverse carpal ligament by a longitudinal incision medial to the thenar eminence and just lateral to the axis of the ring finger. Serial MRI scanning confirmed that postoperative relief was associated with an increase in volume of the carpal tunnel (Pierre-Jerome *et al.*, 1997). According to a prospective study (Mackinnon *et al.*, 1991), neurolysis adds no benefit to the postoperative outcome. The same applies to epineurotomy (Leinberry *et al.*, 1997), or lengthening of the transverse carpal ligament (Karlsson *et al.*, 1997). Endoscopic division of the carpal ligament is becoming increasingly popular, despite an increased risk of complications (Murphy *et al.*, 1994). A randomized multi-centre trial confirmed the risk of complications with the endoscopic technique (in 4 of 87 patients: damage to median or ulnar nerves, haematoma or pseudoaneurysm from damage to the superficial palmar arch); whereas the efficacy of both methods was excellent, the only advantage of the endoscopic method was a quicker return to previous activities, and slightly less tenderness of the wound (Brown *et al.*, 1993).

Also, open surgical treatment has its complications and failures. Necrotizing fasciitis may follow the operation, especially in diabetic patients (Greco and Curtsinger, 1993), and insufficient attention to anatomical details may damage the palmar cutaneous branch of the median nerve (Carroll and Green, 1972), or the recurrent thenar motor branch, which may pierce the transverse carpal ligament rather than leaving the main stem of the median nerve a few millimetres distal to it (Lilly and Magnell, 1985). Persistence or recurrence of paraesthesia may be caused by incomplete sectioning of the retinaculum, closing of the fibres of the retinaculum, excessive scar formation, or an underlying lesion.

A 50-year-old man had been operated upon for Dupuytren's contracture of the right hand. Several months later he developed painful paraesthesia in all fingers of the operated hand, together with progressive weakness. On examination there was partial thenar atrophy with marked weakness of the abductor pollicis brevis and opponens pollicis muscles, with equivocal sensory loss; forced hyperflexion of the wrist increased the tingling sensations. Both sensory and motor conduction velocities of the right median nerve were markedly decreased at the level of the wrist. Disappointingly, surgical decompression was entirely unsuccessful. Re-exploration after several months showed that the retinaculum had been divided completely, but further distally in the palm an arteriovenous malformation was found to compress the median nerve and its branches. Extirpation of the malformation proved feasible; several months later a slow but definite recovery had set in.

Nowadays MRI scanning is an important technique in helping to establish anatomical factors that may explain persistent symptoms and thereby to assess the need for re-exploration (Murphy *et al.*, 1993). In such cases a second operation is often successful (Cobb *et al.*, 1996). In the case of residual pain without paraesthesia, it is usual to find that nerve conduction abnormalities have improved. Yet some permanent increase in latency is to be expected, because in the process of remyelination relatively short internodal segments are formed, with more mini-delays caused by depolarization at the nodes of Ranvier. Occasionally, patients complain after the operation about loss of manual strength or of subluxation of the tendons on flexing the wrist. So-called 'sympathetic reflex dystrophy' has important psychological components and should be treated with behaviour therapy rather than with blocks of the stellate ganglion (Schott, 1995).

Lesions of the palmar cutaneous branch of the median nerve

This sensory branch of the median nerve is rarely injured in isolation. The symptoms consist of pain, paraesthesia and numbness in the palm, especially in the thenar region. The Hoffmann–Tinel sign (distal tingling on percussion of the nerve) may be present. Possible causes are a ganglion of the flexor carpi radialis tendon, just proximal to the wrist flexion crease (Buckmiller and Rickard, 1987; Haskin, 1994), entrapment within the antebrachial fascia (Semer *et al.*, 1996), an atypical palmaris longus muscle (Stellbrink, 1972), or iatrogenic injury following carpal tunnel release (Carroll and Green, 1972).

Lesions of digital branches of the median nerve

Injury to a common digital nerve in the palm causes sensory impairment in the adjoining halves of two fingers and in the web space between them, whereas injury to a cutaneous nerve after the division between the two fingers (proper digital nerve) causes sensory loss in one-half of a single finger. Sensation at the tip of the finger may be spared, depending on the overlap with the proper digital nerve of the other half-finger. A common cause is the frequent use of scissors, for instance by orthopaedic surgeons (Roberts and Allan, 1988). Another typical source of pressure is the rim of the hole in bowling balls ('bowler's thumb') (Dobyns *et al.*, 1972). Digital nerves may be compressed by a variety of other objects (Howell and Leach, 1970; Rayan and O'Donoghue, 1983), including a cheerleader's baton (Shields and Jacobs, 1986) or bowstrings in archers, as well as by intrinsic lesions of skin, tendons or bony structures close to the digital nerves (Rosenbaum and Ochoa, 1993).

The *ulnar digital nerve of the thumb* may be compressed by a splint (Rayan and O'Donoghue, 1983), or by hooking the thumbs into a suspender or other straps.

A 71-year-old retired professor of neurology, who regularly walked in the mountains of Austria, had the habit of hooking his thumbs into the front straps of his rucksack. After several hours he regularly noticed tingling and numbness in both thumbs. Each time the symptoms immediately disappeared when he took his hands from the straps.

The *radial digital nerve of the thumb* may be compressed by a fibrous band from the flexor pollicis brevis to the sheath of the flexor pollicis longus muscle (Berlemann and Dunkerton, 1994). Iatrogenic laceration of this nerve may occur during release of a trigger finger (Carrozzella *et al.*, 1989).

Chapter 9
The ulnar nerve

Anatomy

The ulnar nerve (Figure 9.1) carries fibres from the roots of C8 and Th1, sometimes also from C7, and passes through the lower trunk and medial cord of the brachial plexus. In the axilla the ulnar nerve runs in close contact with the median nerve and with the axillary artery and vein. Halfway down the humerus it pierces the intermuscular septum and then runs downwards between the intermuscular septum and the medial head of the triceps muscle, at the dorsomedial side of the upper arm. At the elbow the ulnar nerve passes into the ulnar groove behind the medial epicondyle of the humerus, a site where

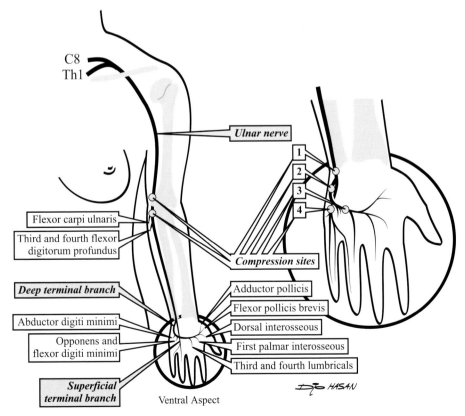

Figure 9.1
Muscles innervated by the ulnar nerve.

the nerve is most easily injured because of its exposed position (see Figure 9.1). Above the elbow the nerve does not give off any branches. On entering the forearm the ulnar nerve passes through the so-called 'cubital tunnel', another well-known point of entrapment; this space is confined by ligaments and the medial epicondyle and becomes reduced in size during flexion of the elbow. Subsequently the ulnar nerve courses between the two heads of the flexor carpi ulnaris muscle, where branches are given off to this muscle and to the flexor digitorum profundus III and IV (that is, of the ring finger and little finger). All other motor branches originate distal to the wrist.

At the level of the wrist the ulnar nerve passes over the transverse carpal ligament (other than the median nerve, which passes under it), and below the palmar fascia of the pisiform bone and the hamulus of the hamate bone. This space, through which the ulnar nerve passes together with the ulnar artery and vein, is called Guyon's canal. The close topographical relationship between the ulnar nerve, the hamulus of the hamate and several carpal joints explains why the ulnar nerve is so often damaged after hand injuries. On leaving Guyon's canal the ulnar nerve divides into its two terminal branches: the superficial terminal branch (almost purely sensory) and the deep terminal branch, which is purely motor.

Motor innervation The only two forearm muscles innervated by the ulnar nerve are the flexor carpi ulnaris and the flexor digitorum profundus III and IV, which flex the terminal phalanx of the ring finger and the little finger. In the palm, the *deep terminal motor branch* innervates consecutively the abductor, opponens and flexor of the little finger, the third and fourth lumbricals, the interossei and, finally, the adductor pollicis (see Figure 9.1). The *superficial terminal branch* consists mainly of sensory fibres but also supplies the palmaris brevis muscle; this small muscle contracts during strong abduction

of the little finger and causes indentation of the skin overlying the hypothenar.

Sensory innervation The *palmar cutaneous branch* arises in the middle of the forearm and supplies the skin of the proximal part of the hypothenar eminence. The *dorsal cutaneous branch* originates at about 5 cm proximal to the wrist crease and innervates on the dorsal side the ulnar part of the hand, the little finger, the proximal phalanx of the ring finger, and some of the base of the middle finger (Figure 9.2; Laroy *et al.*, 1998). At the inner side of the pisiform bone, within Guyon's canal, the *superficial terminal branch* originates to supply first the skin of the distal part of the hypothenar and then, ending in digital nerves, the palmar side of the little finger and ring finger and also the dorsal side of the tips of these two fingers, distal to the parts supplied by the dorsal cutaneous branch. Thus, as a rule, ulnar nerve entrapments proximal to the wrist show motor and sensory signs, whereas entrapments distal to the wrist mostly cause motor deficits only.

Ulnar nerve lesions at the axilla and upper arm

Because the ulnar nerve does not give off branches in the upper arm, lesions at that level and at the elbow will result in similar neurological deficits. Signs of concomitant involvement of the median or radial nerve point to a lesion in the upper arm. Localisation of the lesion can usually be achieved by nerve conduction studies.

Causes

Isolated lesions of the ulnar nerve in the axilla are extremely uncommon; one of these rare conditions is the existence of a chondroepitrochlaris muscle, arising from the pectoralis major, crossing over the neurovascular bundle in the axilla, and inserting into the brachial fascia and medial epicondyle of the humerus (Spinner *et al.*, 1991). Other causes are related to trauma,

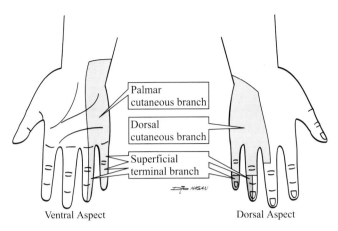

Palmar
cutaneous branch

Dorsal
cutaneous branch

Superficial
terminal branch

Ventral Aspect

Dorsal Aspect

Figure 9.2
Approximate skin area innervated by the ulnar nerve.

such as aneurysms of the axillary or brachial artery (see under median nerve), or to pressure from long crutches or inappropriately applied tourniquets. Isolated sleep paralysis from prolonged pressure after excessive intake of alcohol or drugs is equally rare. The importance of asking 'What have you been doing with your arm?' is underlined by the example of a veterinary surgeon who for many hours of the day had his arm inside cows for performing artificial insemination; during these manipulations his ulnar nerve was chronically injured at the upper arm (Mumenthaler and Schliack, 1993).

Management

As a rule, the treatment of ulnar nerve lesions in the axilla or upper arm is self-explanatory: surgical exploration in case of damage to the axillary artery or brachial artery (Staal *et al.*, 1966; Staal and van Voorthuisen, 1969), or avoidance of any source of external compression such as long crutches.

Compression of the ulnar nerve at the elbow

History

The elbow is by far the most common site of entrapment of the ulnar nerve. In an authoritative monograph, Mumenthaler (1961) described 354 patients with ulnar neuropathy not caused by direct injury; in 317 of these the lesion was at the elbow (256 with an identifiable cause), against three with lesions in the forearm and 34 at the wrist or the palm of the hand (26 with a known cause). It is not exceptional to find ulnar neuropathy at the elbow on both sides. In the elbow region there are two sites where the ulnar nerve may be compressed: the shallow condylar groove, a vulnerable spot known to most lay people where the nerve lies directly under the skin, and slightly distal to this, in the cubital tunnel. In the condylar groove the ulnar nerve can be damaged not only by external pressure but also by deformities of the elbow joint. The cubital tunnel has the medial ligament of the elbow joint as its floor, and the roof is formed by the aponeurosis of the flexor carpi ulnaris muscle. Flexion of the elbow increases pressure in the cubital tunnel. Distinction between the two potential compression sites is often difficult, if not impossible, unless the history clearly points to compression of the ulnar nerve in the condylar groove. Even during surgical exploration exact localisation may be difficult and intra-operative nerve conduction studies may be necessary to resolve the question (Brown *et al.*, 1980; Campbell *et al.*, 1988a).

At the level of the elbow the ulnar nerve carries motor, sensory and autonomous fibres. Sensory symptoms are usually the first to appear, but strangely enough there may be only motor symptoms in other patients, probably depending on which fascicles are compressed. Patients complain about pins and needles and of numbness and sometimes also of a burning pain in the ring finger and little finger, with or without extension to the hypothenar region. Occasionally, the nerve itself in the ulnar groove or even the entire elbow region may be extremely painful to touch. In contrast with the carpal tunnel syndrome, symptoms do not occur outside the sensory area of the ulnar nerve in the hand, except with anomalies of innervation, which are not uncommon. Unlike the history of carpal tunnel syndrome, patients are not woken up at night by pins and needles ('brachialgia paraesthetica nocturna'). Symptoms may increase while the patient is leaning on the elbow (such as a driver who finds that when his car window is lowered the groove of the elbow fits nicely in the lower ridge), and by sitting or lying with the elbows flexed (as with reading in bed). Although pain in the elbow is not uncommon, it rarely spreads to the upper arm; if it does, it may even give rise to precordial pain (Luyendijk, 1960). If symptoms progress to impairment of motor function these consist of clumsiness and weakness of fine finger movements, especially on buttoning and unbuttoning garments. Closing a belt and zipping trousers require unimpaired function of the adductor pollicis and of the first interosseous. Of course any loss of power and dexterity is discovered most rapidly in needleworkers, musicians, surgeons and similar professions.

Examination

Sensory findings consist of disturbed sensation at the palmar and dorsal sides of the little finger, the ulnar half of the ring finger, and often also the adjoining parts of the hand; the abnormalities are most conspicuous on the palmar side of the little finger. However, sensory findings may be restricted to the tips of the fourth and fifth fingers. In exceptional cases of ulnar neuropathy sensory impairment may be minimal or even absent, which makes it difficult to localize the lesion without taking recourse to nerve conduction studies.

Autonomic findings are uncommon and consist of furrowed or atrophic nails in the two last fingers, with or without trophic skin lesions in the distribution of the ulnar nerve (Mumenthaler, 1961).

Motor signs rarely involve the flexor carpi ulnaris or the flexor digitorum profundus muscles, at least in the early stages. Initially, weakness may be confined to the first dorsal interosseous, diminished adduction of the little finger, or both. Diminished adduction of the little finger as an isolated finding in the arm may also occur in patients with supranuclear lesions (Alter, 1973). In severe ulnar nerve palsy inspection alone strongly suggests the diagnosis. This so-called 'ulnar claw' hand shows guttering of the dorsum from atrophy of the interosseous muscles and the third and fourth lumbricals. An effect on finger posture is hyperextension of the fourth and fifth metacarpophalangeal joints, together with slight flexion of the interphalangeal joints, and abduction of the little finger (Figure 9.3). The index and

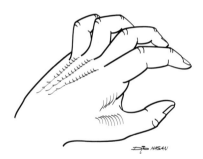

Figure 9.3
Claw hand (ulnar nerve lesion).

middle fingers also show some hyperextension of the metacarpophalangeal joints, but much less marked because of their intact lumbricals, innervated by the median nerve. The loss of muscle bulk in the hand is most marked between the thumb and index finger, and the hypothenar eminence is also flattened, by atrophy of the abductor, short flexor and opponens muscle of the little finger. Typically, the thenar region does not show atrophy, in contrast with lesions of the T1 root, which are associated with atrophy of all the muscles in the hand.

For testing the strength of the muscles innervated by the ulnar nerve we prefer the following limited repertoire of tests. Examination is most easily performed while sitting opposite the patient, with a table in between. Testing in the *horizontal plane* concerns abduction and adduction of the individual fingers; 'abduction' of the thumb in the horizontal plane is, by convention, called extension, for which movement the relevant muscles are innervated by the radial nerve. The muscles necessary for abduction and adduction of the fingers are the interossei, the abductor and opponens digiti quinti, and the adductor pollicis. After having asked for maximal and strong abduction of the fingers, one should look at the width of the interspaces between the fingers that is attained; in ulnar nerve dysfunction these will be smaller than in the normal hand. Even slight weakness will be readily detected with this manoeuvre. If there happens to be a radial nerve lesion (alone or in combination), precise testing of abduction of the fingers is impossible, since more or less intact finger extensors are required to make the 'horizontal' movements possible. In such a case abduction of the fingers should be tested with the fingers resting in an extended position upon a hard surface, with the palm facing downwards, although even then the movements will not be quite normal despite the ulnar nerve being intact. With complete ulnar nerve paralysis adduction and abduction of the fingers is virtually impossible. In a unilateral, mild lesion the power of finger abduction should be compared with that of the normal hand. If a bilateral lesion is suspected a sensible method is to compare the strength of finger abduction with that of a healthy person of more or less the same age, since even normal strength in these muscles can often easily be overcome by the examiner (although office workers should not be compared with blacksmiths). Abduction and adduction should be tested separately for all the long fingers (Figures 9.4 to 9.6) and for adduction of the thumb (Figure 9.7); normal strength in the adductor pollicis muscle is not easily overcome by the examiner, if at all. A useful test for thumb adduction is to ask the patient to squeeze a sheet of paper between the base of the thumb and the index finger; weakness of the adductor pollicis is evident if the patient resorts to flexion of the distal phalanx of the thumb, a movement subserved by the median nerve (Froment's sign). Contraction of the palmaris brevis muscle is visible on extreme abduction of the little finger and results in a dimple at the base of the hypothenar. Normal action of this muscle is helpful in localizing an ulnar nerve lesion as distal to the wrist (together with normal sensation, see Table 9.2).

Examination in the *vertical plane* consists, firstly, of flexion of the distal

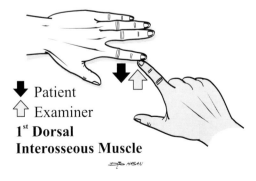

Figure 9.4
The palm of the patient's hand and fingers rest on a flat surface, while the index finger is abducted against resistance at the metacarpophalangeal joint.

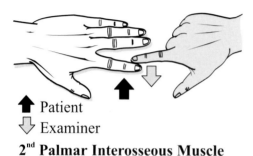

↑ Patient
⇩ Examiner

2nd Palmar Interosseous Muscle

Figure 9.5
The palm of the patient's hand and fingers rest on a flat surface, while the index finger is adducted against resistance at the metacarpophalangeal joint.

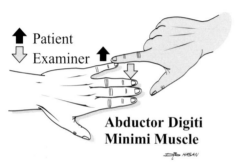

↑ Patient
⇩ Examiner ↑

Abductor Digiti Minimi Muscle

Figure 9.6
The palm of the patient's hand and fingers rest on a flat surface, while the little finger is abducted against resistance at the metacarpophalangeal joint.

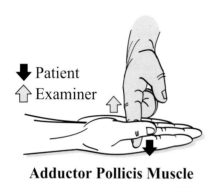

⬇ Patient
⬆ Examiner ⬆

Adductor Pollicis Muscle

Figure 9.7
The thumb is pressed against the index finger against resistance.

phalanx of the ring finger and little finger. These movements are exclusively executed by the flexor digitorum profundus III and IV; these muscles are tested by flexion of each distal interphalangeal joint against resistance, while the middle phalanx is fixed (Figure 9.8). Wasting may be visible at the medial border of the forearm. Interpretation of muscle strength is not easy, as in many individuals these two muscles may be normally overcome by the examiner. The lumbricals III and IV and the corresponding flexor digiti minimi brevis (Figure 9.9) contribute to flexion of the proximal phalanges of the fourth and fifth finger, but their action cannot be distinguished from that of the (median-innervated) flexor digitorum superficialis muscle in the arm, which has its insertion at the middle phalanges of all four long fingers. Finally, part of wrist flexion (flexor carpi ulnaris) is subserved by the ulnar nerve. However, this muscle often escapes with compression of the ulnar nerve at the elbow; even if this is not the case, wrist flexion remains largely unaffected through the action of the (median-innervated) flexor carpi radialis;

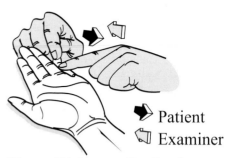

➤ Patient
◁ Examiner

Flexor Digitorum Profundus Muscle of the Little Finger

Figure 9.8
The dorsum of the hand rests on a flat surface and the little finger is flexed against resistance at the distal interphalangeal joint, while the middle phalanx is fixed by the left index finger of the examiner.

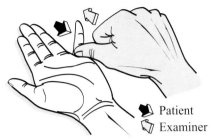

Patient
Examiner

Flexor Digiti Minimi Brevis and 4ᵗʰ Lumbrical Muscle

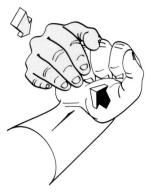

Flexor Carpi Ulnaris Muscle

Patient

Examiner

Figure 9.9
The dorsum of the hand rests on a flat surface and the little finger is flexed against resistance at the metacarpophalangeal joint.

Figure 9.10
The hand is flexed and adducted at the wrist against resistance.

a slight radial deviation of the hand on flexion of the wrist may be the only sign. The testing of this muscle is shown in Figure 9.10.

Differential diagnosis of ulnar nerve lesions at the elbow

Concomitant involvement of the median nerve obviously indicates a lesion in the upper arm, axilla or even higher. Given there are no clinical differences between (rarely occurring) instances of isolated ulnar nerve damage in the axilla or upper arm and the much more common compression at the elbow, only neurophysiological studies can allow a distinction to be made between them. If sensory involvement is slight or absent, which is most unusual, the clinical picture may be confused with spinal muscular atrophy. If the tendon jerks happen to be brisk, then a suspicion of amyotrophic lateral sclerosis may even be raised. In that case the history, together with neurographic studies, must be used to differentiate between a disorder of anterior horn cells, ulnar nerve compression at the elbow with minimal sensory involvement, and ulnar nerve

compression at the palm, in which case the deficit is purely motor (see below).

Electrophysiological and radiological studies

Motor nerve conduction studies are performed by recording from an ulnar-innervated intrinsic hand muscle and stimulating the nerve at the wrist and below and above the elbow. Slowing across the elbow segment and/or amplitude reduction of the compound muscle action potential (CMAP) with proximal stimulation indicate a lesion at the elbow. Conduction velocity at the elbow is best compared with that in the forearm. A relative slowing of more than 10 or 11 m/s has been found to be abnormal (Kincaid *et al.*, 1986; Kothari and Preston, 1995). In these studies the elbow was flexed to 135° and 90°, respectively. If the arm is extended (~0°) the length of the nerve segment at the elbow is underestimated. It has indeed been shown that conduction studies with

The ulnar nerve

a flexed elbow position are more sensitive in localizing ulnar neuropathy at the elbow (Kothari and Preston, 1995). Because nerve fibres to the abductor digiti minimi and the first dorsal interosseous may be unevenly involved, it is advisable to record from both muscles (Stewart, 1987).

Most authors have used distances across the elbow of at least 10 cm. Within a nerve segment of this length a moderate focal slowing may remain unnoticed ('dilution effect'). Shorter conduction distances, however, were found to be susceptible to considerable error in velocity calculation due to inaccuracies in measuring distance and latencies (Maynard and Stolov, 1972). In order to increase sensitivity and to localize the lesion to the ulnar groove or the cubital tunnel an 'inching' technique (see page 10) may be used (Miller, 1979; Campbell *et al.*, 1992). Knowledge of the exact site of compression is important if surgical treatment is considered. More precise information can be obtained by intraoperative conduction studies (Brown *et al.*, 1980; Miller and Hummel, 1980; Campbell *et al.*, 1988). Surface-recorded sensory conduction studies have been found to be more sensitive than standard motor conduction studies (Raynor et al., 1994).

Even when no conduction abnormalities are found, ulnar nerve lesions may lead to axonal damage which can be recognized by needle EMG. For localization of the lesion, the EMG is less informative than conduction studies because lesions at the elbow often cause no signs of axonal damage in the ulnar-innervated forearm muscles.

Cervical arthrosis on plain radiographs is such a common finding in middle age that one should be extremely cautious in attributing any importance to 'foraminal narrowing'; if clinical and neurographical findings point to a lesion at the elbow, ordering radiographs of the cervical spine tends to confuse rather than to clarify the issue.

Causes of ulnar nerve compression at the elbow

Causes of ulnar nerve compression at the elbow are listed in Table 9.1. Simple bed rest with the elbows in flexion, whatever the reason, is an underestimated cause, also in non-comatose patients (Ciulla *et al.*, 1996). Not surprisingly, the risk increases with the duration of bed rest (Warner *et al.*, 1994). Malpositioning of elbows on the operating table is an equally underrated problem. In a retrospective series from the Mayo Clinics, 414 cases of persistent ulnar neuropathy occurred over 34 years (Warner *et al.*, 1994). This complication was not related to intraoperative positioning or the duration of the operative procedure. Perhaps the risk of nerve damage is equally great in the recovery room. In more than half of the patients in this series the symptoms did not occur until 24 hours or more after the operation. It seems rational to try and prevent damage to the nerve by padding and by placing the patient's arms in supination during anaesthesia, although there is no evidence that such measures are indeed effective (Stoelting, 1993).

In May 1990, a 57-year-old building site supervisor underwent coronary artery bypass grafting, because of anginal pain. He also suffered from insulin-dependent diabetes mellitus. As soon as he could remember, two days after the operation, he noted an ache in his left arm. The pain remained more or less the same for the next two months, radiating from the left shoulder to the outer side of the upper arm and the extensor side of the forearm to the fifth and fourth fingers. The only change was that after two months these two fingers had become numb rather than painful. On specific questioning it emerged that the left hand had also become weak and looked thinner than usual. On examination (December 1990) there was weakness and atrophy of the interosseous muscles and the adductor pollicis, and also weakness of the flexor carpi ulnaris and the flexor digitorum profundus III and IV. Conduction studies confirmed marked slowing in the ulnar nerve at the level of the elbow. Because of persisting pain and deficit he was operated on, in July 1991. Exploration of the ulnar groove revealed adhesions and evidence of previous haemorrhage in this area; the nerve was dissected free and transposed to the ventral side of the arm. Recovery was slow and incomplete.

Table 9.1
Causes of ulnar nerve lesions at the elbow

External pressure (non-iatrogenic)
- Prolonged bed rest (Mumenthaler, 1961; Warner *et al.*, 1994; Ciulla *et al.*, 1996)
- Prolonged leaning with the elbow on a desk, for example in telephone operators (Mumenthaler, 1961) or shoe workers (Agnesi *et al.*, 1993)
- 'Drivers's elbow': resting the elbow against the lower edge of a car window (Abdel Salam *et al.*, 1991; Mansukhani and D'Souza, 1991)

Iatrogenic
- Malpositioning during general anaesthesia (Dawson and Krarup, 1989)
- Haemodialysis shunt, with proliferating granulation tissue (Konishiike *et al.*, 1994)
- Median sternotomy, probably with traction at the brachial plexus (Casscells *et al.*, 1993)
- Steroid injection for medial epicondylitis, with undetected dislocation of the nerve (Stahl and Kaufman, 1997)

Occupational movements
- Repeated flexion/extension of the elbow, such as by operating the handle of a mounted drill (Mumenthaler, 1961) or in diamond sorters (Mansukhani and D'Souza, 1991)
- Operating chain-saws (Stefenelli *et al.*, 1990)

Acquired abnormalities at the elbow joint
- Arthrosis of the elbow joint (Mumenthaler, 1961)
- Arthritis, chondromatosis (Mumenthaler, 1961)
- Forestier's disease: diffuse idiopathic skeletal hyperostosis (Haskard and Panayi, 1988)
- Heterotopic calcifications (Vorenkamp and Nelson, 1987; Varghese *et al.*, 1991)
- Ganglia (Mumenthaler, 1961)
- Gout (Akizuki and Matsui, 1984)
- Rheumatic synovial cyst (Mainard *et al.*, 1991)
- Epineural cyst (Ferlic and Ries, 1990)
- Hypertrophic ulnar neuropathy (Phillips *et al.*, 1991; Taras and Melone, 1995)

Table 9.1 (continued)
Causes of ulnar nerve lesions at the elbow

- Snapping of the medial head of the triceps muscle (Hayashi *et al.*, 1984)

Traumatic injury
- Acute, with or without fractures (of the joint or supracondylar) (Uchida and Sugioka, 1990; Dormans *et al.*, 1995)
- Delayed, with or without fractures or luxations (Mumenthaler, 1961), for example by callus formation after supracondylar fracture of the humerus (Lalanandham and Laurence, 1984), or aneurysm of the ulnar collateral artery (Bruijn and Koning, 1992)

Congenital abnormalities
- Spontaneous (sub)luxation of the nerve from the ulnar sulcus (Mumenthaler, 1961)
- Hereditary liability to pressure palsies (Earl *et al.*, 1964; Staal *et al.*, 1965)
- Presence of epitrochleo-anconeus muscle (Mumenthaler, 1961; Hodgkinson and McLean, 1994)
- Struther's arcade: supracondylar spur and ligament (Ochiai *et al.*, 1992)
- Abnormal insertion of the triceps muscle (Matsuura *et al.*, 1994)

Hypertrophic neuropathy (Phillips *et al.*, 1991; Taras and Melone, 1995) (see Chapter 30)

Tumours (Patel *et al.*, 1996) (see Chapter 30)

Leprosy (Schmutzhard *et al.*, 1984) (see Chapter 26)

Bony alterations of the elbow joint, arthrotic or post-traumatic, are another frequent cause. With arthrotic elbow joints the ulnar nerve can not be palpated in the ulnar sulcus. Spontaneous luxation or subluxation during flexion of the elbow can be palpated and even seen. The phenomenon may lead to paraesthesia, pain and sensory or motor deficits (Mumenthaler, 1961), but it may also be entirely asymptomatic.

Fractures of the elbow may lead to ulnar nerve damage even years after the event (tardy ulnar nerve palsy), particularly if the fracture is associated with deformity of the elbow joint, for instance an abnormal valgus position.

Management of ulnar nerve lesions at the elbow

First of all, a detailed history-taking should explore all possible causes of external compression, such as peculiar sitting habits. These questions should be asked repeatedly, since patients tend to forget such things, and unnecessary operations can sometimes be avoided.

> A 72-year-old musicologist developed, over several months, a slowly progressive, severe motor and sensory ulnar neuropathy with marked muscle wasting in both hands. Playing the piano became impossible, as did buttoning his garments. Altogether this vital man was severely handicapped in his professional and social life. Only after persistent questioning in which we also involved his spouse, did it become evident that in the period between six and three months before he had been extremely busy with writing music, in preparation for a student class. The music paper was positioned at an angle on a reading stand, while he leaned with both elbows on the supporting table. In this fashion he had been writing for six to eight hours each day, for three months. Motor and sensory conduction velocities in both ulnar nerves were markedly decreased across the elbows. Although he had actually been referred to the neurosurgeon for a decompressive operation and we were only asked to perform a 'neurological screening' the obvious treatment was strong advice to stop leaning on his elbows. It took some time to convince him to change his habit, but four months later he could again manage an octave on the piano and on formal examination the muscle power had also improved considerably, although wasting of the hand muscles was still visible.

In a prospective study of 128 patients with ulnar neuropathy at the elbow in whom conservative management was initially preferred by the physician (because there was no neurological deficit) or by the patient, it often proved possible

to avoid operation in the next few years, especially in patients without electrophysiological abnormalities (Dellon *et al.*,1993). On the other hand, this 'conservative treatment' implied an impressive change in life style: keeping the elbow extended as much as possible, avoiding leaning on the elbows or crossing the arms while sitting, holding the telephone receiver with the other hand, wearing a towel or a thermoplastic splint at night to prevent flexion of more than 30°, placing a pillow under the arm at work, and using a book stand if extensive reading was required. Yet a substantial minority of patients remain who are candidates for surgical treatment, if continuing compression of the elbow region has, within reasonable limits, been ruled out as a causal factor, and if there is no improvement or even deterioration of symptoms and signs; in particular, the presence of disabling paraesthesia, severe pain or invalidating motor deficits may hasten the decision to operate. Another reason for performing an operation is habitual luxation or subluxation of the nerve, for which reason the examination should include palpation of the nerve in the ulnar groove on extension and flexion; nevertheless, sometimes the presence of luxation is revealed only during surgical exploration (Nigst, 1983). The most common type of operation is anterior transposition of the nerve from the ulnar sulcus, often combined with decompression of the cubital tunnel (Leffert, 1982; Rettig and Ebben, 1993). Others have made a strong case for simple decompression of the ulnar nerve, mostly within the cubital tunnel or otherwise at the epicondylar groove, for all forms of idiopathic compression at the elbow (that is, after exclusion of habitual luxation or acquired disease conditions). These opinions are based on uncontrolled observations – some with limited series (Le Roux *et al.*, 1990; Manske *et al.*, 1992) others with almost 500 consecutive patients (Assmus, 1994) – or on the basis of non-randomized comparisons (Davies *et al.*, 1991; Bimmler *et al.*, 1993). Sometimes improvement occurred only after a second operation, consisting of transposition after failure of simple decompression at the ulnar groove (Gabel and Amadio, 1990); success, at least alleviation of pain and paraesthesia, may follow even renewed exploration when initially no relief was obtained after combined decompression and transposition (Rogers *et al.*, 1991). Clearly there is great need for randomized controlled trials in this field, with comparisons between simple decompression, transposition of the nerve, and decompression of the cubital tunnel.

Specific anatomical abnormalities, such as nerve compression by an arthrotic elbow joint, form an undisputed indication for operation. In the past, soft-tissue masses (ganglia, cysts, tumours) were often unexpected findings during operation, but nowadays this will be shown preoperatively by MRI scanning.

In the case of severe deficits by compression of the ulnar nerve at the elbow recovery may take six to twelve months after the operation, or may not occur at all.

In January 1989, a 79-year-old man, a former timber-cutter, underwent an elective operation for aneurysmal dilatation of the abdominal aorta, at another hospital. As soon as he regained his memory, a few days later, he felt pain at the inside of both elbows, with some weakness of the left hand. Over the course of the next few weeks the pain increased in both arms, but most severely on the left, radiating from the elbow to the ulnar side of the forearm, with pins and needles in the little finger and the ring finger. At the same time the weakness became worse and swelling of the left hand developed. When we saw him in May, after an unsuccessful decompression of the left carpal tunnel, examination was consistent with motor and sensory

---

deficits consistent with compression of the ulnar nerve at the elbow, although examination of the left hand was limited by swelling and pain. Nerve conduction studies confirmed the diagnosis. In June, and then in July, both ulnar nerves were transposed to the volar side, and after a few weeks the pain disappeared. Two years later the use of the right hand had returned to normal, but on the left side the patient still had residual weakness, as well as paraesthesia of the last two fingers.

In closing this section, it should be stressed that neurologists can contribute much, not only by treating but even more by preventing ulnar nerve compression at the elbow, by adequate support of the arms in bedridden patients, especially when these are paralysed. Time and again nurses and also residents need to be convinced of the importance of this simple measure. Repeated checking by the physician in charge is, therefore, not superfluous.

Compression of the ulnar nerve in the forearm

Compression of the ulnar nerve in the forearm is uncommon, accounting for approximately 1% of all ulnar neuropathies, against 87% at the elbow and 12% at the wrist or palm (Mumenthaler, 1961). The motor and sensory deficits are often the same as with compression at the elbow, since the flexor carpi ulnaris and the flexor digitorum profundus muscles are often spared not only with lesion at the forearm but also with lesions at the elbow (Stewart, 1987). Therefore, without the help of neurophysiological studies the distinction between these two sites is difficult or even impossible, although local tenderness or swelling may indicate the forearm as the site of entrapment.

The ulnar nerve

Causes of ulnar nerve lesions in the forearm

Compression of the ulnar nerve in the forearm has been reported at the distal part of the flexor carpi ulnaris muscle by fibrous or fibrovascular bands (Holtzman *et al.*, 1984; Campbell *et al.*, 1988; Campbell, 1989), with a greenstick fracture of the ulna (Prosser and Hooper, 1986), a compartment syndrome of the forearm (Shields and Jacobs, 1986), with haemorrhage in the forearm associated with haemophilia (Silverstein, 1964), and as a result of local hypertrophic neuropathy (see the case history in Chapter 30).

The two sensory branches of the ulnar nerve that originate in the forearm may both be selectively damaged by pressure: the *palmar cutaneous branch*, in two young men who rested the flexor side of their forearm against the edge of a table while engaged in directing the mouse of a computer (Deleu, 1992); and the *dorsal cutaneous branch*, arising some 5 cm proximal to the wrist crease, in a female grocery-store clerk who had to perform repeated movements of wrist flexion and pronation on running food items over a code-sensing machine at the checkout counter ('pricer palsy'; Wertsch, 1985). Handcuffs may occasionally also compress the dorsal cutaneous branch (Sheean and Morris, 1993), although entrapment neuropathies with these devices usually involve the superficial branch of the radial nerve.

Compression of the ulnar nerve at the wrist and the palm

Four sites of compression, with distinct clinical syndromes

In the region of the wrist and the hand the ulnar nerve may be injured at four anatomically distinct levels (see Figure 9.1), each level being associated with a separate clinical syndrome (Table 9.2); some overlap is not unusual (Mumenthaler, 1961; Olney and Hanson, 1988).

1. *Deep and superficial branch: just proximal to or within Guyon's canal.* Compression at the level of Guyon's canal (which has the flexor retinaculum as its floor, while it is covered by the fascia bridging the pisiform bone and the hamulus of the hamate bone), usually causes a pure weakness of all hand

Table 9.2
Syndromes of ulnar nerve lesions at the wrist and palm

Syndrome of the deep and superficial branch, at the wrist (Guyon's canal)

Weakness (and possibly atrophy) of:
- adductor pollicis
- interosseous muscles
- hypothenar muscles (most typical movement: abduction of little finger)
- palmaris brevis muscle (no skin dimple on extreme abduction of little finger)

Sensory loss of:
- palmar surface of little finger and ulnar half of fourth finger

Syndrome of the proximal part of the deep branch, at the level of pisiform bone (Ramsay Hunt syndrome)

Weakness (and possibly atrophy) of:
- adductor pollicis
- interosseous muscles
- hypothenar muscles (most typical movement: abduction of little finger)

(normal function of palmaris brevis muscle; no sensory loss)

Syndrome of the distal part of the deep branch, at or distal to the hamate bone

Weakness (and possibly atrophy) of:
- adductor pollicis
- interosseous muscles

(normal function of palmaris brevis muscle and hypothenar muscles; no sensory loss)

Syndrome of the superficial branch (at or distal to Guyon's canal)

Weakness of:
- palmaris brevis muscle (no skin dimple on extreme abduction of little finger)

Sensory loss of:
- palmar surface of little finger and ulnar half of fourth finger

muscles innervated by the ulnar nerve, including the palmaris brevis. The flexor carpi ulnaris and the flexor digitorum profundus of course remain intact but, as these muscles are often spared with lesions at the elbow, their value in localisation is greatest if they are weak and only modest if they are intact. Eventually the wasted 'ulnar hand' may develop. With regard to sensation, there is little pain but often there is sensory loss at the palmar side of the fifth and the ulnar half of the fourth finger, corresponding to the skin area of the superficial terminal branch. Sensation of the skin over the proximal part of the hypothenar and the dorsal part of the fourth and fifth fingers is typically normal.

2. *Deep branch: at the pisiform bone.* Entrapment may also occur distal to Guyon's canal, between the distal border of the pisiform bone and the point where the superficially running ulnar nerve rounds the hook of the hamate bone, before traversing the palm to innervate the interosseous, lumbrical and adductor pollicis muscles. The superficial terminal branch goes off within the canal and, accordingly, the palmaris brevis muscle functions normally and there is no sensory loss. In summary, if the palmaris brevis muscle proves intact, whereas all other hand muscles innervated by the ulnar nerve are involved and sensation is normal, the site of compression lies distal to the fibres going to the palmaris brevis muscle and just proximal to where the deep terminal fibres divide into branches to the interossei and to the hypothenar muscles. This syndrome has been termed the Ramsay Hunt syndrome (Hunt, 1908).

3. *Deep branch: at (or distal to) the hamate bone.* At this site of ulnar nerve compression, the branches to the hypothenar muscles are spared. This results in a remarkable contrast

between the intact function of the hypothenar muscles and the weakness and atrophy of the more radial hand muscles innervated by the ulnar nerve.

4. *Superficial branch: distal to Guyon's canal.* Rarely, the superficial branch may be involved in isolation, resulting in hypaesthesia of the fourth (ulnar half) and fifth finger on the palmar side, as well as weakness of the palmaris brevis muscle.

Especially in occupational palsies, transitional syndromes may occur between the proximal and distal syndromes of the palm of the hand.

Nerve conduction studies and needle EMG are useful, for localisation of the site of the nerve lesion as well as for differentiation from other disorders. Sensory conduction in the segment between wrist and ring finger (superficial branch) can be compared with that in median nerve fibres to the same finger. Slowing of conduction in the deep branch can be demonstrated by comparing median and ulnar distal motor latencies to the second interosseous space (Kothari *et al.*, 1996). An ulnar neuropathy at the elbow may cause a reduced or absent SNAP at the little finger, while the SNAP of the dorsal cutaneous branch is spared. Therefore, this combination cannot reliably be used alone to localize the site of the lesion at the wrist (Venkatesh *et al.*, 1995).

Differential diagnosis of ulnar neuropathy at the wrist or palm

Motor neurone disease (spinal muscular atrophy and amyotrophic lateral sclerosis) always comes up as a diagnostic possibility in pure motor ulnar neuropathy. A thorough history-taking may already have uncovered unusual postures as a precipitating cause (see case history of an 18-year-old boy on page 83). Motor deficit exclusively in the distribution of the ulnar nerve (that is, with largely intact muscle contour of the thenar eminence) should always raise a suspicion of ulnar nerve disease. Conversely, atrophy of muscles innervated by the ulnar nerve is often more conspicuous than that of other hand muscles, and involvement of other nerve territories may therefore be missed. Neurophysiological investigations are essential in difficult cases.

Syringomyelia, even in its early stages, often leads to dissociated sensory loss (impairment of skin sensation with intact position and vibration sense), which is most often found at the hands and forearms and sometimes also on the trunk. Moreover, in syringomyelia the motor signs and atrophy of the hand muscles are almost invariably associated with decreased or absent reflexes of the arm, and less often with long tract signs. MRI of the cervical cord will readily demonstrate a syrinx or a spinal tumour, but on the other hand cavitation of the spinal cord may sometimes be asymptomatic.

Lesions of the lower brachial plexus (especially the T1 root) caused by a cervical rib and band, a Pancoast tumour or other abnormality are associated with sensory symptoms and signs outside the distribution of the ulnar nerve, at the ulnar side of the forearm. Also, the motor deficit often exceeds that of the small hand muscles innervated by this nerve, a difference that may be immediately apparent on inspection of the palm. The presence of a cervical rib is often an incidental finding, unless accompanied by a characteristic syndrome of the first dorsal root: pain and sensory loss at the ulnar side of the forearm, with partial thenar atrophy (Gilliatt *et al.*, 1978). Compression of the T1 root by a hypertrophic scalenus anticus muscle has been reported in a competitive athlete (Katirji and Hardy, 1995), but must be exceedingly rare.

Cervical radiculopathy resulting from intervertebral disc prolapse usually affects the C7 or C6 root, with motor deficits more proximal than the fingers, and even in the relatively rare case that the C8 root is affected (by a lateral disc prolapse between the vertebrae of C7 and T1) the finger flexors rather than the intrinsic hand muscles are weak. Spondylotic myelopathy may definitely cause weakness and atrophy of intrinsic hand muscles, but is usually associated with long tract signs.

In all these diagnostic considerations neurophysiological or neuroradiological investigations may be decisive, but will not always be necessary.

Causes of ulnar nerve lesions at the wrist or palm

A variety of extrinsic and intrinsic causes may underlie lesions of the ulnar nerve at the wrist or in the hand (Table 9.3). External pressure is by far the most common cause.

Table 9.3
Causes of ulnar nerve lesions at the wrist and palm

External pressure
- Occupational (profession or hobby): handling pneumatic drills, shears, screwdrivers, pliers, knives, etc. (Mumenthaler, 1961; Jones, 1988); meat packing (Streib and Sun, 1984)
- Cyclist's palsy: pressure from handlebars (Guillain *et al.*, 1940; Noth *et al.*, 1980; Hankey and Gubbay, 1988; Maimaris and Zadeh, 1990)
- use of canes or crutches
- handcuffs (Scott *et al.*, 1989)

Hereditary liability to pressure palsies (Earl *et al.*, 1964; Staal *et al.*, 1965; Behse *et al.*, 1972) (see Chapter 25)

Acute injury
- Penetrating wounds (Mumenthaler, 1961)
- Carpo-metacarpal luxation (Gore, 1971)
- Fractures of the radio-ulnar joint (Coccurollo and Galvagno, 1984)
- Fractures of the hamulus of the hamate bone (Mumenthaler, 1961; Shea and McClain, 1969)
- Fractures of the fifth metacarpal bone (Murphy and Parkhill, 1990; O'Rourke and Quinlan, 1993)

Delayed, after acute injury
- Aneurysm of the ulnar artery (Kalisman *et al.*, 1982; Vandertop and van't Verlaat, 1985; Kay *et al.*, 1988)
- Malunion after Colles' fracture (Aro *et al.*, 1988)

Table 9.3 (continued)
Causes of ulnar nerve lesions at the wrist and palm

Acquired lesions in the wrist or palm
- Ganglion (Brooks, 1952; Richmond, 1963; Olney and Hanson, 1988; Subin *et al.*, 1989; Giuliani *et al.*, 1990; Feldman *et al.* 1995)
- Benign giant cell tumour (Bronisch, 1960; Foucher *et al.*, 1993)
- Thrombo-angiitis of the ulnar artery (Dupont *et al.*, 1965)
- Benign chondroblastoma of the hamate (Daly *et al.*, 1993)
- Nodular synovitis (Budny *et al.*, 1992)
- Pathologic calcifications, idiopathic (Sharara and Nairn, 1983), or associated with scleroderma (Thurman *et al.*, 1991; Chammas *et al.*, 1995)
- Pyrophosphate arthropathy (Pattrick *et al.*, 1988)
- Lipoma, with haemorrhage (Zahrawi, 1984)

Congenital anomalies
- Anomalous course of ulnar nerve, under flexor retinaculum (Galzio *et al.*, 1987)
- Duplication of the tendon of the flexor carpi ulnaris muscle, with splitting of the ulnar nerve (Zook *et al.*, 1988; al Qattan and Duerksen, 1992; Kang *et al.*, 1996)
- Reversed palmaris longus muscle (Regan *et al.*, 1988)
- Accessory palmaris longus muscle (Regan *et al.*, 1991)
- Accessory palmaris brevis muscle (Robinson *et al.*, 1989)
- Accessory abductor digiti minimi muscle (Luethke and Dellon, 1992)
- Anomalous origin of the flexor digiti minimi muscle (Spinner *et al.*, 1996)
- Thickened piso-hamate ligament (Ebeling *et al.*, 1960)
- Fusion between pisiform and hamate bones (Berkowitz *et al.*, 1992)
- Tortuosity of the ulnar artery (Segal *et al.*, 1992)

Infections (see Chapter 26)
- Leprosy (Carayon *et al.*, 1966);
- Tuberculoma (Nucci *et al.*, 1988);
- Phlegmon of the palm (Mumenthaler, 1961);

hypothenar. There was marked weakness (MRC 3/5) of the interosseous muscles and of the abductor, opponens and flexor of the little finger; skin sensation was unimpaired. Spontaneous improvement occurred within another three months.

In 'cyclists' palsy' the ulnar nerve is sometimes compressed at the level of the wrist, in Guyon's canal, in which case there are warning paraesthesiae, but most often it is the palm of the hand that bears most of the weight, especially with low handlebars of the type usually found on racing bikes. The problem typically occurs in amateurs; on specific questioning the condition proved to be unknown in a team of professional cyclists. Probably, inexperienced sportsmen and -women lean too heavily on their arms, instead of mainly using the back muscles to maintain the flexed posture of the trunk. Other measures that may help to prevent damage to the ulnar nerve consist of frequently changing the position of the hands, wearing special gloves (that keep the fingers free but have cushions to protect the palm), or covering the handlebars with soft material. In some cases more than one causal factor exists.

A 60-year-old man had a three-month history of weakness in the right hand, most marked in the little finger, without sensory changes. He had first noticed this after he had changed the locks in the doors of his house, which had involved strenuous work with chisels and screwdrivers. On examination the fingers of the right hand were clawed, with atrophy of the

A healthy 18-year-old boy had rather suddenly developed severe weakness of both hands, about one week before. There were no sensory symptoms. Inspection showed slight guttering of both hands, and impressive weakness of finger abduction and adduction; adduction of the thumbs was also weak. The palmaris brevis muscles were intact, and the hypothenar muscles were neither atrophic nor weak. Tendon jerks were brisk and symmetrical. In spite of his young age and the subacute progression, juvenile amyotrophic lateral sclerosis was initially considered. Later, after a conversation with his father it turned out that his hand function had really been completely normal until his recent birthday, when he had been given a racing bicycle. One week before he had made his first tour, of about 100 km. Two days later he repeated the exercise with another 150 km. Between the two tours he noticed for the first time that something was wrong with his hands. On further questioning it emerged that his father had twice suffered a dropping foot after having worked in a kneeling position for one whole day (agricultural work). On both occasions full recovery had ensued after several weeks. Fortunately the diagnosis in the boy could now be changed to 'hereditary liability to pressure palsies' (see Chapter 25). This disease had manifested itself with bilateral and purely motor ulnar nerve palsies, from compression of the palms by tight gripping of the handlebars of the bicycle. As expected the boy made a full recovery in six weeks, during which he was advised not to use his new bicycle. Afterwards, with cushioned gloves and a better cycling technique, there were no further difficulties.

Management of ulnar nerve lesions at the wrist or palm

In some cases with a distal lesion to the ulnar nerve the cause remains unsolved, as in 8 of 34 patients in Mumenthaler's series (Mumenthaler, 1961). In this era of MRI scanning this proportion will now be smaller. Surgical exploration is indicated also in these remaining cases, and more often than not this intervention will reveal the cause (Chaise and Sedel, 1984). Even if no abnormalities are found, opening Guyon's canal may bring relief, despite the lack of a rational explanation.

Chapter 10

The intercostal nerves

Anatomy

Twelve pairs of intercostal nerves, derived from the ventral rami of the thoracic spinal nerves, innervate the intercostal and abdominal muscles as well as the overlying skin. Before continuing as the first intercostal nerve, the first ventral ramus gives off a branch to the brachial plexus. The motor fibres of the first six intercostal nerves run closely under and medial of the ribs (Figure 10.1) and innervate only the corresponding intercostal muscles, whereas the last six intercostal nerves also contribute fibres to the abdominal muscles. The corresponding skin areas are supplied by the *lateral and anterior cutaneous branches* of the intercostal nerves.

The *intercostobrachial nerve* originates from the lateral cutaneous branch of the second or third intercostal nerve, or both, to supply the posterior part of the axilla. It often forms anastomoses with the *medial cutaneous nerve of the upper arm*, which arises from the medial cord of the brachial plexus.

Lesions of intercostal nerves

History and examination

Damage to an intercostal nerve leads to local pain, paraesthesia or both. Sensory loss may involve the entire strip of skin at the level in question, or only part of it. Muscle weakness does not lead to symptoms, but with involvement of a

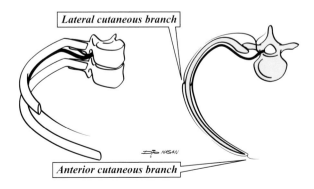

Figure 10.1
Intercostal nerve.

The intercostal nerves

lower intercostal nerve examination may show slight bulging of abdominal muscles.

Electrophysiological studies

Intercostal nerve conduction is studied infrequently. Deep paravertebral stimulation with surface or needle electrodes (Caldwell et al., 1968; Pradhan and Taly, 1989) is difficult to perform and uncomfortable for the patient. Magnetic stimulation, however, is an almost painless technique which can be used very well to stimulate thoracic roots at the intervertebral foramina. Responses can be recorded from the intercostal and abdominal muscles with surface electrodes (Chokroverty et al., 1995). Needle EMG of the intercostal and abdominal muscles can be useful to supplement studies of the paravertebral thoracic muscles. In the abdominal musculature there is always overlap between myotomes so that the exact level of a possible root or nerve lesion cannot be determined. With investigation of the intercostal muscles one should be aware of the risk of pneumothorax.

Causes

Lesions of intercostal nerves may be a complication of operations involving the wall of the chest or abdomen, or during thoracostomy (Abel and Ali, 1992). There may also be local causes such as a schwannoma, diabetic neuropathy, or herpes zoster (Table 10.1). Similar symptoms may be caused by compression of the root of a thoracic nerve, mostly from metastatic disease, but occasionally from a thoracic disk protrusion (Love and Schorn, 1967). *Notalgia paraesthetica*, or burning pain around the scapula with a paravertebral sensory deficit, has been attributed to idiopathic involvement of cutaneous branches of the dorsal rami (Pleet and Massey, 1978); in some cases diabetes may be the underlying cause (Stewart, 1989). Pain in the axilla or at the

Table 10.1
Causes of lesions of intercostal nerves

Iatrogenic

- Thoracostomy, mastectomy (Moore, 1982; Abel and Ali, 1992)
- Abdominal surgery (Teitze et al., 1979; Montagna et al., 1985)

Diabetes (Ellenberg, 1978; Stewart, 1989)

Tumours, especially schwannomas (see Chapter 30)

Herpes zoster (see Chapter 26)

medial side of the upper arm may follow surgery for breast cancer, and accompanying sensory deficits implicate a lesion of the intercostobrachial nerve (Vecht et al., 1989).

In the so-called 'slipping rib syndrome' (or Cyriax syndrome), upper abdominal pain is attributed to irritation of the intercostal nerve by incomplete dislocation of the costal cartilage of the eighth, ninth, or tenth rib; local injection of an anaesthetic is said to relieve the pain (Monnin et al., 1988). Equally contentious is the existence of an entrapment syndrome of endings of the intercostal nerve in the abdominal fascia, as an explanation for severe upper abdominal pain; also in these cases local anaesthesia is claimed to bring relief, even for months or years (Meier, 1989). It is typical of the dubious nature of these entities that advocates have reported scores of patients, whereas most neurologists will have seen none. As in many similar 'syndromes' for which no objective criteria exist and that are diagnosed only in certain pain clinics, somatisation disorder underlies the symptoms in most, if not all, cases, but an anatomical explanation is preferred by physician and patient alike.

Treatment

This varies according to the underlying cause and may range from local surgery or radiation for a local mass lesion to management of diabetes mellitus.

Part two

Mononeuropathies in the leg

Chapter 11
The iliohypogastric nerve

Anatomy

The iliohypogastric nerve (Figure 11.1) originates together with the ilioinguinal nerve from the first lumbar spinal root, sometimes with a contribution from the T12 root as well. After emerging from the lateral border of the psoas muscle, the nerve curves downwards and laterally along the ventral surface of the quadratus lumborum muscle, crossing the lower border of the kidney; then it continues along the lateral abdominal wall. The transverse abdominal muscle is traversed just above the iliac crest, after which the iliohypogastric nerve passes between the transverse abdominal and oblique internal abdominal muscles; both these muscles derive their innervation partly from the iliohypogastric nerve. Finally, the nerve branches into the lateral and anterior cutaneous nerve. The *lateral cutaneous nerve* innervates a small area of the skin of the buttock, at its upper part, and the *anterior cutaneous nerve* supplies a small and rather variable area of skin above the symphysis (Figure 11.2).

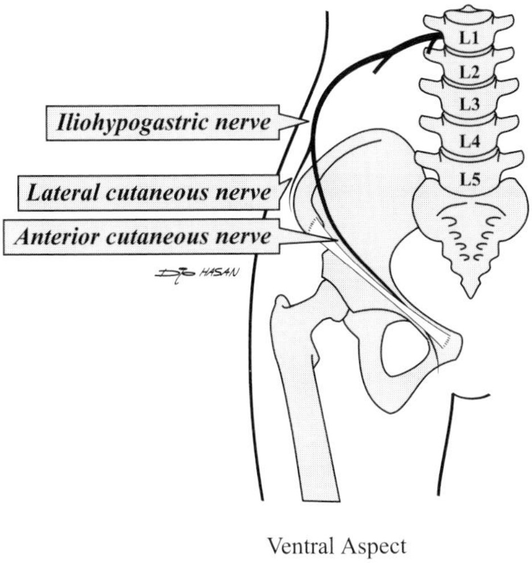

Iliohypogastric nerve

Lateral cutaneous nerve

Anterior cutaneous nerve

Ventral Aspect

Figure 11 .1
The iliohypogastric nerve.

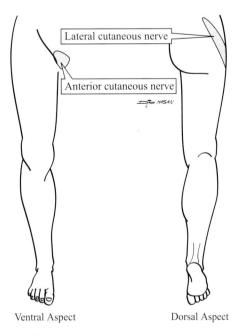

Lateral cutaneous nerve

Anterior cutaneous nerve

Ventral Aspect   Dorsal Aspect

Figure 11.2
Approximate skin areas innervated by the iliohypogastric nerve.

Lesions of the iliohypogastric nerve

History and examination

The main complaint with a lesion of the iliohypogastric nerve is neuralgic pain in the skin area above the symphysis. Examination may reveal a sensory deficit only, since the motor innervation of the muscles of the abdominal wall is partly supplied by the ilioinguinal nerve. Some bulging of the abdominal muscles above the inguinal ligament may be detectable, especially after Valsalva's manoeuvre, but only when both nerves are damaged is this unequivocally clear.

Electrophysiological evaluation of the iliohypogastric nerve has not been described.

Causes

Isolated iliohypogastric nerve damage is rare. Its close anatomical relationship with the ilioinguinal nerve explains why the two nerves may be damaged together. The cause is mostly iatrogenic, by a variety of operations in the lower abdomen, from appendectomies (Stulz and Pfeiffer, 1982) to abdominoplasty (Liszka *et al.*, 1994). Lesions are especially common with Pfannenstiel (transverse) incisions for gynaecological operations (Sippo *et al.*, 1987). The symptoms may develop immediately after the operation or only after many months, after scar tissue has formed (Stulz and Pfeiffer, 1982). Habitual leaning against a bench or wearing tight jeans has been observed to cause injury of the iliohypogastric nerve (Mumenthaler and Schliack, 1993). Some believe they have identified an entrapment syndrome of the iliohypogastric nerve, in patients with pain at the lateral aspect of the hip (Touzard *et al.*, 1989); the pain could be reproduced by local pressure, but there were no objective neurological deficits. The therapeutic effect provided by local infiltration or, if this failed, by neurolysis, is insufficient evidence for the existence of such an entrapment syndrome.

Treatment

Treatment is the same as for the ilioinguinal and genitofemoral nerves; that is, mostly by neurolysis or resection of the nerve (Stulz and Pfeiffer, 1982).

Chapter 12
The ilioinguinal nerve

Anatomy

The ilioinguinal nerve carries fibres from the first and sometimes the second lumbar root (Figure 12.1). After emerging from the lateral border of the psoas muscle the nerve follows the inner side of the abdominal wall, much like an intercostal nerve. When it reaches a point somewhat medial to the anterior superior iliac spine, it turns medially and passes through the inguinal canal and the superficial inguinal ring, where it runs together with the

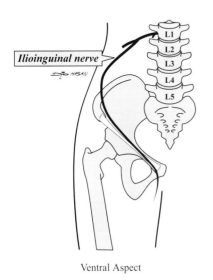

Ventral Aspect

Figure 12.1
The ilioinguinal nerve.

genitofemoral nerve and the spermatic cord in men or the round ligament in women. To reach the spermatic cord the nerve pierces the transverse and internal oblique muscles, which are the only muscles to which this nerve sends its fibres (together with the iliohypogastric and genitofemoral nerves, and some intercostal nerves). The sensory fibres of the ilioinguinal nerve supply a narrow strip of skin that extends from the superior anterior spine across the inguinal ligament, to the base of the penis and the upper part of the scrotum in men, or to the labium maius in women. Finally, the nerve innervates the uppermost medial part of the thigh (Figure 12.2).

Lesions of the ilioinguinal nerve

History

The main symptoms in lesions of the ilioinguinal nerve are burning and stabbing pains in the inguinal region, which may radiate towards the genitals. The pain may also radiate to the hip region. Symptoms are worse with walking and are less intense on flexion of the hip. In the supine position the hip is also kept in flexion (Mumenthaler *et al.*, 1965), and if the pain is severe patients adopt this posture even while standing and move about on crutches (Kopell *et al.*, 1962).

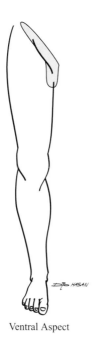

Ventral Aspect

Figure 12.2
Approximate skin areas innervated by the ilioinguinal nerve.

had continuous pain in the region of the scar and the right groin, radiating downwards to the medial side of the thigh. Coughing or sneezing caused stabbing pain in the same region. Four operations were subsequently performed without success (for possible inguinal hernia, tenotomy, or cleaving of adhesions). Injection of anaesthetics around the scar or physiotherapy was equally ineffective, and a psychological cause for the symptoms was eventually postulated. On examination in 1989 it was found that he stood with slight flexion of the right hip. Valsalva's manoeuvre resulted in some bulging of the lower abdominal wall on the right. There was hyperaesthesia on the medial side of the right thigh. Injection with local anaesthetic at the level of the anterior superior spine abolished the pain for about 90 minutes. Maintenance treatment with carbamazepine and amitryptiline reduced the pain to an acceptable degree.

Examination

It is difficult to test the muscles of the abdominal wall. In ilioinguinalis neuropathy there may be some spontaneous bulging of the abdominal wall, medial to the anterior superior spine; this is seen most clearly if there is associated damage of the iliohypogastric nerve, with which it runs together in a large part of its course (Mumenthaler and Schliack, 1993). Weakness of the abdominal muscles does not cause symptoms. A sensory deficit may be present in the skin area described above. A Tinel sign over an appendectomy site or other surgical scar may suggests a neuroma.

In 1968, a 41-year-old man underwent laparotomy for suspected Crohn's disease; the diagnosis was not confirmed and only appendectomy was performed. Ever since the operation he

Differential diagnosis

Lesions of the first lumbar root or genitofemoral neuropathy are the main conditions to be considered. The preferred position with the hip in flexion assumed by patients with ilioinguinal neuropathy may simulate a disorder of the hip joint.

Causes

Spontaneous entrapment at the outlet through the abdominal wall does occur (Kopell *et al.*, 1962). However, this idiopathic variety of ilioinguinal neuropathy is a less common cause than are surgical interventions in the inguinal region, with or without associated damage to the iliohypogastric nerve (Stulz and Pfeiffer, 1982). Examples are herniorrhaphy (Starling *et al.*, 1987), appendectomy (Purves and Miller, 1986), abdominoplasty (Liszka *et al.*, 1994) or bone grafting (Smith *et al.*, 1984). Other operations associated with ilioinguinal neuropathy are needle suspension procedures for stress incontinence (Miyazaki and Shook, 1992; Monga and Ghoniem, 1994) or nephrectomy (Mumenthaler *et al.*, 1965). Finally, endometriosis may be to blame (Purves and Miller, 1986).

Electrophysiological studies

Neurophysiological studies do not contribute much to the evaluation of ilioinguinal nerve lesions. A technique for motor nerve conduction studies has been described (Ellis *et al.*, 1992), but so far its diagnostic value has not been evaluated. Needle electromyography of the paraspinal musculature is helpful to differentiate this lesion from an L1 radiculopathy.

Treatment

Injection of a local anaesthetic agent around the nerve or at the level of a painful trigger point is often informally reported to be helpful. Sometimes hydrocortisone is injected as well. Medication with carbamazepine, hydantoin or imipramine may also bring relief. However, if scar tissue compresses the nerve or if a neuroma has developed after surgical trauma these lesions should, as a rule, be removed. To be certain of the diagnosis the extirpated tissue should be carefully examined by the pathologist. Serial sections may be necessary to identify a microscopic neuroma (personal observation by one of us). Neurolysis may be sufficient (Mumenthaler *et al.*, 1965), but often resection of the nerve is necessary (Starling *et al.*, 1987; Hahn, 1989).

Chapter 13
The genitofemoral nerve

Anatomy

After arising from the first two lumbar spinal roots the genitofemoral nerve runs downward through the psoas muscle and emerges on its ventral side to run further on the surface of the psoas muscle, down to the inguinal ligament (Figure 13.1). Here it divides into a *femoral branch* and a *genital branch*. In the inguinal canal the genital branch runs together with the ilioinguinal nerve; these two nerves overlap in their skin supply of the mons pubis and the scrotum or labium majus. The genital branch also innervates the cremaster muscle; therefore, in lesions of

the genitofemoral nerve, the cremaster reflex may be abolished. The femoral branch crosses under the inguinal ligament and innervates a tiny part of the skin on the anterior surface of the thigh, just distal to the inguinal ligament (Figure 13.2).

Lesions of the genitofemoral nerve

History

Damage of the genitofemoral nerve may give rise to continual and severe pain and paraesthesia. Mumenthaler and Schliack (1993) call this 'Spermatikusneuralgie'. Damage is often not confined to the genitofemoral nerve, and often also involves the fibres of the ilioinguinal nerve, since the two nerves are so close. Some amalgamate a lesion of this pair of nerves under the term 'postoperative inguinal neuralgia' (Purves and Miller, 1986; Stewart, 1993).

Examination

There may be a sensory deficit in the (overlapping) skin areas innervated by the ilioinguinal and genitofemoral nerves, and the cremaster reflex may be absent on the affected side.

To our knowledge no electrophysiological technique for

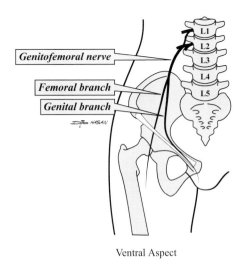

Ventral Aspect

Figure 13.1
The genitofemoral nerve.

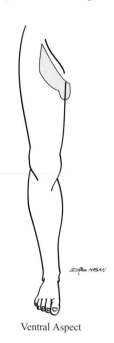

Ventral Aspect

Figure 13.2
Approximate skin area innervated by the genitofemoral nerve.

studying the genitofemoral nerve has been described.

Causes

Spontaneous entrapment does not seem to occur; the potential causes are the same as for ilioinguinal neuropathy, since the nerves are so close together. Leading

causes are previous herniorraphy, appendectomy, or nephrectomy, removal of bone grafts from the inner table of the iliac crest, and blunt trauma (Starling and Harms, 1989; Benini, 1992). Tumours are a relatively uncommon cause:

> A 46-year-old man with the acquired immune deficiency syndrome and non-Hodgkin lymphoma stage IV had for two months had an increasingly severe, stabbing pain in the right scrotal area. In the last three or four weeks he had also had stabbing pain in the region of the right hip, especially on lying down. On examination there was hypaesthesia and hypalgesia in the right half of the scrotum and in the right groin. Computed tomography scanning of the pelvis showed an enlarged paraaortal lymph node on the right, at the level of the intervertebral disc L2–L3. After local radiotherapy the pain resolved completely.

Treatment

The management does not differ from that of ilioinguinal neuropathy. Neurectomy proximal to the point of compression is advocated (Starling and Harms, 1989).

Chapter 14

The lateral cutaneous nerve of the thigh

Anatomy

This sensory nerve carries fibres from the second and third spinal lumbar nerves. It emerges from the lateral border of the psoas muscle and then crosses the iliacus muscle (Figure 14.1). Just medial to the anterior superior iliac spine it is usually enclosed between two folds of the lateral attachment of the inguinal ligament. The nerve may leave the pelvis in different ways: through a notch between the anterior superior and the inferior area of the iliac spine; through the inguinal ligament, sometimes with two or three separate branches; or at the medial side of the inguinal ligament, close to the femoral nerve. On entering the thigh the lateral cutaneous nerve runs in a fibrous canal within the fascia lata, and thereby abruptly changes its course from a more or less horizontal to a more or less vertical position. The degree of angulation is influenced by extension and flexion of the hip, and this anatomical arrangement makes the nerve vulnerable to entrapment. A few centimetres distal to the inguinal ligament, but sometimes earlier, the nerve divides into several twigs to innervate the skin of the lateral part of the thigh. This area extends as far down as the knee, but not beyond the upper ridge of the patella (Figure 14.2).

Lesions of the lateral cutaneous nerve (meralgia paraesthetica)

History

The first descriptions of a disorder of the lateral cutaneous nerve of the thigh were reported in 1895 (Bernhardt, 1895; Roth, 1895). In that same year Sigmund Freud, still in his 'neurological period', reported about his own '*Bernhardt'sche Sensibilitätsstörung am Oberschenkel*' (Schiller, 1985). The symptoms, for which Roth coined the term 'meralgia

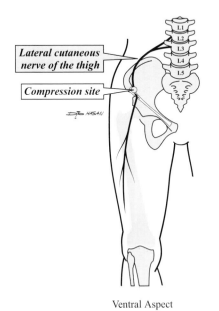

Ventral Aspect

Figure 14.1
The lateral cutaneous nerve of the thigh.

The lateral cutaneous nerve of the thigh

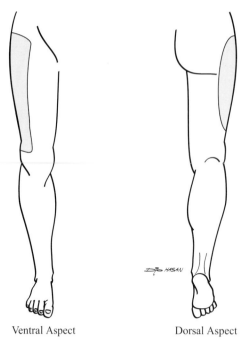

Ventral Aspect   Dorsal Aspect

Figure 14.2
Approximate skin area innervated by the lateral cutaneous nerve of the thigh.

paraesthetica' (*mèros* is Greek for thigh), consist of pain, tingling, a burning sensation, and often also numbness in the skin territory of the nerve. For unknown reasons the symptoms rarely extend as far down as the knee, whereas with involvement of other nerves sensory symptoms often first appear in the most distal part of the area supplied by the nerve. In some instances the patient cannot even bear the touch of clothes or sheets, but in other cases there is only numbness. Standing or walking may aggravate the unpleasant sensations, and flexion of the hip may alleviate them. Infrequently, the syndrome is bilateral.

Examination

Sensory examination often shows a deficit of superficial sensation, mostly in the centre of the territory of the lateral cutaneous nerve. Touch may be unpleasant or even painful. The

symptoms may be precipitated or increased by hyperextension of the hip, or by pressure on the presumed point of entrapment, somewhat medial of the anterior superior iliac spine. Frequent rubbing of the skin or dysfunction of autonomous innervation may lead to hypertrichosis or, conversely, to local alopecia (Aranoff *et al.*, 1985; Krause *et al.*, 1987).

Causes

In many patients the cause remains unknown, even after extensive investigations. Obesity is often mentioned in connection with meralgia paraesthetica, as bulging of the abdomen would increase the angulation of the nerve as its exits the pelvis (Keegan and Holyoke, 1962), but the condition is also found in lean subjects. It may even occur in children and adolescents (Edelson and Stevens, 1994). Diabetes is not a predisposing condition either. It is unknown how often an abnormal anatomic course or a neuroma underlies this most common, unexplained form of meralgia paraesthetica. Possible factors other than dependent abdominal fat include attachment of the fascia lata or the sartorius muscle to the inguinal ligament, the muscle fibres from the internal oblique and tranversus abdominis muscles originating from the inguinal ligament, or the external oblique muscle inserting on it (Keegan and Holyoke, 1962).

Apart from the idiopathic form, numerous separate causes are known to lead to meralgia paraesthetica (Williams and Trzil, 1991). These may damage the nerve at the level of the pelvis, at the inguinal ligament, or in the thigh (Table 14.1). After the idiopathic syndrome the most common causes are pregnancy, tight clothing or belts, scars, iliac bone grafts, and intrapelvic masses compressing the nerve.

Table 14.1
Causes of meralgia paraesthetica

Idiopathic entrapment

Exercise or postural factors
- Pregnancy (Van Diver and Camann, 1995)
- Falling asleep in siddha yoga position (Mattio *et al.*, 1992)
- Body building (Szewczyk *et al.*, 1994)
- Gymnastics (Macgregor and Moncur, 1977)

Iatrogenic lesions
- Misplaced injections (Ecker and Woltman, 1938)
- Laparoscopic repair of inguinal hernia (Kraus, 1993; Darzi *et al.* 1994; Broin *et al.* 1995)
- Laparoscopic cholecystectomy (Yamout *et al.* 1994)
- Transfemoral angiography (Sommer and Ferbert, 1992)
- Abdominoplasty (Floros and Davis, 1991)
- Gastroplasty for morbid obesity (Grace, 1987)
- Lithotomy position for gynaecological operations (Heidenreich and Lorenzoni, 1983)
- Groin flap in plastic surgery (Moscona and Hirshowitz, 1980)
- Rotational osteotomy of acetabulum for congenital dysplasia of the hip (Azuma and Taneda, 1989)
- Removal of bone graft from ileum (Weikel and Habal, 1977; Garlipp, 1979; Daupleix and Dreyfus, 1984)
- Renal transplantation (Jindal *et al.* 1993)

Trauma
- Avulsion fracture of the anterior superior iliac spine (Buch and Campbell, 1993; Thanikachalam *et al.*, 1995)
- Injury to the anterolateral thigh (Moscona and Sekel, 1978)

Tumours or other mass lesions
- Malignant tumour of psoas muscle (Amoiridis *et al.*, 1993)
- Osteoid osteoma of the hip, in children (Goldberg and Jacobs, 1975)
- Haemorrhage in haemophilia (Ehrmann *et al.*, 1981)

External compression
- Seat-belt trauma (Beresford, 1971)
- Pocket watch (Mack, 1968)
- Tight trousers (Boyce, 1984; Schärli and Ayer, 1984)
- Pregnancy (Rhodes, 1957)

Familial form
- Autosomal dominant meralgia paraesthetica (Malin, 1979)

Differential diagnosis

If the abnormalities are clearly confined to a sensory deficit in the appropriate area, without weakness and with symmetrical knee jerks, alternative diagnoses are limited to involvement of the second lumbar root. Collapse of thoracic vertebral bodies is a rare cause (Liveson, 1984b); more common are metastases in the L2 vertebra (Rinkel and Wokke, 1990), or retroperitoneal tumours at that level (Suber and Massey, 1979).

A 51-year-old physician complained of numbness on the outer side of the right thigh, for two months. He came to see one of us when, in addition, he had suffered a sudden and severe backache after some heavy lifting on his yacht; in the past two years he had had four similar episodes of backache, though less severe. On examination there was an area of hypaesthesia and hypalgesia at the lateral part of the thigh, approximately the size of the examiner's hand, with a thin strip extending down to a midpatellar level. Two weeks later the backache had largely cleared, but another two months later he developed abdominal pain, and an unoperable carcinoma of the pancreatic tail was diagnosed.

Electrophysiological and imaging studies

Needle EMG may be helpful in the differentiation between a lesion of the lateral cutaneous nerve of the thigh and lumbar radiculopathy, plexopathy or femoral neuropathy. Nerve conduction studies have limitations because it is often not possible to stimulate or record at a short distance proximal to the supposed site of compression. Therefore nerve conduction studies are usually performed in a more distal nerve segment (Butler *et al.*, 1974; Sarala *et al.*, 1979; Po and Mei, 1992; Spevak and Prevec, 1995). This means that any slowing of conduction implies loss of the thickest nerve fibres; such a finding is therefore accompanied by a reduced amplitude of sensory nerve action potentials. As the course of the nerve is rather variable, the correct site for stimulation or recording should be determined by eliciting maximal sensations in the lateral aspect of the thigh. Results should always be compared with findings on the unaffected side. Bilateral absence of sensory nerve action potentials has been found in some normal subjects (Flügel *et al.*, 1984). Somatosensory evoked potentials may also be used as a diagnostic test for a lesion of the lateral cutaneous nerve of the thigh (Lagueny *et al.*, 1991; Po and Mei, 1992). To distinguish a lesion of the nerve itself from a plexopathy or a radiculopathy, the dermatomal sensory evoked potential of the ilioinguinal nerve can be used for comparison (Wiezer *et al.*, 1996).

It is generally wise to order radiographs of the lumbar spine, certainly if there are associated symptoms or if the area of numbness extends too far anteriorly or downwards to correspond with the area innervated by the lateral cutaneous nerve. If this is abnormal it should be followed by MRI scanning of the upper lumbar vertebrae, or otherwise by an echogram of the abdomen and pelvic region. If these investigations are normal the patient can be reassured that the condition is benign and self-limiting.

Treatment

Any therapeutic claims should take account of a sizeable proportion of patients showing spontaneous recovery within months or years; this proportion has been estimated at one-quarter

(Mumenthaler and Schliack, 1993). In the impressive series of 277 patients reported by Williams and Trzil (1991), surgical intervention was necessary in only 24 of these. Conservative measures consisted of removing constrictive items around the waist, cooling with ice packs (three times daily), or non-steroidal anti-inflammatory drugs. In persistent cases the pain was often relieved by an injection with steroids and an analgesic agent at the presumed trigger point at the inguinal ligament (Williams and Trzil, 1991). Such injections were also successful in another series, where it was the first-line treatment (Prabhakar *et al.*, 1989), and more specifically in patients with AIDS (Myers and George, 1996). Some have claimed success for transcutaneous electrical nerve stimulation (Fisher and Hanna, 1987). Surgical resection is only the last resort and usually involves removal of a 4 cm segment of the nerve, at its passage through the inguinal ligament. In the series reported by Williams and Trzil (1991), a pathologically verified neuroma was found in 16 of the 24 patients who underwent surgery; the procedure was successful in 23, and in the single failure a pelvic neoplasm was ultimately detected (Williams and Trzil, 1991). The resulting sensory deficit did not lead to anaesthesia dolorosa or other problems. An alternative procedure is neurolysis; in observational studies this was slightly to markedly less effective than transection of the nerve (Antoniadis *et al.*, 1995; van Eerten *et al.*, 1995), but these comparisons were not based on randomized treatment allocation. Re-exploration after an initially unsuccessful neurolysis is usually fruitless (Macnicol and Thompson, 1990).

Chapter 15
The posterior cutaneous nerve of the thigh

Anatomy

The posterior cutaneous nerve of the thigh (Figure 15.1) arises from the lower part of the lumbosaral plexus, carrying fibres from the roots S1-S3. Together with the inferior gluteal nerve it passes through the greater sciatic notch, below the piriform muscle. At the lower border of the gluteus maximus muscle it enters the thigh, close to the sciatic nerve; here branches are given off to the skin of the perineum and scrotum (or labium majus). The nerve then descends superficially over the hamstring muscles to the politeal fossa, supplying fibres to the lower part of the buttock, the dorsal side of the thigh and the proximal third of the calf (Figure 15.2).

Lesions of the posterior cutaneous nerve of the thigh

History and examination

Patients complain about paraesthesia and numbness over the lower part of the

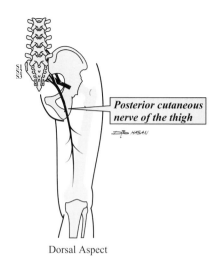

Figure 15.1
The posterior cutaneous nerve of the thigh.

Dorsal Aspect

Posterior cutaneous nerve of the thigh

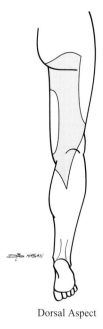

Dorsal Aspect

Figure 15.2
Approximate skin area innervated by the posterior cutaneous nerve of the thigh.

The posterior cutaneous nerve of the thigh

buttock and the posterior aspect of the thigh. A sensory deficit may or may not be found.

It is possible to perform nerve conduction studies of the posterior cutaneous nerve of the thigh (Dumitru and Nelson, 1990). Needle EMG can be useful in the differentiation from an S2 radiculopathy or a plexopathy.

Causes

Apart from wounds at the dorsal aspect of the thigh, the nerve is most often damaged by compression: by prolonged gymnastic exercises performed on the buttocks, by a sedentary occupation, or by extensive bicycle riding (Arnoldussen and Korten, 1980). Mass lesions that may involve the nerve include colorectal tumours (LaBan et al., 1982), haemangiopericytoma (Stewart et al., 1983), and a venous malformation (Chutkow, 1988). Iatrogenic causes are intramuscular injections in the buttock (Iyer and Shields, 1989), or gluteal thigh flaps for reconstruction of the vagina following resection of infiltrating carcinoma (Achauer et al., 1984).

Treatment

The management of posterior femoral cutaneous neuropathy depends on the cause and will often consist of either removal of the responsible mass lesion or advice to avoid pressure to the lower buttock and dorsal thigh.

Chapter 16
The femoral nerve

Anatomy

The femoral nerve arises from the spinal roots L2–L4 within the psoas muscle (Figure 16.1). Initially it runs at the lateral border of the psoas muscle, within the fascia between the psoas and iliacus muscles. More distally it passes under the inguinal ligament, where it lies lateral to the femoral artery. Proximal to the inguinal ligament branches go to the iliopsoas muscle, and at the level of this

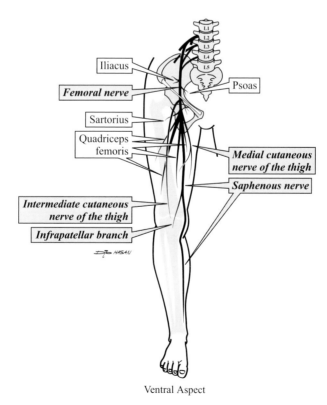

Iliacus

Femoral nerve

Sartorius

Quadriceps femoris

Psoas

Medial cutaneous nerve of the thigh

Saphenous nerve

Intermediate cutaneous nerve of the thigh

Infrapatellar branch

HASAN

Ventral Aspect

Figure 16.1
Muscles innervated by the femoral nerve.

ligament branches are given off to the sartorius and the four parts of the quadriceps muscle.

Sensory branches, the *intermediate cutaneous nerve of the thigh* and the *medial cutaneous nerve of the thigh*, leave the nerve distal to the inguinal ligament, to innervate the skin on the anterior and medial sides of the thigh (Figure 16.2). The terminal branch of the femoral nerve is the purely sensory *saphenous nerve*, which courses within the quadriceps muscle through Hunter's canal. About 10 cm above the knee it leaves this canal and gives off the *infrapatellar branch*, which supplies the skin on the medial side of the knee down to the tuberositas of the tibia (see Figure 16.2). More distally the saphenous nerve descends along the medial side of the tibia and the anterior surface of the medial malleolus, to innervate the skin at the medial and anterior surface of the knee, and the medial side of the lower leg, including the ankle and the arch of the foot (see Figure 16.2).

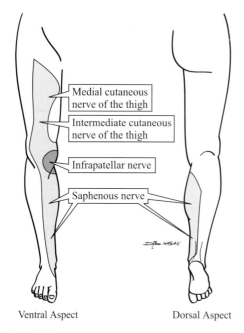

Figure 16.2
Approximate skin area innervated by the femoral nerve.

Lesions of the femoral nerve

History

Patients with motor deficits caused by a lesion of the femoral nerve may initially complain only of sudden falls caused by buckling of the knee. This may already occur when there is only slight weakness of the quadriceps muscle. Falls are induced especially if patients walk on an uneven road surface, step up the pavement or come down a staircase, in other words as soon as the body weight has to be supported with some flexion of the knee. When the weakness progresses the knee is locked in a hyperextended position (genu recurvatum) during walking. Depending on the cause and the location of the lesion there may be deep, severe nerve trunk pain with or without numbness and paraesthesia on the anterior side of the thigh or the inner side of the leg. Pain is common in psoas haematoma and in diabetic amyotrophy, in which condition the deficits may resemble those of femoral neuropathy (see below); to relieve the pain as much as possible the patient will often keep the leg fully flexed in the hip. Acute pain in the flank is especially reported with haematomas in the iliacus muscle that compress the femoral nerve.

Examination

Testing the iliopsoas muscle can be done with the patient sitting on the edge of the couch with the knee flexed, or preferably in the supine position (Figure 16.3). The quadriceps muscle is one of the few exceptions to the rule that the power of a particular muscle is best tested in a shortened position, when force is maximal. Because the quadriceps is a massive muscle, so much stronger than the opposing force of the examiner's arm muscle (usually the triceps), it is best to put the quadriceps muscle at a mechanical disadvantage and

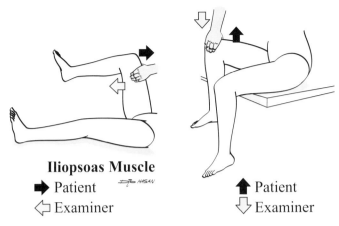

Iliopsoas Muscle

➡ Patient
⇦ Examiner

⬆ Patient
⬇ Examiner

Figure 16.3
Left: the thigh is flexed against resistance, with the hip and knee in flexion.
Right: the thigh is flexed against resistance, with the patient sitting on a couch.

test it with the knee in flexion. Also, testing the quadriceps with the knee extended (or, by the same token, the triceps brachii muscle with the elbow extended) would mean that a locked joint has to be wrenched open; this is not only painful but also misleading, because mild weakness can easily be missed. The quadriceps muscle can be tested in the supine position (Figure 16.4), but this method is a bit more awkward and is less reliable than with the patient sitting and trying to bring the leg forward against resistance (see Figure 16.4). Both

muscles, the iliopsoas and the quadriceps, are very strong and should not be overcome by the investigator in adolescent and adult patients. The most reliable proof of the normal power of the quadriceps is when a patient, after getting down on one knee, can rise from the floor by extending the other leg, but with advancing age one can be less and less certain that weakness is present if a patient fails this test.

A decreased or absent knee jerk is another early sign in femoral nerve involvement, although of course it is not

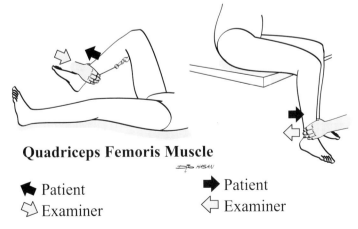

Quadriceps Femoris Muscle

⬆ Patient
⬁ Examiner

➡ Patient
⇦ Examiner

Figure 16.4
Left: the leg is extended against resistance, with the hip and knee in flexion.
Right: the leg is extended against resistance, with the patient sitting on a couch.

specific (see below). In the case of severe weakness, wasting of the anterior aspect of the thigh will invariably occur after some time, and sensory loss may be found over the anterior and medial aspect of the thigh and the medial side of the lower leg.

Differential diagnosis

It is vital to examine carefully the power of the adductor muscles in suspected femoral neuropathy: if weakness is also found in the adductor muscles the lesion is proximal to the femoral nerve, in the lumbosacral plexus or the lumbar roots 2–4. In such cases the brunt of the weakness often falls on the quadriceps muscle. This pitfall occurs especially in so-called 'diabetic amyotrophy', which on careful examination usually can be shown to result from a disorder of the lumbar plexus or lumbar roots. This condition has many other names, the most common of which are 'lower limb proximal motor neuropathy', 'asymmetrical proximal motor neuropathy', 'diabetic plexopathy', 'diabetic radiculoplexopathy' and (incorrectly) 'diabetic femoral neuropathy'. Needle EMG studies are very helpful in making the distinction. The disease process is characterized by loss of axons rather than by demyelination. Signs of denervation are commonly found in the quadriceps as well as in the adductor muscle, outside the supply area of the femoral nerve, and also in the paravertebral muscles, indicating a proximal root lesion (Bastron and Thomas, 1981; Wilbourn and Aminoff, 1988).

CT scanning is a reliable tool for detecting mass lesions in the pelvis; it should always be performed in a patient with femoral neuropathy (Eustace *et al.*, 1994).

Causes

Causes of femoral neuropathy are manifold (Table 16.1); the nerve is most often compressed in the iliac fossa, and less often in the inguinal region. Entrapment of a distal motor branch (to the vastus lateralis muscle) has been reported in a body building champion (Padua *et al.*, 1997). Iatrogenic factors are often present, such as retroperitoneal haematomas resulting from treatment with anticoagulant drugs; remarkably, this may occur bilaterally (Barontini and Macucci, 1986; Niakan *et al.*, 1991; Jamjoom *et al.*, 1993). Occasionally, the underlying cause may be an intrinsic disorder of coagulation.

> A 20-year-old man suddenly experienced severe pain in his right flank after a friendly bout of wrestling with his younger brother. The pain radiated to the anterior aspect of his right thigh. Two days later his knee buckled on attempted walking, which then proved impossible. On examination he preferred to lie down with the right hip in flexion, because of the pain. The iliopsoas muscle was weak (MRC grade 3) and the quadriceps muscle was almost paralytic (grade 1). The right knee jerk was absent. CT scanning showed an impressive haematoma in the psoas muscle (Figure 16.5). After needle aspiration of the haematoma the pain promptly disappeared, but the motor deficits took several months to recover. Haematological analysis showed von Willebrand's disease.

Surgical trauma of the femoral nerve may occur with a variety of abdominal operations, including gynaecological and obstetrical procedures; in these cases the nerve is compressed by retractor blades or stretched by a position of extreme abduction and exorotation of the thighs.

Table 16.1
Causes of lesions of the femoral nerve

Spontaneous haematoma in the psoas or iliacus muscle
- As a complication of anticoagulant treatment (Young and Norris, 1976; Mastroianni and Roberts, 1983; Wooten and McLaughlin, 1984; King and Bechtold, 1985; Ganglani *et al.*, 1991; Puschmann *et al.*, 1991; Rosset *et al.*, 1991)
- In haemophilia (Goodfellow *et al.*, 1967);
- Rupture of abdominal aortic aneurysm (Wilberger, 1983)
- Traumatic (Berlusconi and Capitani, 1991; Kumar *et al.* 1992)

Compression or stretch during surgical or obstetrical procedures
- Catheterization via the femoral artery, with retroperitoneal haematoma (Sreeram *et al.*, 1993), or pseudoaneurysm in the groin (Jacobs *et al.*, 1992)
- Haematoma after nerve block (Johr, 1987)
- (Self-retaining) retractor blades in abdominal surgery (Kvist-Poulsen and Borel, 1982; Massey and Tim, 1989; Walsh and Walsh, 1992; Helbling *et al.*, 1994; Brasch *et al.*, 1995; Hall *et al.*, 1995)
- Vaginal hysterectomy, in lithotomy position (Hopper and Baker, 1968)
- Laparoscopy (Hershlag *et al.*, 1990; al Hakim and Katirji, 1993)
- Stapling in laparoscopic hernia repair (Seid and Amos, 1994)
- Inadvertent suturing (Schottland, 1996)
- Kidney transplantation, associated with pressure from retractor blades (Pontin *et al.*, 1978; Vaziri *et al.*, 1981), haematoma (Sisto *et al.*, 1980; Probst *et al.*, 1982) or ischaemia from 'stealing' (Jog *et al.*, 1994)
- Hip arthroplasty (Hudson *et al.* 1979; Schmalzried *et al.*, 1991)
- Abdominal hysterectomy (Kvist-Poulsen and Borel, 1982)
- Hip abscess after parturition (Brandenberger *et al.*, 1992)
- Vaginal delivery (Vargo *et al.*, 1990; al Hakim and Katirji, 1993)

Prolonged pressure on the abdomen, after intoxication (Bernard *et al.*, 1991)

Vincristine toxicity (Levitt and Prager, 1975)

Irradiation (Laurent, 1975; Mendes *et al.*, 1991)

Inflammatory conditions
- Heterotopic ossification (Brooke *et al.*, 1991)
- Rheumatoid bursitis of the iliopsoas muscle (Letourneau *et al.*, 1991)
- Inflamed lymph nodes in the inguinal region (Khella, 1979)

Synovial cyst of the hip (Stadelmann *et al.*, 1992)

Penetrating injuries (Gousheh and Razian, 1991).

A 72-year-old physician underwent an abdominal operation for carcinoma of the prostate. One day after the operation he noticed pins and needles on the anterior aspect of both thighs and on the inner side of the calves. He also experienced difficulty in rising from his chair. On examination there was bilateral weakness of the iliopsoas and quadriceps muscles (MRC grade 4), and the knee jerks were practically absent. We diagnosed bilateral femoral neuropathy from compression by retractor blades; as expected the surgeon disagreed. After two months the weakness and sensory symptoms had completely disappeared.

Compression of the femoral nerve by tumours is decidedly uncommon. It is questionable whether there is a place in the nosological system for so-called 'idiopathic femoral neuropathy'. Diabetic 'neuropathy' of the femoral nerve often turns out on meticulous clinical examination and neurophysiological study to be a plexopathy, while in non-diabetics appropriate imaging of the pelvis will often uncover a structural lesion. Only in exceptional cases can a diagnosis of idiopathic, progressive, painless femoral neuropathy with axonal degeneration be made with confidence, when not only intensive investigations but even surgical exploration was negative (Engstrom *et al.*, 1993).

Surgical dissection in the femoral triangle, for reconstruction of the femoral artery, may lead to paraesthesia and numbness limited to the territory of the intermediate cutaneous nerve of the thigh (Belsh, 1991).

Treatment

Femoral neuropathy after operation, from stretch or compression, tends to be followed by spontaneous recovery,

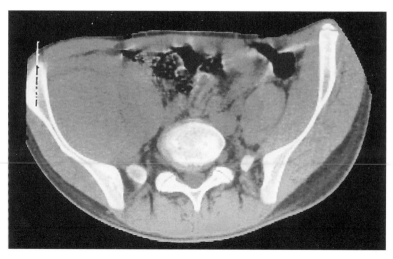

Figure 16.5
Computed tomography of abdomen showing haematoma in right psoas muscle.

although this may take weeks or even months. Retroperitoneal haematomas are often operated on or aspirated as an emergency; as a rule this quickly relieves the pain, but there is no firm evidence to support the impression that operative treatment improves the chance of recovery. Painful paraesthesia are often alleviated with phenytoin or carbamazepine, although this is also merely a clinical impression without the backing of a controlled study.

Lesions of the saphenous nerve

This main sensory branch of the femoral nerve may be affected at the level of thigh, the knee, or more distally. This results in pain, paraesthesia and a sensory deficit in the skin territory (or part of it) supplied by the nerve; with procedures around the knee joint only the infrapatellar branch may be involved. The causes are, again, mostly iatrogenic (Table 16.2), for example with operations for varicose veins, or harvesting of the saphenous vein for arterial grafting, but sometimes no precipitating factors can be identified (Luerssen *et al.*, 1983; Worth *et al.*, 1984).

Different segments of the saphenous nerve can be examined using peripheral

nerve conduction studies (Stöhr *et al.*, 1978; Wainapel *et al.*, 1978) and with somatosensory evoked potentials (Vogel and Vogel, 1982; Tranier *et al.*, 1992).

Table 16.2
Causes of lesions of the saphenous nerve

Surgical procedures
- Meniscectomy or arthroscopy (Worth *et al.*, 1984; Senegor, 1991; Abram and Froimson, 1991; Mochida and Kikuchi, 1995)
- Arterial reconstruction in the thigh (Jones, 1978; Roder *et al.*, 1984)
- Saphenous vein grafting (Lederman *et al.*, 1982; Dimitri *et al.*, 1987)
- Operations for varicose veins: stripping, of the saphenous vein (Holme *et al.*, 1990; Creton, 1991; Sarin *et al.*, 1992); endoscopic dissection of perforating veins (Lang *et al.*, 1995; Jugenheimer and Junginger, 1992); or cryosurgery (Etienne *et al.*, 1995)

Following irradiation (Mendes *et al.*, 1991)

Compression by neighbouring structures
- Entrapment in the subsartorial canal (House and Ahmed, 1977; Luerssen *et al.*, 1983)
- Entrapment at the medial side of the knee (Worth *et al.*, 1984)
- Entrapment by a branch of the femoral artery (Murayama *et al.*, 1991)
- Bursitis of the pes anserinus, distal to the adductor canal (Hemler *et al.*, 1991)
- Neurilemmoma (Edwards *et al.*, 1989)

Special postures
- Straddling a surfboard (Fabian *et al.*, 1987)
- Playing viola de gamba (Howard, 1982)

Chapter 17
The obturator nerve

Anatomy

The obturator nerve originates by the union of the ventral branches of the spinal nerves L2, L3 and L4 within the belly of the psoas muscle (Figure 17.1). It emerges on the medial side of the psoas muscle and passes downwards over the sacroiliac joint along the wall of the pelvis to the obturator canal. Here *anterior branches* and *posterior branches* are given off, which enter the thigh to innervate the adductor muscles of the thigh, consisting of the adductor brevis, adductor longus and adductor magnus muscles.

The anterior branch of the obturator nerve ends as a sensory nerve supplying a skin area on the inner side of the thigh (Figure 17.2).

Lesions of the obturator nerve

History and examination

The adductor muscles stabilize the hip; therefore, patients with obturator nerve damage complain of weakness in the leg

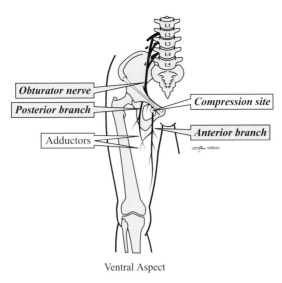

Ventral Aspect

Figure 17.1
Muscles innervated by the obturator nerve.

The obturator nerve

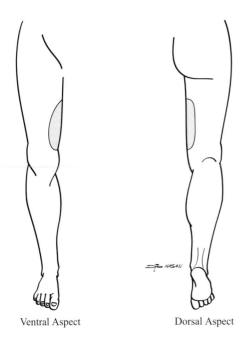

Ventral Aspect   Dorsal Aspect

Figure 17.2
Approximate skin area innervated by the obturator nerve.

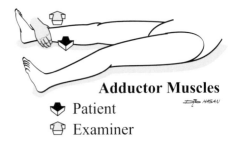

Adductor Muscles

⬇ Patient
⬆ Examiner

Figure 17.3
The extended leg is adducted against resistance, with the patient lying on his back.

the obturator nerve by impingement of neighbouring structures seems to occur only with an obturator hernia (Somell *et al.*, 1976; Hannington-Kiff, 1980; Bjork *et al.*, 1988). Other causes are almost always evident (Table 17.1); these often consist of pelvic masses and may result in involvement of both the obturator and femoral nerves. If labour is complicated by

and the gait may be broad-based. The weakness may be accompanied by paraesthesia and pain high at the medial side of the thigh. The adductor muscles are tested as illustrated in Figure 17.3. The tendon jerk of the adductor muscles should be tested as well, as this reflex will be decreased on the side of an affected nerve or root (Hannington-Kiff, 1980).

Electrophysiological studies

No nerve conduction technique for the obturator nerve has been described. Needle EMG may indirectly confirm the diagnosis of a lesion of this nerve by demonstrating denervation activity confined to the hip adductors.

Causes

Isolated palsies of the obturator nerve are rare; weakness of the adductor muscles of the hip is most often caused by lesions of the lumbar roots or plexus. Entrapment of

Table 17.1
Causes of lesions of the obturator nerve

Obturator hernia (Somell *et al.*, 1976; Hannington-Kiff, 1980; Bjork *et al.* 1988)

Scar formation in the thigh (Fettweis, 1966)

Normal labour (Hopf, 1974)

Pelvic masses (often in combination with a lesion of the femoral nerve)
- Haematoma in the psoas muscle (Fletcher and Frankel, 1976)
- Endometriosis (Redwine and Sharpe, 1990)
- Retroperitoneal schwannoma (Brady *et al.*, 1993)

Iatrogenic causes
- Prolonged hip flexion in urologic surgery (Pellegrino and Johnson, 1988)
- Hip surgery, with damage by retractor blades, overstretching, cement, or fixation screws (Weber *et al.* 1976; Melamed and Satya Murti, 1983; Siliski and Scott, 1985; Schmalzried *et al.* 1991; Fricker *et al.* 1997)
- Fixation of acetabular fracture (Cole and Bolhofner, 1994)
- Intrapelvic surgery (Bischoff and Schonle, 1991)
- Laparoscopic dissection of pelvic nodes (Mazeman *et al.*, 1992; Burney *et al.*, 1993; Fishman *et al.*, 1993; Kavoussi *et al.*, 1993; Doublet *et al.*, 1994)
- Gracilis flap operations (Deutinger *et al.* 1995)

compression of an obturator nerve the patient may feel a sharp pain in the groin and inner thigh (Hopf, 1974).

Differential diagnosis

Isolated weakness of the adductor muscles of the thigh, with or without sensory changes, conclusively indicates obturator neuropathy. However, since the roots from which the obturator nerve originates also contain fibres to the femoral nerve, special attention should be paid to the power of the quadriceps muscle and to the knee jerk; both should be normal in obturator neuropathy. Neuralgic pain in obturator neuropathy may be confused with osteitis or other disorders of the symphysis, in which pain is experienced in the groin and in the medial part of the thigh.

Chapter 18
The gluteal nerves

Anatomy

The *superior gluteal nerve* (Figure 18.1), carrying fibres from roots L4 to S1, passes over the piriform muscle, through the suprapiriform foramen, and then courses between the gluteus medius and minimus muscles; it innervates both these muscles, and also the tensor fasciae latae muscle. The *inferior gluteal nerve* carries fibres from roots L5 to S2 and leaves the pelvis through the infrapiriform foramen, dorsolateral to the sciatic nerve; it innervates the gluteus maximus muscle.

Lesions of the gluteal nerves

History

The main symptoms of involvement of the gluteal nerves are pain in the buttock and weakness. In the case of the superior gluteal nerve the deficit is manifested as difficulty in walking, as defective tilting of the pelvis (gluteus medius and minimus muscles) interferes with swinging the contralateral leg forward. With involvement of the inferior gluteal nerve the weakness affects extension of the hip joint (gluteus maximus muscle), leading to

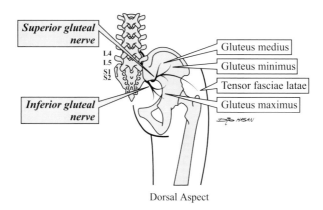

Dorsal Aspect

Figure 18.1
Muscles innervated by the superior and inferior gluteal nerves.

an impairment of gait and to special difficulties in descending stairs or getting up from a chair.

Examination

On the examination couch the muscles of the superior gluteal nerve (gluteus medius, gluteus minimus, and tensor fasciae latae) can be tested together by having the patient abduct the thigh against resistance (Figure 18.2), whereas the gluteus medius and minimus muscles can be tested separately by internal rotation of the thigh against resistance while the knee is flexed, the patient being prone (Figure 18.3) or supine. When the patient is in a standing position and is asked to stand on one leg, weakness of the gluteus medius and minimus muscles can be inferred from tilting of the pelvis towards the healthy side (Trendelenburg sign); this weakness can be compensated for by bending the trunk towards the affected side.

The gluteus maximus muscle is tested with the patient in a prone position, in which he is asked to lift the thigh against resistance (Figure 18.4). Aged or obese patients may find this position very uncomfortable; in such patients the power of the gluteus maximus can be tested by the examiner slipping a hand under the knee and asking the patient to press the leg into the couch, against resistance (Figure 18.5).

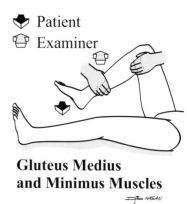

**Gluteus Medius
and Minimus Muscles**

Figure 18.3
The thigh is internally rotated against resistance, while the patient lies on his back with the hip and knee flexed.

Electrophysiological studies are limited to needle EMG, which may show denervation activity in the relevant muscles (LaBan *et al.*, 1982). Nerve conduction tests are not feasible.

Causes

A fall on the buttocks may lead to an acute but transient entrapment of the superior gluteal nerve between the piriform muscle and the major sciatic incisure (Tesio *et al.*, 1990), or to secondary muscle fibrosis and more permanent damage to the superior gluteal nerve (Rask, 1980). Inaccurately placed intramuscular injections in the buttock may lead to damage not only of

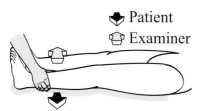

**Tensor Fasciae Latae,
Gluteus Maximus, Medius,
and Minimus Muscles**

Figure 18.2
The extended leg is abducted against resistance, while the patient lies on his back.

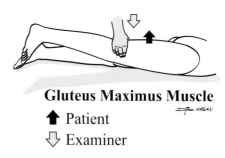

Gluteus Maximus Muscle

**↑ Patient
⇩ Examiner**

Figure 18.4
The patient is lying prone and is elevating the leg against resistance.

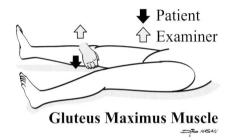

Gluteus Maximus Muscle

Figure 18.5
The leg is extended at the hip against resistance, while the patient lies on his back.

the sciatic nerve but also of the superior gluteal nerve (Obach *et al.*, 1983), but a partial lesion, with weakness of only the tensor fasciae latae muscle, may also occur after correctly placed injections, in the upper outer quadrant of the buttock (Muller-Vahl H., 1985). Compression during coma or anaesthesia may involve the gluteal nerves as well as the sciatic nerve (Stöhr, 1976). Hip surgery by techniques with a posterior approach (the so-called 'Hardinge approach') may lead to damage of the superior gluteal nerve in about a quarter of all cases (Ramesh *et al.*, 1996).

The inferior gluteal nerve may be compressed by colorectal tumours, in which case there is often simultaneous involvement of the posterior cutaneous nerve of the thigh, with a sensory deficit over the inferior lateral buttock (LaBan *et al.*, 1982). Both gluteal nerves can be damaged together by prolonged labour (Mumenthaler and Schliack, 1993), or by spondylolisthesis of L4 on L5, possibly through entrapment within the piriform muscle (de Jong and van Weerden, 1983).

Differential diagnosis

The only category to be considered is proximal weakness from myopathies (dystrophinopathy, acid maltase deficiency, polymyositis, limb girdle dystrophy, to name only a few). However, all these conditions are symmetrical and are slowly progressive. Disorders of the hip joint bear only a slight resemblance to gluteal neuropathies.

Treatment

If a nerve lesion is more or less total and there is no tendency to recovery, a surgical approach should be considered, depending on the cause and on the results of MRI scanning.

Chapter 19
The sciatic nerve

Anatomy

The sciatic nerve (Figure 19.1) carries fibres from L4 to S3 and leaves the pelvis through the sciatic foramen. Subsequently it usually passes below the piriformis muscle, although the division that eventually will form the peroneal nerve (and sometimes even the entire nerve) may pierce the piriformis muscle, or even pass over it (Pecina, 1979). In the gluteal region the nerve courses first laterally and then downwards. Under the gluteus maximus muscle it is situated between the greater trochanter and the ischial tuberosity, just posterior to the hip joint. At the inferior part of the buttock the nerve lies superficially, embedded in loose collagen and fat tissue, the subgluteal space. Wrongly applied injection fluids or an inflammatory process may easily spread here and damage the nerve. From there the sciatic nerve runs at the dorsal side of the femoral bone, between the flexor muscles of the knee, to terminate at the proximal part of the popliteal fossa. Here it divides into the tibial nerve and common peroneal nerve. Nevertheless, as

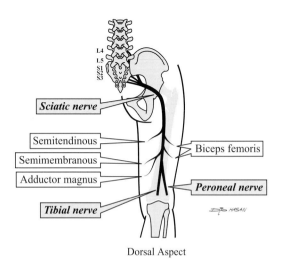

Dorsal Aspect

Figure 19.1
Muscles innervated by the sciatic nerve.

proximal as the gluteal region, or even in the pelvis, the fibres for the tibial and common peroneal nerves are arranged in two separate divisions: the medial and the lateral trunk, respectively.

In the thigh the medial division of the sciatic nerve consecutively innervates the semitendinous, biceps femoris (long head) and semimembranous muscles. It also participates in the innervation of the adductor magnus muscle, which is mainly supplied by the obturator nerve. The short head of the biceps femoris is the only thigh muscle supplied by the lateral division of the sciatic nerve.

The main sciatic trunk does not have sensory branches, but the nerve is accompanied by the posterior cutaneous nerve of the thigh (S1–S3), which innervates the skin of the dorsal side of the thigh and the proximal part of the calf (see Figure 15.2).

Lesions of the sciatic nerve

Examination

The examination of the 'hamstring muscles' (semitendinous, semimembranous and biceps femoris muscles) is illustrated in Figure 19.2.

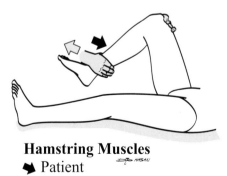

Hamstring Muscles
🠖 Patient
🖑 Examiner

Figure 19.2
The patient lies on his back, while the hip and knee are flexed. The leg is flexed in the knee against resistance.

The arrangement in separate divisions of tibial and common peroneal fibres within the sciatic nerve explains why partial lesions of the sciatic nerve may appear as isolated tibial or common peroneal lesions. The peroneal nerve fibres within the lateral division of the sciatic nerve are more prone to compression than the medial division, which will form the tibial nerve; the clinical features may be indistinguishable from those of a peroneal nerve palsy in the leg, including preservation of the ankle jerk (Katirji and Wilbourn, 1994). However, if weakness of muscles innervated by the peroneal nerve is accompanied by a diminished or absent ankle jerk, a lesion of the sciatic nerve or of spinal roots should certainly be suspected. Other signs indicating sciatic nerve damage are weakness of the flexors of the knee and a decreased tendon jerk of the biceps femoris. Isolated lesions of the medial division of the sciatic nerve are much less common; the cause is usually not compression but, for example, a neurilemmoma. The clinical manifestations of such a nerve tumour may mimic a tarsal tunnel syndrome (Persing *et al.*, 1988; Wolock *et al.*, 1989). If lesions of the sciatic nerve are associated with damage of the posterior cutaneous nerve of the thigh, there will be diminished sensation at the back of the thigh and calf. With complete lesions of the sciatic nerve all movements of the foot and toes are impossible, and there is also paralysis of knee flexion.

Differential diagnosis

Lesions of the L5 and S1 roots are a far more common cause of sciatica than are lesions of the sciatic nerve itself, and these should therefore be considered first. Important clues indicating a root lesion are paraesthesia or sensory deficits in the typical distribution of a dermatome, most often the dorsum of the foot and the big toe (L5), and the lateral border of the foot (S1), or motor and reflex deficits pertaining to one of these two roots (the calf muscle and ankle jerk for S1, the anterior and posterior tibial muscles for L5). If appropriate imaging studies fail to show the expected herniation of an intervertebral disc (or a paraspinal mass), inflammatory conditions such as borreliosis should not be forgotten.

Electrophysiological studies

Needle EMG is the most helpful method for distinguishing sciatic nerve lesions from lesions at other levels. Demonstration of denervation activity in the paraspinal muscles at the lumbosacral level is typical of a radiculopathy. Even with negative findings in the paraspinal muscles the distribution of the denervation activity can still be typical for a root lesion. EMG abnormalities outside the supply area of the sciatic nerve indicate a lesion at the level of the plexus. Demonstration of denervation activity in the short head of the biceps femoris is essential for the distinction between a lesion of the lateral division of the sciatic nerve and a common peroneal nerve palsy (Katirji and Wilbourn, 1994). In a series of 100 patients with sciatic nerve lesions Yuen *et al.* (1995) found EMG signs of axonal loss to be much more common than signs of demyelination. The lateral division was more severely affected than the medial division in 64% of patients.

Sciatic nerve tumours may damage only a single, or very few, fascicles with correspondingly limited EMG abnormalities; this makes it difficult to localize the lesion correctly.

Because the sciatic nerve lies deeply, motor nerve conduction studies are hard to perform (only if needle electrodes are used for stimulation). Abnormal late responses (soleus H-reflex, foot muscle F-waves) may result from a radiculopathy or a plexopathy as well as from a lesion of the sciatic nerve. Reduced sensory nerve action potentials of the sural and/or

superficial peroneal nerve argue against a radiculopathy (see page 10).

Causes

Compression of the sciatic nerve may occur in the pelvis, in the gluteal region and in the thigh. On the basis of the neurological examination it is difficult to distinguish between these three possibilities. In some cases of chronic compression the clinical features consist of sciatica only, without neurological deficits.

In the pelvis, the sciatic nerve may be involved by tumours (Figure 19.3), endometriosis or a variety of vascular lesions, mostly aneurysms or false aneurysms (Table 19.1). Syphilitic sciatica is nowadays very rare.

> A 30-year-old waiter had a two month history of severe pain in the dorsal aspect of the right thigh. Straight-leg raising was painful at 60°. Pain sensation was diminished and delayed in both calves, and strong pressure on the testicles was not painful. Serological tests for syphilis were strongly positive in the serum as well as in the cerebrospinal fluid, while the white cell count in the cerebrospinal fluid was only slightly raised (7×10^6/l). The most probable diagnosis was spirochaetal neuritis of the sciatic nerve, although radiculitis could not be excluded.

The gluteal region is the most common site of entrapment, if only because the nerve is relatively exposed in this area and may be compressed by sitting on hard surfaces or in peculiar positions, usually in association with intoxication or anaesthesia. A typical patient we saw had drunk 10–20 glasses of beer, then fell asleep while he was sitting on a rail, and woke up with a bilateral sciatic nerve palsy. Some unusual postures may lead to sciatic nerve compression in the absence of intoxication:

A 30-year-old healthy woman fell asleep while sitting tailor-wise, in a cross-legged position. When she woke up three hours later her left leg felt numb. She went to bed, and on getting up found that the left leg was also weak. Examination a few days later showed paralysis of all foot and toe muscles and marked weakness (MRC grade 3) of the hamstring muscles. Skin sensation was diminished on the lateral side of the calf and the dorsal side of the leg and thigh. The left ankle jerk was absent. Six weeks later only slight recovery had occurred, and there was some wasting of the left calf (3 cm difference); after another two months only mild weakness of the foot muscles remained.

Table 19.1
**Causes of sciatic nerve lesions in the pelvis
tumours**

- Metastatic carcinoma (for example of the prostate)
- Schwannoma, neurofibroma (Caplan *et al.*, 1983)
- Lipoma (Vanneste *et al.*, 1980)

Endometriosis
- Symptoms varying with menstrual cycle (Baker *et al.* 1966; Salazar Grueso and Roos, 1986; Richards *et al.*, 1991; Jelk and Estape, 1995; Dhôte *et al.*, 1996)
- With permanent symptoms (Bergqvist *et al.*, 1987)

Vascular abnormalities
- Arteriovenous malformation (Vos *et al.*, 1995)
- Ruptured aneurysm, of the hypogastric artery (Bacourt *et al.*, 1994)
- False aneurysm, of the abdominal aorta (Ashleigh and Marcuson, 1993)
- Unruptured aneurysm, of the common iliac artery (Levy, 1977; Mohan and Grimley, 1987), or the internal iliac artery (Geelen *et al.*, 1985)

Childbirth, by caesarean section with epidural analgesia (Silva *et al.*, 1996)

Infection
- *Clostridium septicum*, with immunoincompetence (Hoefnagels *et al.*, 1991)

If local pressure has caused rhabdomyolysis of the gluteal compartment, fasciotomy may be indicated (Shields and Jacobs, 1986; Schmalzried *et al.*, 1992). Iatrogenic lesions are a relatively frequent cause of sciatic nerve lesions in the gluteal region (Table 19.2). Misdirected intramuscular injections are most notorious in this category; to avoid nerve damage, injections should be given only in the upper and outer quadrant of the buttock.

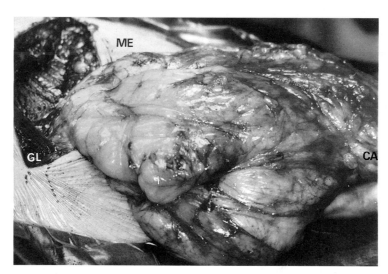

Figure 19.3
Intrapelvic lipoma compressing the sciatic nerve, just before its removal. ME, medial side of patient; CA, caudal side; GL, gluteal muscle. (From Vanneste et al. (1980), with permission of the authors and the publisher.)

Table 19.2
Causes of sciatic nerve lesions in the gluteal region

Prolonged compression
- Sitting in alcoholic- or drug-induced stupor on a toilet, with wedging of buttocks (Tyrrell *et al.*, 1989), or on a hard rail (personal observation; bilateral lesions)
- Anaesthesia, in sitting position (Stewart and Aguao, 1984)
- Rhabdomyolysis after drug-induced coma (Schmalzried *et al.*, 1992);
- Meditating or sleeping in a cross-legged position (Vogel *et al.*, 1991); see also the case history of the 30-year-old healthy woman on page 120
- 'Backpocket sciatica', from credit cards (Collier, 1985), or coins (Berlit, 1993)

Vascular lesions
- Persistent sciatic artery (Martin *et al.* 1986; Gasecki *et al.*, 1992)
- False aneurysm of the superior gluteal artery (Proschek *et al.*, 1983), or inferior gluteal artery (Papadopoulos *et al.*, 1989), or loop of abnormal collateral of inferior gluteal artery (Merlo *et al.*, 1997)
- Spontaneous haematoma, under warfarin treatment (Wallach and Oren, 1979; Rogers *et al.* 1983; Palliyath and Buday, 1989)

Tumours
- lipoma (Wouda and Vanneste, 1993)
- Schwannoma, neurofibroma (Caplan *et al.*, 1983)
- Lymphoma (Pillay *et al.*, 1988);
- Hemangiopericytoma (Young *et al.*, 1991; Harrison *et al.* 1995)

Iatrogenic lesions
- Intramuscular injections
- Ipsilateral hip surgery (Weber *et al.*, 1976; Dhillon and Nagi, 1992; Yuen *et al.*, 1994), especially with trochanteric wiring (Mallory, 1983)
- Rhabdomyolysis after contralateral hip surgery (Lachiewicz and Latimer, 1991)
- Harrington's operation for scoliosis (Guillemin *et al.*, 1991)
- Closed nailing of femoral fracture (Britton and Dunkerley, 1990)
- Catheterization or occlusion of femoral artery, in association with heart surgery (McManis, 1994)
- Mechanical compression, during heart surgery (Kempster *et al.*, 1991)
- In children: operations in the lithotomy position, or closed reduction of hip dislocation (Jones, *et al.*, 1988)
- In neonates: inadvertent injection into umbilical artery (San Augustin *et al.*, 1962)

Delayed, after acute trauma or operation
- After fracture-dislocation of the hip (Gadelrab, 1990), or the femur (Reinstein and Eckholdt, 1983)
- After hip surgery, by extruding cement (Casagrande and Danahy, 1971; Oleksak and Edge, 1992), or by pieces of broken wire (Glover and Convery, 1989)
- Ectopic bone formation, after stabbing (Kaplan and Challenor, 1993)

'Piriformis syndrome' (see text)

A 25-year-old woman received a poorly placed intramuscular injection of an analgesic drug in her left buttock. During the injection she immediately felt an intense pain, with the sensation of an electric current radiating from the back of her thigh down to the sole of the foot. At the same time her foot had become paralysed. Examination showed complete loss of function of all motor and sensory fibres of the left sciatic nerve. Six months later not a trace of recovery had occurred; subsequently, this unfortunate woman was lost to follow-up.

Injections in the buttocks may give rise to sciatic nerve damage even if they are well placed, if the injected drug causes muscle necrosis (Hornig and Dorndorf, 1983) or muscle fibrosis, via repeated injections (Rousseau *et al.*, 1979). The most common iatrogenic lesion of the sciatic nerve occurs with total hip arthroplasty (Yuen *et al.*, 1994).

Sciatic nerve compression in the thigh is relatively uncommon; reported causes are lipomas, neurofibromas, schwannomas and aneurysms (Table 19.3).

A 69-year-old woman had, over the course of three or four years, and gradually developed a continuous ache in the right leg, initially only as a sensation of a tight band around the ankle, gradually evolving into mild pain, radiating from the lower back via the lateral part of the thigh and the shin to the dorsum of the foot. The ache increased on walking or prolonged sitting; it continued at night, but did not interfere with sleep. Also, she occasionally had some difficulty in supporting her leg while climbing stairs. On examination the most striking finding was an increased circumference of the right thigh (difference 4 cm, measured 15 cm above the medial border of the knee joint. There were no motor or sensory

The sciatic nerve

deficits, apart from minimal weakness of the right knee flexors and bilaterally absent ankle jerks. The straight-leg raising test was normal. MRI scanning of the pelvis and thighs showed a large lipoma dorsal to the femur (Figure 19.4). Operation was successful (despite an unexpected episode of anaphylactic shock after administration of albumin) and the pain disappeared.

The piriformis syndrome

The piriformis syndrome is presumed to be caused by an anatomical variation in which the piriformis muscle compresses the sciatic nerve as it emerges from the pelvis through the greater sciatic notch. The existence of the syndrome has for a long time been controversial, because lumbar disc herniation was not always adequately excluded, certainly not in the era before CT and MRI scanning, or even before the introduction of water-soluble contrast agents for myelography. The original publication about the piriformis syndrome reported two patients (Robinson, 1947). Both patients had sciatica with a positive straight-leg raising test, and also in both a 'tender sausage-like mass was palpable, extending from the sacrosciatic notch to the greater trochanter of the femur'. Atrophy of the gluteal muscles was found in one of the two patients. Myelography was not mentioned. Treatment consisted of

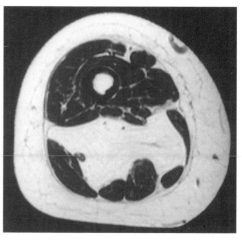

Figure 19.4
MRI scan (transverse section) of the right upper leg; a lipoma separates the hamstring muscles from the femur, and compresses the sciatic nerve.

removal of the adhesions between the piriformis muscle and the sciatic nerve, with partial transection of the piriformis muscle; both patients had immediate relief of pain, without recurrence in a period of more than five years. The same miraculous recovery by this intervention was reported by Mizuguchi (1976) in 12 of his 14 patients, but six of these patients had been operated on before for a disc lesion and the follow-up period averaged only 12 weeks (range 5–40 weeks). The author's conclusion that 'in well selected patients with sciatica due to herniated lumbar discs at lumbar 4–5 and lumbar 5–sacral 1 levels sectioning of the piriformis could be beneficial' is not supported by his observations. An accompanying editorial rightly commented that 'almost any form of treatment, including placebo injections, results in 70–80% of good short term results in low back pain, with and without sciatica' (Stauffer, 1976).

A very first requirement for a firm diagnosis of the piriformis syndrome is that there should be objective signs of sciatic nerve involvement, and not just pain in the buttock (Dawson *et al.*, 1990), even with reproduction of the pain on

Table 19.3
Causes of sciatic nerve lesions in the thigh

Tumours
- Schwannoma, neurofibroma (Caplan *et al.*, 1983; Persing *et al.*, 1988; Wolock *et al.*, 1989)
- Lipoma (Chiao *et al.*, 1987); see also the case history of a 69-year-old woman on page 121

Vascular lesions
- Aneurysm of persistent sciatic artery (Simon and Rosenberg, 1992);
- Aneurysm of the popliteal artery (Beaudry *et al.*, 1989).

deep palpation via the gluteal or rectal route (Durrani and Winnie, 1991). This should be supported by electrophysiological evidence of damage to the nerve, with negative EMG findings in the paraspinal muscles. Appropriate neuroradiological studies should exclude root compression and masses in the paravertebral area, lower pelvis, and sciatic notch. Finally, the cerebrospinal fluid should show no signs of inflammation, reflecting root involvement by infections such as borreliosis. The ultimate test is, of course, the confirmation by operation and subsequent relief. Very few patients meet or even approach these criteria. One such patient has been seen by one of us, and subsequently reported by our neurosurgical colleagues (Vandertop and Bosma, 1991).

A 51-year-old man had a six month history of pins and needles radiating from the left hip region to the posterolateral part of the thigh and calf to the fourth and fifth toes. The symptoms increased on walking and on standing on the affected leg. Examination showed fasciculations in the left calf and hamstring muscles. There was some wasting and weakness of the left gluteus maximus muscle. The left ankle jerk was absent. Skin sensation was diminished at the inferior half of the left buttock, on the lateral side of the thigh and calf, and on the dorsal side of the fourth and fifth toes. Straight-leg raising was not painful but led to an increase of paraesthesia. CT scanning and plain radiographs of the lumbosacral spine, myelography, bone scintigraphy and an intravenous digital subtraction angiogram of the legs were all normal. Needle EMG showed signs of denervation in the lateral head of the gastrocnemius, but not in any of eleven other leg muscles or in the paraspinal muscles. The spinal fluid was normal. On exploration of the sciatic notch the expected compression due to the piriformis muscle was not found, but instead the nerve was compressed by a fibrous band between the tendon of the piriform muscle and the inferior gluteal vessels, 1–1.5 cm in width and containing small vessels. Both this band and the tendon of the piriformis muscle were sectioned. Eight weeks later the paraesthesia had disappeared, the patient had resumed his former occupation as a bar-bender at construction sites; fasciculations could no longer be seen. Four years later the patient was still doing well.

A fibrovascular band constricting the sciatic nerve has also been found in a child (Venna *et al.*, 1991). A fibrous band association with an anomalous piriformis muscle was reported in two patients, the muscle being located anterior to the nerve (Sayson *et al.*, 1994), or with a bipartite structure (Chen, 1994). Sectioning of the abnormal structures was reported to be successful.

Chapter 20
The tibial nerve

Anatomy

The tibial nerve (Figure 20.1) carries fibres from the roots L4 to S3. It originates from the sciatic trunk at a variable level above the knee. Regardless of where it originates, in a large segment of the thigh these fibres run in a separate trunk, located in the ventral part of the sciatic nerve. In the popliteal fossa and in the calf the tibial nerve has a deep, well-protected position. In the lower leg it innervates both heads of the gastrocnemius muscle, the soleus, the posterior tibial, the flexor digitorum longus and the flexor hallucis longus muscles. Behind and below the

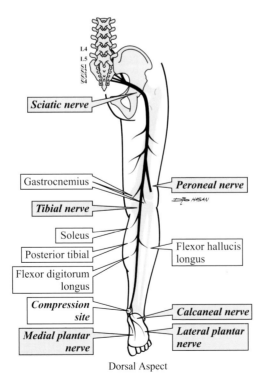

Dorsal Aspect

Figure 20.1
Muscles innervated by the tibial nerve.

medial malleolus the tibial nerve passes through the tarsal tunnel. This superficially located space is roofed by the laciniate ligament, or flexor retinaculum, which extends between the malleolus and the medial side of the calcaneus. Apart from the tibial nerve, the tarsal tunnel contains the posterior tibial artery and the tendons of the posterior tibial muscle, the flexor digitorum longus and the flexor hallucis longus muscles. Within or just after the tarsal tunnel the tibial nerve branches into the *medial and lateral plantar nerves*. The medial plantar nerve supplies the abductor hallucis and the short flexor digitorum muscles; the lateral plantar nerve innervates the flexor and abductor digiti minimi, the adductor hallucis muscle and the interossei.

Sensory fibres from both plantar nerves innervate the sole of the foot and end in six terminal branches to the toes: the *medial plantar proper digital nerve* (to the great toe), the *lateral plantar proper digital nerve* (to the little toe), and four terminal branches, the *interdigital nerves* (Figure 20.2). After passing between the distal ends of the metatarsal bones, the interdigital nerves divide each into two digital nerves. At the point near the tarsal

tunnel where the lateral and medial plantar nerves separate, a purely sensory branch, the *calcaneal nerve*, originates from the tibial nerve to innervate the medial part of the heel. In the popliteal fossa the medial cutaneous nerve arises from the tibial nerve, whereas the peroneal nerve gives off the lateral sural cutaneous nerve. In the calf these two branches unite to form the *sural nerve* (see Chapter 22).

Examination

The gastrocnemius and soleus muscles are often tested together, although the soleus muscle can be more or less selectively activated by testing plantar flexion against resistance with the leg flexed in the hip and the knee (Figure 20.3); with the leg extended plantar flexion is mainly mediated by the gastrocnemius muscle (Figure 20.4). Because the calf muscles are very strong, even marked weakness can easily be missed if the power of foot plantar flexion is tested only against the examiner's hand and arm muscles, with the patient supine. If the patient is ambulant he should first be asked to walk on the toes, without the heel touching the floor. Slight weakness is found only when

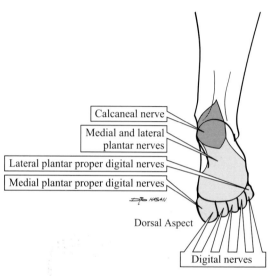

Figure 20.2
Approximate skin areas innervated by the tibial nerve.

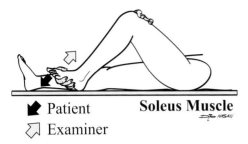

Soleus Muscle

◀ Patient
◁ Examiner

Figure 20.3
The patient lies on his back, while the hip and knee are flexed. The foot is plantar flexed against resistance.

the patient is asked to stand on one leg and then to support the body weight on the toes only, or to hop around on the forefoot, during which the heel should remain free from the floor. Aged but normal patients may not be able to perform this manoeuvre. The posterior tibial muscle and the flexor digitorum muscle should be tested as indicated in Figures 20.5 and 20.6. Normally the strength of the toe flexors can be overcome by the examiner's finger flexors without much difficulty.

Lesions of the tibial nerve proximal to the ankle

Lesions of the tibial nerve proximal to the ankle are uncommon. The signs follow simply from the anatomy and consist of weakness of plantar flexion and inversion of the foot, as well as of flexion of the toes, sensory deficits of the sole of the foot (with or without the lateral border supplied by the sural nerve) and a decreased or absent ankle jerk.

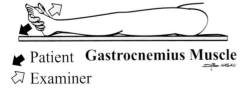

◀ Patient **Gastrocnemius Muscle**
◁ Examiner

Figure 20.4
The patient lies on his back, with the leg extended. The foot is plantar flexed against resistance.

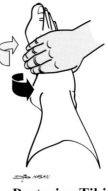

Posterior Tibial Muscle

🖑 Patient
☞ Examiner

Figure 20.5
The foot is inverted against resistance.

Causes

Ankle sprains may cause stretch injury not only of the common peroneal nerve but also of the tibial nerve. Other potential causes of compression in or just below the popliteal fossa are haematoma, congenital bands, cysts and tumours, especially of the nerve sheath (Table 20.1). MRI is very helpful in identifying any mass lesion.

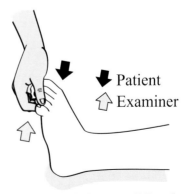

▼ Patient
⬆ Examiner

Flexor Digitorum Muscles

Figure 20.6
The toes are flexed against resistance.

Table 20.1
Causes of lesions of the tibial nerve proximal to the ankle

Entrapment
- Idiopathic (Ekelund, 1990)
- Under a transverse fibrous band between the gastrocnemius muscles (Psathakis and Psathakis, 1991)
- Under a tendinous arch at the origin of the soleus muscle (Costigan *et al.*, 1991; Iida and Kobayashi, 1997)

Haematoma in the popliteal fossa
- By blunt injury (Logigian *et al.* 1989)
- By rupture of the popliteus muscle (Geissler *et al.* 1992)

Synovial cyst
- Of the knee joint (Baker's cyst) (Nakano, 1978; Kashani *et al.*, 1985; DiRisio *et al.*, 1994)
- Of the superior tibio-fibular joint (Groulier *et al.*, 1987)

Stretch injury, from ankle sprain (Nitz *et al.*, 1985)

Nerve sheath tumours (Thiebot *et al.*, 1991; Suh *et al.*, 1992)

Lesions of the tibial nerve at the ankle: (posterior) tarsal tunnel syndrome

The tarsal tunnel syndrome is rare, but well recognized and treatable (DeLisa and Saeed, 1983). The main symptom is pain in the sole of the foot, often with a burning character and accompanied by paraesthesia in the toes. The syndrome is mostly unilateral, but may occur on both sides (Denislic and Bajec, 1994). Some patients have symptoms only while standing and walking, jogging or playing tennis, which may falsely suggest lumbar spinal stenosis. In others the symptoms are especially nocturnal; mixed patterns also occur.

Examination

The Hoffmann–Tinel sign may be present, paraesthesia being provoked by percussion or constant pressure of the tarsal tunnel (under the medial malleolus), especially with the foot held in eversion. Apart from local pain, an electric sensation

is felt radiating over the sole of the foot towards the toes, most often the medial toes. One should look carefully for painful trigger points over the sole of the foot in order to distinguish the tarsal tunnel syndrome from Morton's neuralgia (see below). Sensory loss usually occurs in the distribution of the medial plantar nerve, but sometimes also, or even exclusively, in the area of the sole supplied by the lateral plantar nerve. Motor signs are hard to assess since the intrinsic muscles at the sole of the foot cannot be tested or seen separately. Comparison with the normal foot may identify the difference. Finally, one should look for abnormal postures of the foot, hypermobility of the ankle joint, or local swellings. In leprosy a perforating ulcer of the foot may be associated with compression of the tibial nerve in the tarsal tunnel (de Coninck *et al.*, 1983).

Electrophysiological studies

Nerve conduction studies. The tibial nerve can be stimulated with surface electrodes in the popliteal fossa and at the ankle. Motor conduction in the medial and lateral plantar nerve can be assessed by stimulating at the ankle and recording from the abductor hallucis and the abductor digiti minimi, respectively (Oh *et al.*, 1979; Fu *et al.*, 1980). Compression at the tunnel may affect one or more branches of the tibial nerve. This means that by measurement of these distal latencies no distinction can be made between lesions within the tunnel and more distal ones. By stimulating the tibial nerve proximal to the tunnel and the plantar nerves distal to the tunnel this problem can be solved (Felsenthal *et al.*, 1992). In a large proportion of patients with a clinically definite tarsal tunnel syndrome, however, motor nerve conduction is within normal limits. Sensory conduction studies have been found to be more sensitive. Good results have been obtained with surface electrodes (Guiloff and Sherratt, 1977; Oh *et al.*, 1979; Ponsford, 1988) as well as with needle electrodes (Behse and Buchthal, 1971; Oh *et al.*, 1979; Oh *et al.*, 1985). Such studies can also be used for the assessment of interdigital nerve lesions (Oh *et al.*, 1984; Falck *et al.*, 1984).

Needle EMG studies may be helpful by revealing signs of denervation and abnormal motor unit potentials in the intrinsic foot muscles. It should be borne in mind, however, that fibrillation potentials may occur in some healthy subjects (Falck and Alaranta, 1983). Intra-individual comparison with EMG findings in other intrinsic foot muscles may help to determine whether there is true abnormality. Fasciculations are frequently encountered in the intrinsic foot muscles of healthy subjects, especially in the abductor hallucis. They may also be numerous in the gastrocnemius muscle, but not in the tibialis anterior (Van der Heijden *et al.*, 1994).

Differential diagnosis

First of all the symptoms should be distinguished from pain secondary to *disorders of bones or ligaments*, such as stress fractures, plantar fasciitis and bursitis. None of these disorders is associated with paraesthesia or with conduction abnormalities of the tibial nerve. *Morton's neuralgia* (see below) consists of shooting pain caused by pressure over one of the metatarsal bones. In *medial plantar neuropathy* (see below) the signs and symptoms do not involve the lateral sole, and the pain is precipitated by pressure more distally than the medial malleolus (Oh and Lee, 1987). Burning feet in *polyneuropathy*, particularly diabetic neuropathy, may have some similarities with bilateral tarsal tunnel syndrome. Even a sciatic nerve tumour may initially mimic a tarsal tunnel syndrome (Wolock *et al.*, 1989).

Causes

The tarsal tunnel syndrome may appear spontaneously but can be precipitated by ill-fitting footwear, hypermobility of the ankle, or previous trauma to the foot. There is a large variety of other causes (Table 20.2), including inflammatory conditions and local mass lesions, in which cases MRI is very helpful (Erickson *et al.*, 1990; Kerr and Frey, 1991). Leprosy deserves special mention. It should be suspected also in white people with sensory mononeuropathies living in

Table 20.2
Causes of lesions of the tibial nerve in the tarsal tunnel

Entrapment
- With ill-fitting footwear (Goodgold *et al.*, 1965; Marinacci, 1968; Mann, 1974)
- Idiopathic (DeLisa and Saeed, 1983)

Trauma
- Fractures or soft tissue injuries (Kerr and Frey, 1991)
- Fibrous scarring after previous trauma of the ankle (Goodgold *et al.*, 1965; Kerr and Frey, 1991)
- Strained flexor digitorum accessorius muscle (Ho *et al.*, 1993)

Hypermobility of the ankle (Francis *et al.*, 1987)

Tumour
- Cyst of the nerve sheath (Edwards and Nilsson, 1969)
- Intraneural ganglion (Poppi *et al.*, 1989)
- Ganglion arising from flexor hallucis longus tendon sheath (Erickson *et al.*, 1990)
- Neurilemmoma (Erickson *et al.*, 1990)
- Lipoma (Chen, 1992)

Inflammation
- Rheumatoid arthritis (Grabois *et al.*, 1981)
- Leprosy (Palande and Azhaguraj, 1975; de Coninck *et al.*, 1983; Chaise and Boucher, 1987)
- Non-specific tenosynovitis (Erickson *et al.*, 1990; Kerr and Frey, 1991)

Dilated veins or varicosity (Kerr and Frey, 1991)

Hypertrophy of the abductor hallucis muscle (Kerr and Frey, 1991)

Metabolic disorders
- Lipid deposition in hyperlipidaemia (Ruderman *et al.*, 1983)
- Hypothyroidism (Schwartz *et al.*, 1983)

countries where leprosy is endemic, especially when nerves are palpable.

A 31-year-old white male in good health had for six months had pain and pins and needles in his right foot when playing lawn tennis. As manager of a building company he worked mainly in Nigeria. On examination during a brief return to Europe the posterior tibial nerve was palpable over the tibial tunnel, and the Hoffmann–Tinel sign was strongly positive with painful paraesthesia in all the toes. Sensory conduction velocity was markedly decreased in the right posterior tibial nerve. A tarsal tunnel syndrome was diagnosed and he was operated on in the usual way. Unfortunately, this had not produced even the slightest relief of his symptoms when a year later he returned on another leave to Europe. This time there was a patch of analgesia over the dorsum of the foot, outside the territory of the tibial nerve. Analgesia was also found in part of the area of the superficial radial nerve on the left. No skin depigmentations were visible. Biopsy of a small branch of the superficial radial nerve showed lepromatous inflammation. He was treated with appropriate medication and his symptoms slowly abated in about six months.

Treatment

In case of local entrapment, surgical decompression of the retinaculum is rapidly and definitively successful, as in the carpal tunnel syndrome. Exceptions do occur (De Stoop *et al.*, 1989; Mumenthaler and Schliack, 1993), but this should lead to a renewed search for conditions requiring specific treatment, from antilepromatous drugs to the change of ill-fitting footwear.

Lesions of the sensory branch of the tibial nerve at the heel

The sensory branch to the medial surface of the calcaneus, the calcaneal nerve, may be compressed below the deep fascia of the abductor hallucis muscle, causing pain in one or both heels (Pace *et al.*, 1991; Schon *et al.*, 1993). The condition occurs especially in athletes (Henricson and Westlin, 1984). Surgical decompression is the treatment of choice (Henricson and Westlin, 1984; Pace *et al.*, 1991).

Lesions of the plantar nerves

Clinical features

Damage to the plantar nerves as they course across the sole is manifested by paraesthesia and sensory loss alone (usually in the medial part of the sole), since weakness of the intrinsic foot muscles causes virtually no symptoms. Even on examination this is difficult to detect, as many normal individuals cannot fan their toes. Palpation of the sole may reveal local swelling or atrophy, and sometimes a Hoffmann–Tinel sign. It should be kept in mind that paraesthesia in the sole may also be caused by more proximal lesions, from the nearby tarsal tunnel up to the S1 root. Muscle power in the calf will be normal and the ankle jerk unaffected with lesions of the plantar nerves or at the tarsal tunnel, but with more proximal lesions these functions will often suffer. Electrophysiological studies will help to make the distinction, and sometimes plain radiographs, ultrasound studies or MRI scanning are necessary to demonstrate a lesion in the sole (see below).

Causes

Mostly the medial plantar nerve is affected (Table 20.3). Idiopathic entrapment may occur just distal to the

Table 20.3
Causes of lesions of the medial plantar nerve

Idiopathic entrapment, at the navicular tuberosity (Oh and Lee, 1987)

Athletic exercise ('jogger's foot') (Rask, 1978)

Tumours
- Cyst of the tibialis posterior tendon (Stewart, 1981)
- Synovial cyst (Pagliughi, 1980)
- Malignant schwannoma (Giannestras and Bronson, 1975)
- Plantar fibromatosis (Boc and Kushner, 1994)

Inflammation
- Leprosy (Guiloff and Sherratt, 1977)

tarsal tunnel, at the entrance of the fibromuscular tunnel behind the navicular tuberosity (Oh and Lee, 1987). Occasionally the lateral plantar nerve may be damaged by fractures or sprains of the foot (Johnson *et al.*, 1992; Hah *et al.*, 1992), or its first branch may become compressed between intrinsic muscles of the sole (Schon and Baxter, 1990). Both plantar nerves may suffer from wearing tight shoes, from standing on the rungs of a ladder with soft shoes (Kopell and Thompson, 1963), immobilization in a hospital bed with prolonged pressure against the footboard, or from local callus, fasciitis or arthritis.

Lesions of the plantar proper digital nerves

Clinical features and causes

The *medial plantar proper digital nerve* may be damaged in isolation, where it crosses the first metatarso-phalangeal joint, or on the medial side of the big toe (Joplin, 1971; Ames *et al.*, 1980; Merritt and Subotnick, 1982). Patients report symptoms on walking, with pain and paraesthesia on the medial side of the big toe that can be very cumbersome. The most common cause is poorly fitting shoes; otherwise

scar tissue after bunion surgery or arthritis of the first metatarsophalangeal joint may be responsible (Meier and Kenzora, 1985). On examination one may find a tender and thickened nerve, often together with sensory loss.

The counterpart on the outer side of the little toe, the *lateral plantar proper digital nerve*, may develop a traumatic neuroma secondary to bunion (Thul and Hoffman, 1985).

Treatment

Better shoes with protective padding are often the first measure. If symptoms persist excision of the nerve may be considered, which often provides dramatic relief, for the medial proper plantar digital nerve (Joplin, 1971; Merritt and Subotnick, 1982) as well as for the lateral counterpart; any associated bunion should be excised at the same time (Thul and Hoffman, 1985).

Lesions of the plantar interdigital nerves (Morton's metatarsalgia)

Morton's metatarsalgia is a lesion of one of the interdigital nerves of the foot, which arise from the medial and plantar nerves, at the point where these course between the heads of the metatarsal bones, just before they divide into two digital nerves (Figure 20.7). These lesions are found mostly between the third and fourth metatarsal bones, especially in women. Not only the heads of the metatarsal bones but also the deep transverse ligament contributes to the compression (Gauthier, 1979). The swelling around the nerve mainly consists of fibrous tissue; the term 'neuroma' is a misnomer from a pathological point of view (Guiloff *et al.*, 1984).

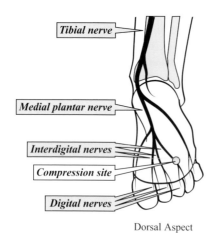

Figure 20.7
Compression site in Morton's metatarsalgia.

History

The patient complains of a severe and burning pain in the sole of the foot, mostly located between the heads of the third and fourth metatarsal bones, the pain often radiating to the third and fourth toes, with paraesthesia and numbness. Initially the discomfort occurs only on standing and walking, but later the symptoms may become continuous, unless the shoes are removed, and the pain may also radiate proximally.

Examination

The symptoms are precipitated or worsened by external pressure between the heads of the metatarsal bones in question, or by passive dorsiflexion of the toes. There may be a sensory deficit of the adjoining sides of two toes, most often the third and fourth. The local swelling can be demonstrated by CT or MRI scanning (Turan *et al.*, 1991).

Differential diagnosis

First of all a tarsal tunnel syndrome should be ruled out. Orthopaedic conditions that may resemble Morton's metatarsalgia are a stress fracture or avascular necrosis of a metatarsal bone, or soft tissue injuries. X-ray studies may be needed to demonstrate or rule out bony changes in the metatarsus. More recently, ultrasound studies have proved helpful in confirming the presence of interdigital neuromas (Shapiro and Shapiro, 1995).

Treatment

Fitting shoes without tight pressure on the sole is a first measure, if necessary supplemented with padding (Gaynor *et al.*, 1989). Local anaesthetics together with corticosteroids may give more than temporary relief: in a series of 65 patients treated by this method one-third recovered and one-third had improved after two years (Greenfield *et al.*, 1984). Carbamazepine orally may also be helpful (Guiloff, 1979). Excision of the abnormal tissue is the most radical approach and is generally successful (Keh *et al.*, 1992). A dorsal route has its proponents because infections would be prevented and mobilization would be faster, but controlled trials have not been performed. However, a new 'neuroma' may form afterwards and the permanent numbness of the toes may be troublesome; some therefore favour neurolysis, by incision of the intermetacarpal ligament above resection (Gauthier, 1979; Dellon, 1992).

Chapter 21
The peroneal nerves

Anatomy

The common peroneal nerve (Figure 21.1) carries fibres from L4 to S1. The nerve is contained in a separate division within the sciatic nerve before this nerve visibly divides into the common peroneal nerve and the tibial nerve; sometimes the actual separation occurs as far proximal as the upper thigh. The *common peroneal nerve* winds around the head of the fibula before entering the compartment of the

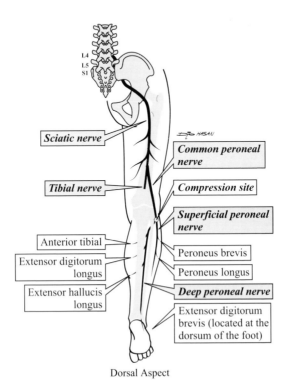

Dorsal Aspect

Figure 21.1
Muscles innervated by the peroneal nerve.

peroneal muscles. At this point the nerve lies directly upon the periost, where it is particularly exposed to compression, stretch or other trauma. The common peroneal nerve then passes through a supposedly more protected fibro-osseous canal between the insertion of the peroneus longus muscle and the fibula (the fibular tunnel). The common peroneal nerve then divides into a deep and a superficial branch. The *deep peroneal nerve* innervates the tibialis anterior, extensor digitorum longus and extensor hallucis longus muscles; the *terminal branch of the deep peroneal nerve* lies superficially at the dorsum of the ankle and foot and innervates the extensor digitorum brevis muscle and a small area of skin, the web between the first and second toes (Figure 21.2). In exceptional cases the extensor hallucis brevis is supplied by the tibial nerve ('all tibial foot') (Linden and Berlit, 1994). The *superficial peroneal nerve* supplies both peroneus muscles (longus and brevis); a

terminal motor branch (*the accessory deep peroneal nerve*) exists in about a quarter of subjects (Neundörfer and Seiberth, 1975). The sensory branch of the superficial peroneal nerve pierces the deep fascia of the lower leg and may be damaged separately (see below).

The skin area innervated by the common peroneal nerve consists of the lateral part of the lower leg and the dorsum of the foot (Figure 21.2). The corresponding sensory fibres arise partly from the common peroneal nerve in the popliteal fossa, as the *lateral cutaneous nerve of the calf* (upper half of the lateral calf), and partly from the superficial peroneal nerve (lower half of the lateral calf and dorsum of the foot). A *sural communicating branch* joins the medial cutaneous nerve of the calf, originating from the tibial nerve, to form the *sural nerve*, which innervates the skin of the lateral side of the heel, the sole, and the fifth toe (see Chapter 22).

Lesions of the common peroneal nerve, at the level of the fibular head

History

Patients with a lesion of the common peroneal nerve complain of foot drop (partial or complete), numbness or paraesthesia of the lateral part of the lower leg, or they may have both motor and sensory symptoms. The extent of the deficits depends on whether the lesion involves the fascicles of the deep or the superficial peroneal nerve, or both, and also on the duration of compression. It is not uncommon for patients to experience paraesthesia in the lateral part of the leg or the dorsum of the foot (superficial peroneal nerve) or at the web between the first two toes (deep peroneal nerve), but pain is a definitely uncommon symptom, at least when the lesion is caused by external compression.

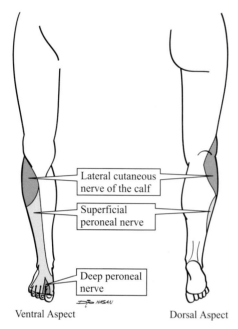

Lateral cutaneous nerve of the calf

Superficial peroneal nerve

Deep peroneal nerve

Ventral Aspect   Dorsal Aspect

Figure 21.2
Approximate skin areas innervated by the common peroneal nerve.

Examination

The muscles innervated by the superficial and deep peroneal nerves are tested as shown in Figure 21.3. For some of these tests a few additional comments are appropriate. To test the peroneal muscles (foot eversion) one should start with the ankle in a position of slight plantar flexion; these muscles are strong and are generally not overcome by the examiner (that is, the examiner's wrist flexors and triceps muscle; see Figure 21.3). The same applies to the tibialis anterior muscle (Figure 21.4). In contrast, on testing the extensors (dorsiflexion) of the toes the examiner easily 'wins' with most individuals (Figure 21.5). The extensor hallucis longus is tested separately (Figure 21.6). Walking with a more or less complete foot drop leads to the typical stepping gait, in which there is compensatory overaction of hip and knee flexors to obtain clearance for the foot during the swing phase. With moderate weakness the foot may still land on the heel but immediately afterwards the foot

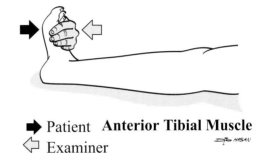

➡ Patient **Anterior Tibial Muscle**
⬅ Examiner

Figure 21.4
The foot is dorsiflexed against resistance.

dorsiflexors give way, causing a characteristic, flat-footed sound. With mild weakness of foot dorsiflexion gait may be more or less normal, but the patient is not able to walk on his heels or, in milder cases, will swing the foot with less clearance from the floor than on the normal side.

The extensor digitorum brevis muscle is tested by extending the proximal phalanges of the toes against resistance. The muscle belly can then be seen and felt as a small bulge on the dorsolateral side of the foot, at least in young people (Figure

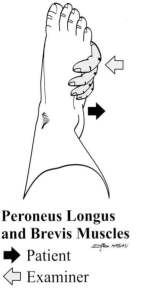

**Peroneus Longus
and Brevis Muscles**
➡ Patient
⬅ Examiner

Figure 21.3
The foot is everted against resistance.

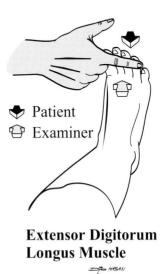

⬇ Patient
⬆ Examiner

**Extensor Digitorum
Longus Muscle**

Figure 21.5
The distal phalanges of the toes are dorsiflexed against resistance.

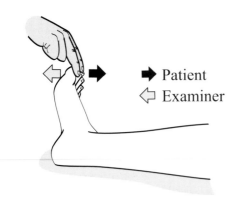

Extensor Hallucis Longus Muscle

Figure 21.6
The distal phalanx of the big toe is dorsiflexed against resistance.

21.7). It is only a small muscle, and it cannot perform any movement on its own. The ankle jerk is typically normal with disorders of the peroneal nerve; if this reflex is decreased in combination with weakness of foot dorsiflexion the lesion should be sought more proximally, in the course of the sciatic nerve or in combined involvement of the roots L5 and S1.

Apart from weakness of foot eversion and dorsiflexion of the foot and toes there

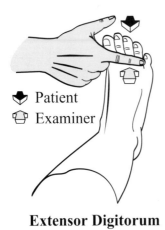

Extensor Digitorum Brevis Muscle

Figure 21.7
The proximal phalanges of the toes are dorsiflexed against resistance.

may be a sensory deficit, but often this is less extensive than might be expected from the anatomical distribution.

Electrophysiological studies

The usual method of performing motor conduction studies of the common peroneal nerve is to stimulate the nerve successively at the ankle, below and above the fibular head while recording from the extensor digitorum brevis muscle. A lesion at the fibular head causes local slowing and/or conduction block (see Figure 1.2) in a majority of patients (Pickett, 1984; Sourkes and Stewart, 1991). Conduction studies are essential, not only to localize the lesion but also to determine to what degree the dorsiflexion weakness is due to axonal loss or to blockade, the latter having a much better prognosis (Berry and Richardson, 1976; Wilbourn, 1986). As dorsiflexion is dependent on the tibialis anterior, and the extensor digitorum brevis has no functional significance, it is important to record CMAPs from the tibialis anterior. Moreover, recording from this muscle increases the chance of demonstrating conduction block (Wilbourn, 1986; Brown and Watson, 1991; Sourkes and Stewart, 1991).

Needle EMG studies should be performed in the muscles supplied by the deep and superficial branches of the peroneal nerve. Especially if no conduction abnormalities are found in the nerve segment across the fibular head, other leg muscles should be examined to differentiate from a sciatic neuropathy, plexopathy or radiculopathy. This study should always include the short head of the biceps femoris (supplied by the lateral division of the sciatic nerve) and the tibialis posterior (supplied by L5 but not by the peroneal nerve). Axonal loss due to a peroneal nerve lesion may also be recognized by a reduced or absent sensory nerve action potential of the superficial peroneal nerve examined in a distal segment (Wilbourn, 1986). Unless there is an obvious cause for a peroneal nerve lesion, it is advisable to extend the study by looking for an underlying polyneuropathy.

Differential diagnosis

Weakness of muscles innervated by the common peroneal nerve may be caused not only by a lesion of the nerve itself; the cause may also be located more proximally (sciatic nerve, the L5 root, anterior horn cells, or the pyramidal tract), or more distally (distal myopathies, compartment syndrome).

Pyramidal tract lesions may result in weakness mainly affecting the flexor muscles of the leg, especially the most distal movement: foot dorsiflexion (confusingly enough the dorsiflexors of the foot and toes are flexor muscles in a physiological sense, as these shorten the leg (van Gijn, 1978), but have been termed extensor muscles by the anatomists). However, the pattern of gait is different: the foot tends to be dragged or there is even circumduction of the foot, because the other flexor muscles of the leg are often also involved, and one does not see the stepping gait seen in peroneal nerve lesions. In addition, muscle tone and tendon reflexes may be increased and the plantar response will often be extensor (van Gijn, 1978).

Disorders of *anterior horn cells* such as motor neurone disease or spinal muscular atrophy may present with weakness of the muscles innervated by the peroneal nerve. Subtle weakness or fasciculations outside the territory of the common peroneal nerve may be important clues in clinching the diagnosis (sometimes the signs are as remote as unequivocally abnormal quivering in the tongue). It should be emphasized, however, that healthy people may have fasciculations in some muscles, especially in the calves and intrinsic foot muscles (Blexrud *et al.*, 1993; van der Heijden *et al.*, 1994). For a definitive diagnosis of motor neurone

disease the disease should involve three of the four regions formed by head, arms, trunk and legs (Swash and Leigh, 1992).

Involvement of the *fifth lumbar root* may also lead to weakness of the extensors of the foot and toes. By far the most frequent cause is protrusion of the disc between the vertebrae L4 and L5; more rarely there is an extremely lateral prolapse of the L5-S1 disc. With lesions of the L5 root weakness of the extensor hallucis longus muscle is most conspicuous, because this muscle is largely innervated by the L5 root. In contrast, a lesion of the L5 root alone will not result in paralysis of foot and toe dorsiflexors, because of overlap in root innervation. Another helpful sign is weakness of the tibialis posterior muscle, which subserves inversion of the foot, with only a minor contribution of the tibialis anterior muscle. With lesions of the peroneal nerve foot inversion is typically normal. Backache and a positive straight leg raising test may also point in the direction of a root lesion, but absence of these features does not exclude this diagnosis. A diminished ankle jerk indicates involvement of the S1 root or the sciatic nerve. Sensory deficits in lumbosacral root lesions are often vaguely demarcated and may not be very helpful in distinguishing between lesions of the peroneal nerve and the L5 root.

EMG studies (see above) are very helpful in making this differential diagnosis. Investigation by CT or MRI scanning may well show a disc protrusion, but such abnormalities are extremely common in asymptomatic people (Boden *et al.*, 1990; Jensen *et al.*, 1994).

Lesions of the *sciatic nerve* may present as an isolated footdrop (Katirji and Wilbourn, 1994); the lateral division largely corresponds with the peroneal nerve, and somehow this is more prone to compression than the portion corresponding to the tibial nerve.

Myopathic weakness of the muscles innervated by the peroneal nerve is almost invariably bilateral and rarely confined to these muscles, features which will usually allow one to make the distinction.

Compartment syndromes (anterior or lateral) often involve the deep or superficial peroneal nerves. These syndromes are discussed below.

Causes

Painless peroneal palsy is one of the commonest mononeuropathies; it may occur also in children (Jones *et al.*, 1993). The large majority of acute and subacute palsies of the peroneal nerve is caused by compression or stretching of the nerve at its superficial site near the head of the fibula, in one or in both legs. Usually the common peroneal nerve is involved, but sometimes only the deep or the superficial branch. There are numerous precipitating causes (Table 21.1), almost invariably involving an unusual posture, in combination with a second factor: intoxication, hereditary predisposition, medical procedures or extremely long duration of the abnormal position.

Table 21.1
Causes (single or in combination) of lesions of the common peroneal nerve

Hereditary liability to pressure palsies (see Chapter 25)

Postural factors
- Habitual sitting with legs crossed (Eaton, 1937; Carney, 1967)
- Bed rest (also without intoxication), especially with a bed rail (Felsenthal, 1983)
- Prolonged squatting or kneeling: for professional reasons, in farmers, gardeners, road menders, strawberry pickers or turnip harvesters (Sandhu and Sandhey, 1976; Seppalainen *et al.*, 1977; Schroter *et al.*, 1990); during delivery (Bademosi *et al.*, 1980); in so-called 'hunkering contests' (Massey *et al.*, 1981)
- Grasping one's own legs, during delivery (Adornato and Carlini, 1992)

Sports
- Running (Leach *et al.*, 1989; Mitra *et al.*, 1995)

Weight loss
- Anorexia nervosa (MacKenzie *et al.*, 1989)

Table 21.1 (continued)
Causes (single or in combination) of lesions of the common peroneal nerve

- Starvation, in prisoners of war (Sprofkin, 1958)
- Voluntary fasting, or 'slimmer's paralysis' (Sprofkin, 1958; Cruz Martinez, 1987)
- Whipple's disease (Cruz Martinez *et al.* 1987)

Trauma
- Fracture of the femur (Sorell *et al.*, 1976)
- Fracture of the fibula (Mino and Hughes, 1984)
- Inversion trauma of the foot (Meals, 1977; Stoff and Greene, 1982; Nitz *et al.*, 1985)

Iatrogenic factors
- Malpositioning during anaesthesia (Britt and Gordon, 1964; Lederman *et al.*, 1982)
- Plaster casts (Weiss *et al.*, 1992)
- Tight bandages (Garland and Moorhouse, 1952)
- Arthroscopic knee surgery (Esselman *et al.* 1993)
- Intramedullary arthrodesis of the knee (Stiehl and Hanel, 1993)
- High tibial osteotomy (Hsu, 1989)
- Rodding of a shaft fracture of the contralateral femur, with the ipsilateral leg in a calf-supported leg holder despite a similar fracture (Carlson *et al.*, 1995)
- Intermittent pneumatic compression, for the prevention of deep venous thrombosis (Lachmann *et al.*, 1992)
- Intravenous fluid infiltration, in newborns (Kreusser and Volpe, 1984)

Congenital abnormalities
- Constriction band (Tada *et al.*, 1984; Brown and Storm, 1994)
- Fabella (Takebe and Hirohata, 1981)

Vascular lesions
- Haemorrhage in the popliteal fossa (Large *et al.*, 1983; Logigian *et al.*, 1989)

Tumours
- Haemangioma (Bilge *et al.*, 1989);
- Exostosis of the fibular head (Rinaldi, 1983), or intraosseous cyst (Donahue *et al.*, 1996);
- Cysts of the lateral meniscus (Leon and Marano, 1987; Edwards *et al.*, 1995), or of the tibio-fibular joint (Evans *et al.*, 1994)
- Intraneural cysts (Katz and Lenobel, 1970; Eiras and Garcia Cosamalon, 1979; Nucci *et al.*, 1990; Marchiodi *et al.*, 1994; O'Brien *et al.*, 1995)
- Osteochondroma (Cardelia *et al.*, 1995)
- Neurofibroma (Dawson *et al.*, 1990)

Other
- Pretibial myxoedema (Siegler and Refetoff, 1976)
- Lipomatosis of the popliteal fossa, steroid-induced (Rawlings *et al.*, 1986)
- Herniation of the gastrocnemius muscle (Alhadeff and Lee, 1995)

A 51-year-old professor of biochemistry had spent most of a Saturday on his knees, in order to cover the roof of his garage with water-resistant material. On getting up he had tingling sensations in his left lower leg and he could not raise his foot. Examination showed moderate weakness of dorsiflexion of the foot and toes, and of foot eversion; there was superficial sensory loss corresponding with the territory of the common peroneal nerve. Nerve conduction studies showed focal slowing and a partial conduction block in the common peroneal nerve at the level of the fibular head; needle EMG demonstrated signs of denervation in the tibialis anterior muscle. Recovery took about three months before it was complete.

Intoxications may not be immediately admitted, and similarly hereditary liability to pressure palsies may not be immediately evident from the history. In cases of neuropathy of the common peroneal nerve after minor trauma such as a brief period of squatting one should never forget to enquire about episodes of foot drop in the past, not only in the patient but also in parents or siblings (see Chapter 25). Prolonged squatting or kneeling may lead to peroneal palsy in patients without such a family history. This posture may be associated with certain professional activities (see Table 21.1). Delivery may cause peroneal nerve palsy by squatting, which is a customary position in Nigeria (Bademosi *et al.*, 1980), or by the mother grasping her own legs in a supine position (Adornato and Carlini, 1992). Another posture associated with compression of the common peroneal nerve is prolonged crossing of the legs, with the patella of the lower leg compressing the region of the fibular head in the upper leg; in obese patients this may be deduced from a local dimple

(Carney, 1967). If bed rest is followed by a peroneal palsy there usually is an associated intoxication, family history or at least a bed rail (Felsenthal, 1983), but sometimes no causal factor can be found:

A 32-year-old physician called one of us in distress, because she had woken up with numbness and weakness of the right foot and thought this might be a stroke, since a niece had suffered a brain infarct in her twenties and in herself a raised level of homocysteine had been found. She had been sleeping in (it was a weekend), but she had already noticed some numbness when she had briefly got up in the middle of the night. She and her partner emphatically denied abuse of alcohol or other drugs, there was no family history of pressure palsies, and no bed rail. On examination there was moderate weakness of foot dorsiflexion and foot eversion, marked weakness of the toe extensors, and normal power with other movements (including foot inversion). Superficial sensation was impaired at the lateral aspect of the leg (distal two thirds) and at the dorsum of the foot. Ten days later the deficits had largely cleared.

Separate sections of this book have been devoted to metabolic and inflammatory causes (see Chapters 26 and 28), nerve tumours (see Chapter 30), and the complications of systemic disease (see Chapter 27).

Lesions of the peroneal nerves between the fibular head and the ankle

Isolated deficits in the distribution of the deep or superficial peroneal nerve are much more likely to result from a lesion of a separate fascicle at the level of the head of the fibula than from a more distal lesion involving a single one of the two branches.

Compartment syndromes have a special place among the lesions of the peroneal nerve below the knee. The *anterior compartment syndrome* may lead to weakness of the tibialis anterior, the extensor hallucis longus and the extensor digitorum longus muscles, with sensory loss at the web between the first and second toes (Reneman, 1975; Iyer and Shields, 1989). In the *lateral compartment syndrome* compression of the superficial peroneal nerve results in weakness of the long and the short peroneal muscles, and sensory loss over the dorsum of the foot and the lower half of the lateral calf (Reneman, 1975). Occasionally swelling of necrotic peroneal muscles may secondarily lead to compression of the deep peroneal nerve (Arancio *et al.* 1985). Both these syndromes are provoked by strenuous exercise, in athletes or in insufficiently trained joggers. Severe pain in the affected part, red discoloration of the skin and sometimes even absence of the pulsations in the dorsal pedal artery are important diagnostic clues in distinguishing a compartment syndrome from other, more frequent causes of peroneal nerve compression. The pain may be severe and rapidly progressive within hours, or may remit. It may be difficult to assess weakness if patients are in severe pain, and the sensory deficits are then helpful in localizing the lesion to either the deep or the superficial peroneal nerve, and thereby to the anterior or the lateral compartment.

The deep peroneal nerve may be compressed in the lower leg by an aneurysm of the anterior tibial artery (Kars *et al.*, 1992). Isolated entrapment of the superficial peroneal nerve may occur as it passes through the deep fascia of the lower leg after having given off its motor branches to the peroneal muscles, about 10 cm proximal to the lateral malleolus. This results in pain and sensory deficits at the dorsum of the foot (Banerjee and Koons, 1981; Kernohan *et al.*, 1985; Sridhara and Izzo, 1985). The most common cause is athletic exercise

(McAuliffe *et al.*, 1985; Styf, 1989); more rarely, the cause is callus formation after midshaft fracture of the fibula (Mino and Hughes, 1984). In idiopathic cases the condition may be bilateral (McAuliffe *et al.*, 1985; Saragaglia *et al.*, 1986; Styf, 1989).

Lesions of the peroneal nerves at the ankle

The *terminal branch of the deep peroneal nerve* may be compressed at the anterior aspect of the ankle, a condition often termed the 'anterior tarsal tunnel syndrome' (Dellon, 1990; Liu *et al.*, 1991). Symptoms consist of painful paraesthesia in the web space between the first two toes; weakness of the extensor hallucis brevis muscle can be detected only by inspection, but in older subjects these muscles will often be atrophic. Among the possible causes are local contusion, tight shoelaces, wearing ski boots (Lindenbaum, 1979), ganglion (Brooks, 1952), talotibial exostoses (Edlich *et al.*, 1987) and entrapment below the extensor hallucis brevis muscle (Reed and Wright, 1995).

The *terminal branches of the superficial peroneal nerve*, supplying the dorsum of the foot, can be compressed distally, leading to pain and numbness in part of the dorsum of the foot. Causes include entrapment during sleep or sitting (Lemont and Cullen, 1984), epidermoid cysts (Nelson *et al.*, 1985), fascial bands (Rubin *et al.*, 1991) or, unavoidably, iatrogenic factors such as cannulation of foot veins (Horowitz, 1984; Preston and Logigian, 1988), arthroscopic knee surgery (Esselman *et al.*, 1993), or intermittent pneumatic compression for the prevention of deep venous thrombosis (Lachmann *et al.*, 1992).

Lesions of the lateral cutaneous nerve of the calf

Isolated compression of this nerve, which arises in the popliteal fossa from the common peroneal nerve to innervate the skin of the upper part of the lateral calf, may rarely cause pain in the popliteal fossa and the lateral part of the calf (Gross *et al.*, 1980).

Treatment

In most cases of external compression of the common peroneal nerve spontaneous recovery through a process of remyelination and perhaps reinnervation can be expected within weeks or months, certainly if the deficits are only partial. Watchful waiting and prevention of further compression (see below) is therefore the most sensible course to follow. Only in cases associated with long-lasting anaesthesia or drug-induced coma may the paralysis be permanent, because of severe axonal damage (which can be established by EMG investigation), and then even surgical decompression is pointless. Idiopathic entrapment of the common peroneal nerve by neighbouring structures is very uncommon; the existence of a 'fibular tunnel syndrome' has been proposed (Maudsley, 1967; Sunderland, 1978), but it is rare enough to make exploratory surgery unwarranted unless a valid indication exists. Only neurolysis of the superficial peroneal nerve may be rational if the signs and symptoms are compatible with compression at the site where the nerve pierces the fascia, 10 cm above the lateral malleolus (Kernohan *et al.*, 1985; McAuliffe *et al.*, 1985; Sridhara and Izzo, 1985; Styf, 1989).

Three good reasons for surgical decompression of the peroneal nerve can be distinguished, apart from this rare entrapment of the distal part of the superficial peroneal nerve. The first is penetrating trauma, which necessitates immediate exploration since the continuity of the nerve may have been disrupted. This includes peroneal palsy after surgery in the region of the knee, immediate or delayed (Vastamäki, 1986). Secondly, exploration is mandatory with local mass lesions such as a nerve tumour, a lipoma, a cyst or a ganglion (see Table 21.1). MRI is an invaluable tool in detecting these local abnormalities (Leon and Marano, 1987). However, with slowly progressive deficits the chance of finding a mass lesion is high even if this investigation is negative. The third reason for surgical treatment is the existence of a compartment syndrome, in which case immediate fasciotomy is the treatment of choice (Rorabeck, 1984; Styf and Korner, 1986).

In all patients with weakness of the extensors of the foot, gait should be made safer and more comfortable by a lightweight plastic orthosis, which should of course not further compress the peroneal nerve at the head of the fibula.

Prevention

In all comatose patients and in those bedridden with paralysed legs, such as may occur in Guillain–Barré syndrome, the common peroneal nerves at the head of the fibula should be protected by soft padding around the head of the fibula. It often proves difficult to convince residents and nurses of the rationale of these measures. Also, in patients with a leg plaster reaching as far as the head of the fibula or higher, the common peroneal nerve should be protected, preferably by an appropriate window in the plaster cast. Such precautions may avert not only pressure palsies but also lawsuits. It makes sense to instruct every patient with a leg plaster to check every day if the strength of the toe extensors is still normal; if there is weakness the plaster should be opened. Finally, medical personnel should be reminded to be careful with sawing or cutting when a lower leg plaster is removed; we have seen severe damage of the common peroneal nerve as a result of this procedure.

Chapter 22
The sural nerve

Anatomy

The sural nerve contains only sensory fibres, with few exceptions (Liguori and Trojaborg, 1990). It originates by the joining of two branches, one from the tibial nerve (medial cutaneous nerve of the calf) and one from the common peroneal nerve. The main branch from the tibial nerve originates at the level of the popliteal fossa (Figure 22.1). From there it runs downwards, first in the middle of the calf region, between the two heads of the gastrocnemius muscle. After it has pierced the fascia, halfway down the calf, it is joined in the subcutaneous region by the branch from the *lateral cutaneous nerve of the calf*, which originates from the

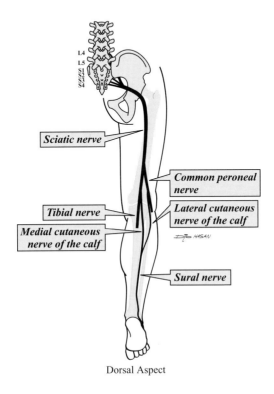

L4
L5
S1
S2
S3
S4

Sciatic nerve

Common peroneal nerve

Tibial nerve

Lateral cutaneous nerve of the calf

Medial cutaneous nerve of the calf

Sural nerve

Dorsal Aspect

Figure 22.1
The sural nerve.

peroneal nerve. From there it courses more laterally, between the Achilles tendon and the outer malleolus; it ends at the lateral border of the foot, by curving around the lateral malleolus. The skin area innervated by the nerve consists of the lateral side of the ankle and the lateral border of the sole, up to the base of the fifth toe (Figure 22.2).

Lesions of the sural nerve

History and examination

Symptoms consist of paraesthesia, pain, or numbness in the lateral ankle or sole. Aggravation by local pressure (Hoffmann–Tinel sign) may indicate the site of the lesion.

Electrophysiological studies

The nerve can be studied very well with surface or needle electrodes (Behse and Buchthal, 1971; Burke *et al.*, 1974; Schuchmann, 1977). The amplitude of the sensory nerve action potential can be used for the differentiation between an S1 radiculopathy and more peripheral lesions. Because sural nerve action potentials are relatively high and easy to obtain, the sural nerve is the most frequently studied leg nerve in the investigation of polyneuropathies.

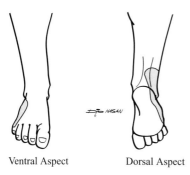

Ventral Aspect   Dorsal Aspect

Figure 22.2
Approximate skin area innervated by the sural nerve.

Causes

The sural nerve may be compressed or damaged at the level of the knee, the calf and, most commonly, at the ankle (Table 22.1). A relatively common iatrogenic cause is persistent pain after sural nerve biopsy, which occurred in 3/60 (5%) in one series, not to mention 22% of patients with infections at the biopsy site or delayed wound healing (Rappaport *et al.*, 1993). Other medical procedures that can lead to a lesion of the sural nerve are muscle biopsies in the calf and a variety of operations in the popliteal fossa (Smith and Litchy, 1989). External compression at the ankle may result from injury to bone or soft tissue, from tumours or cysts, or from special postures (see Table 22.1). Hard ridges or tightly fitting high-topped footwear may cause compression of the sural nerve in the calf (see Table 22.1 and below).

Table 22.1
Causes of lesions of the sural nerve

In the popliteal fossa
- Baker's cyst (Nakano, 1978)
- Arthroscopy, or operation for varicose veins (Smith and Litchy, 1989)

In the calf
- Tight lacing of high-topped footwear (Gross *et al.*, 1980; Heuser, 1982; Smith and Litchy, 1989)
- Calf muscle biopsy (Smith and Litchy, 1989)
- Compression by elastic socks (Shaffrey *et al.*, 1992)
- Pressure against a hard ridge, or wearing of tight chain (Reisin *et al.*, 1994)

At the ankle
- Chronic or acute ankle sprains (Smith and Litchy, 1989)
- Avulsion fracture of the base of the fifth metatarsal bone (Gould and Trevino, 1981)
- Adhesions after soft tissue injury (Colbert *et al.*, 1975; Docks and Salter, 1979)
- Ganglion (Pringle *et al.* 1974)
- Fractured sesamoid bone in the peroneus longus tendon (Perlman, 1990)
- Osteochondroma (Montgomery *et al.* 1989)
- Sitting with crossed ankles (Gross *et al.* 1980) or sitting on crossed ankles (Bruyn, 1994)
- Idiopathic neuroma (Pasternack and Lipp, 1992)
- Persistent pain after diagnostic biopsy of the sural nerve (Rappaport *et al.* 1993)

Treatment

In the case of compression by post-traumatic fibrosis or tumours, operative treatment is often necessary, with neurolysis or sectioning of the nerve (Docks and Salter, 1979; Pasternack and Lipp, 1992). Simple advice is sufficient if the causal factor is external compression; for example, special postures with crossed ankles (Gross *et al.* 1980; Bruyn, 1994), or with the calves against hard ridges (Reisin *et al.*, 1994), or wearing of tight chains (Reisin *et al.*, 1994) or high-topped boots (Gross *et al.*, 1980; Heuser, 1982; Smith and Litchy, 1989).

Chapter 23
The pudendal nerve

Anatomy

The pudendal nerve arises from the roots S2, S3 and S4 and supplies most of the perineum. It emerges from the pelvis below the piriformis muscle, crosses the sacrospinous ligament and enters the perineal area through the lesser sciatic notch. With its associated vascular branches, the nerve passes anteriorly along the intrapelvic wall within a tunnel-shaped passway in the dense obturator fascia, called the obturator canal or Alcock's canal. The pudendal nerve terminates by dividing into three branches (Figure 23.1).

The first branch is the *inferior rectal (haemorrhoidal) nerve*. It innervates the external anal sphincter, the perianal skin and the mucosa of the lower anal canal. The inferior rectal nerve may also arise independently from the third and fourth sacral nerves.

The second branch, the *perineal nerve*, supplies the muscles of the perineum (among which is the bulbocavernosus muscle), the erectile tissue of the penis, the external urethral sphincter, the distal

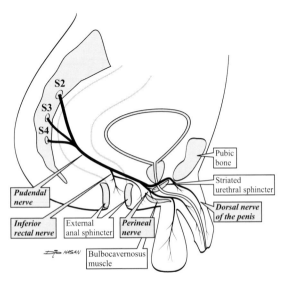

Figure 23.1
Schematic overview of the course of the left pudendal nerve and its branches.

part of the mucous membrane of the urethra, and the skin of perineum and scrotum/labia.

The final branch of the pudendal nerve is the *dorsal nerve of the penis/clitoris*. It runs forward in Alcock's canal, pierces the urogenital diaphragm and gives a branch to the corpus cavernosum. Subsequently it passes forward on the dorsum of the penis (or clitoris) to supply skin, prepuce and glans.

Symptoms

A one-sided or double-sided pudendal nerve lesion may cause faecal and/or urinary incontinence, impotence and sensory disturbances in the area supplied by the pudendal nerve.

Physical examination

The function of the external anal sphincter can be assessed by inspection, digital examination and reflexes. The classical anal reflex is elicited by pricking the perianal skin; the response consists of contraction of the external anal sphincter which can be observed as a dimpling of the perianal skin (Pedersen *et al.*, 1978). The bulbocavernosus reflex consists of contraction of the bulbocavernosus muscle or anal sphincter on compression of the glans penis. Clinically, contraction of the bulbocavernosus can best be assessed by palpation (Bors and Blinn, 1959). Both reflexes indicate integrity of the pudendal nerve and the roots S3 and S4.

To some degree the function of the pudendal nerve may be assessed by anorectal manometry (Read and Sun, 1992) and by urodynamic investigations (van Waalwijk van Doorn *et al.*, 1992). Moreover a battery of electrophysiological tests can be applied.

Electrophysiological studies

Needle EMG, conduction studies, reflex responses and evoked potentials may all

be helpful in detecting and localizing the lesion.

Needle EMG studies can be performed in the external anal sphincter, the external urethral sphincter, the bulbocavernosus and the puborectalis muscle (Chantraine, 1973; Swash, 1992). Investigation of the urethral sphincter is rather difficult and unpleasant to the patient. Therefore in cases of urinary incontinence often the anal sphincter and/or the bulbocavernosus muscle are examined. If, however, the site of the lesion is in the terminal nerve branches to the urethral sphincter the information obtained in this way is not relevant. Normally, sphincter muscles are active at rest so that it may be difficult to detect fibrilliation potentials in a partially denervated sphincter.

Motor nerve conduction of the terminal parts of the pudendal nerves can be studied by intrarectal nerve stimulation and recording the evoked muscle potential from the external anal and urethral sphincters, innervated by the inferior rectal nerve and the perineal nerve, respectively. This can be accomplished with disposable surface electrodes mounted on the index finger of a disposable glove (Snooks *et al.*, 1984). Responses of the external urethral sphincter can be recorded with electrodes mounted on a Foley catheter.

Reflex responses on stimulation of the dorsal nerve of the penis (or clitoris) can be obtained from the anal sphincter (Figure 23.2) and the bulbocavernosus muscle (Vodusek *et al.*, 1983). These studies give information on the total course of the nerve. Perianal stimulation is not advisable because of large stimulus artifacts and direct muscle responses (Pedersen *et al.*, 1982; Vodusek *et al.*, 1983). The external urethral sphincter is not commonly used in reflex studies because of technical difficulties.

Somatosensory evoked potentials and motor evoked potentials can be used to study peripheral as well as central nervous conduction from and to the perineal

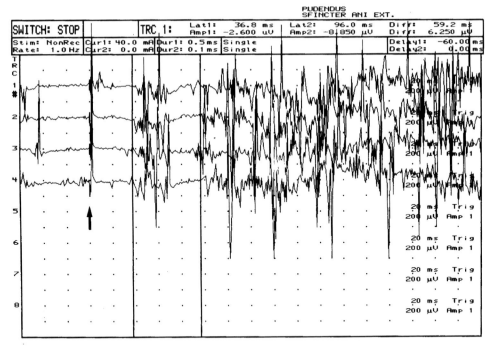

Figure 23.2
Normal pudendo-anal reflex. The dorsal nerve of the penis was stimulated with surface electrodes and responses were recorded from the external anal sphincter with a concentric needle electrode. The arrow indicates the stimulus artifact. The first reflex response may be followed by a second one (onset of both responses marked with a line). The reflex has been repeated a few times to show reproducibility

region, respectively (Opsomer *et al.*, 1989; Loening-Baucke *et al.*, 1994).

Causes of pudendal nerve lesions

Lesions of the pudendal nerve may be due to external compression, stretch injuries and polyneuropathies (Table 23.1). During operations for hip fractures a perineal post is sometimes used. If the polstering of this post is insufficient, forceful traction at the relevant leg during reposition of the fracture may lead to pudendal nerve damage (Schulak *et al.*, 1980; Lindenbaum *et al.*, 1982; Hofmann *et al.*, 1982; Kao *et al.*, 1993). This may result in sensory disturbances, incontinence and erectile impotence.

Perineal nerve compression in Alcock's canal may result from long bicycle rides. This leads to numbness of half or all of the

Table 23.1
Causes of pudendal nerve lesions

External compression
- Perineal post used in operation on hip fractures (Schulak *et al.*, 1980; Hofmann *et al.*, 1982; Lindenbaum *et al.*, 1982; Kao *et al.*, 1993)
- Long bicycle rides (Weiss, 1985; Oberpenning *et al.*, 1994)
- Suturing through the sacrospinal ligament during colposcopy, with subsequent entrapment of the nerve (Alevizon and Finan, 1996)

Stretch injuries
- Repeated straining during defaecation, or faecal incontinence (Roig *et al.*, 1995)
- Childbirth (Snooks *et al.* 1984; Snooks *et al.*, 1985; Allen *et al.*, 1990; Sultan *et al.*, 1994)
- Pelvic fractures
- Pelvic surgery

Polyneuropathies
- Diabetic polyneuropathy (Haldeman *et al.*, 1982)
- Alcoholic polyneuropathy (Fabra *et al.*, 1993)

penis/labia majora and perineum, and even to erectile impotence (Weiss, 1985; Oberpenning *et al.*, 1994). In other cases repeated microtrauma has been postulated (Pisani *et al.*, 1997).

Pudendal neuropathy is perhaps the most common cause of faecal incontinence. In series of patients with idiopathic anorectal incontinence 70–80% of cases were found to have a pudendal neuropathy (Snooks *et al.*, 1984; Roig *et al.*, 1995). The lesions are mainly localized in the distal segment of the pudendal nerve or in the inferior rectal nerve; they are often asymmetrical (Lubowski *et al.*, 1988).

Childbirth may cause anal sphincter muscle division. In up to 60% of cases there is additional damage to the pudendal nerves (Snooks *et al.*, 1985). Also, without obvious damage to the anal sphincter, vaginal delivery has been shown to cause compressive lesions of the pudendal nerves. It seems that most of these lesions initially recover to a sufficient degree, but that later in life, possibly through additional ageing of the neuromuscular apparatus, they may lead to incontinence (Snooks *et al.*, 1984; Allen *et al.*, 1990). Urinary incontinence could be caused in this way (Snooks *et al.*, 1986).

Differential diagnosis

Neurogenic disturbances in the sacral area may also be caused by polyneuropathies and by lesions of the cauda equina and the conus medullaris. In these cases clinical and/or electrophysiological studies will demonstrate that the abnormalities are not limited to the supply area of the pudendal nerve.

Dysfunction of the anorectal and urogenital structures may also result from disturbances of vascular supply or autonomic innervation, or from structural abnormalities of the pelvic floor and the relevant viscera themselves.

Part three
Causes of mononeuropathies other than focal lesions

Chapter 24
Neuralgic amyotrophy

Neuralgic amyotrophy is a rather vague term, coined fifty years ago (Parsonage and Turner, 1948), but this opacity still accurately reflects the incompleteness of our knowledge about the condition. Typically, the condition affects the brachial plexus, on one side, as a single episode in the patient's life. The incidence has been estimated at 1.64 per 100 000 population (Beghi *et al.*, 1985). Before explaining the clinical features of the classical form in more detail, we should point out that many rare variants exist, such as with involvement of separate nerves, cranial nerves, or even the lumbosacral plexus; also, there are hereditary and recurrent forms (see below). As the clinical spectrum is so wide, the term 'brachial plexus neuropathy' is far from synonymous with 'neuralgic amyotrophy' and should not be used to describe the entire syndrome.

History

The classical story involves a healthy person, male or female, sometimes a child (Figure 24.1; Zeharia *et al.*, 1990). The patient experiences rather suddenly a severe, deep and sometimes excruciating pain in the shoulder and neck. The pain may radiate to the medial part of the scapula or throughout the arm (Favero *et al.*, 1987), and it may even remain restricted to a part of the upper arm or forearm. The pain often starts in the

evening or during the night and may last from a few hours to several days or even weeks. Slight numbness may be present, often over the deltoid muscle, more or less in the distribution of the axillary nerve. Paraesthesia occur rarely, if ever.

During the episode of pain, or more often just after it has more or less subsided, severe and mostly unilateral weakness develops within a matter of hours, often overnight, in muscles of the shoulder, arm or both. Eventually the pain disappears entirely or lingers as a vague ache. The weakness reaches its peak soon after the beginning, but uncommonly there is some progression. In unusual instances the pain is only slight or is admitted only after repeated questioning.

A 65-year-old dean of a faculty of medicine almost casually told one of us he had been unable to lift his left arm for about two weeks, with rather sudden onset. Only after insistent questioning did it emerge that one week before onset he had had a slight ache in the neck and around the scapula, but not severe enough to interfere with sleep. Examination showed slight weakness (MRC grade 4) of the rhomboid, supraspinatus, biceps and brachioradialis muscles, and more severe weakness (MRC 2–3) in the deltoid, infraspinatus and supinator muscles. The biceps jerk and supinator jerk were slightly diminished on the left. Sensation was normal. The cerebrospinal fluid showed an elevated level of protein (0.73 g/l) but was otherwise normal. Four weeks after the onset, muscle power started to improve, and another two weeks later he had made a complete recovery.

Examination

As a rule the patient is in good general health, without neck stiffness or fever. There is a flaccid paralysis and early atrophy of any combination of muscles of the shoulder and arm: serratus anterior, rhomboids, supra- and infraspinatus, deltoid, latissimus dorsi, or one or more arm muscles innervated by major nerves or their branches. Weakness may be restricted to the serratus anterior muscle, suggesting isolated involvement of the long thoracic nerve. The tendon jerks of the arm may be diminished or remain normal. Sensory loss is much less evident

and, if present, it is mostly in the area of the axillary nerve.

Causes

Sometimes neuralgic amyotrophy is preceded by vaccination, especially against tetanus, but it is difficult to prove a cause-and-effect relationship in individual cases (Fenichel, 1982). Other associations are summarized in Table 24.1. Although this list of causes might suggest that the condition is mostly iatrogenic or preceded by infectious disease, in fact most often it occurs in healthy individuals with no antecedent events (Tsairis *et al.*, 1972).

The pathogenesis of neuralgic amyotrophy is essentially unknown, although the occasional relationship with preceding immunization or infection suggests an autoimmune disorder. Indeed, high levels of complement-fixing antibodies against peripheral nerve myelin in the acute phase of the illness were reported in three patients with neuralgic amyotrophy (compared with 25 controls) (Vriesendorp *et al.*, 1993). These

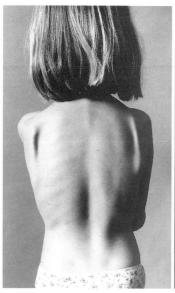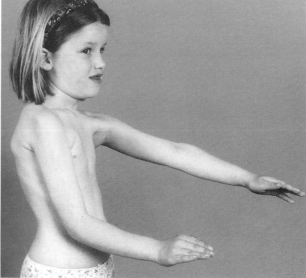

Figure 24.1
Young girl with bilateral neuralgic amyotrophy of the brachial plexus.

Table 24.1
Causal factors implicated in the pathogenesis of neuralgic amyotrophy

Injections with foreign material
- Vaccination (Allen, 1931; Gersbach and Waridel, 1976)
- Treatment with botulinum toxin A (Loh *et al.*, 1992)

Infections
- Salmonella (Neundorfer *et al.*, 1984)
- Parvovirus B19 (Pellas *et al.*, 1993), also in combination with cytomegalovirus (Maas *et al.*, 1996)
- Yersiniosis (Sotaniemi, 1983)
- Leptospirosis (Cumming *et al.*, 1978)

Surgery (Martin, 1989; Malamut *et al.*, 1994)

Parturition (Lederman and Wilbourn, 1996)

Strenuous exercise (Tsairis *et al.*, 1972)

values fell during subsequent recovery. Biopsy from the brachial plexus showed abundant, multifocal mononuclear inflammatory cell infiltrates in four patients with typical clinical features, but in whom concern about a malignant disorder had been raised by focal enlargement or enhancement of lesions on CT or MRI scans of the plexus, or by the severity or the progressive course of the disorder (Suarez *et al.*, 1996). Similar findings were reported in two patients with recurrent episodes, in one patient together with evidence of microvasculitis (Cusimano *et al.*, 1988).

Clinical variants

Neuralgic amyotrophy may involve separate nerves or their branches rather than a large part of the brachial plexus, although of course the diagnosis is then more difficult because a variety of local causes has to be considered. In most of these cases the affected nerves have their origin in the brachial plexus: examples are the long thoracic nerve (Foo and Swann, 1983), the anterior interosseous nerve (Wertsch, 1992), the lateral antebrachial cutaneous nerve, the median nerve trunk, the median palmar cutaneous branch, the

suprascapular nerve, and the axillary nerve (England and Sumner, 1987; Serratrice *et al.*, 1992).

A 47-year-old man, a manual worker in the harbour of Rotterdam but currently unemployed, experienced a rather sudden and severe pain in the neck and the right shoulder and arm. The pain decreased after a fortnight. On the fifth day he could not stretch his fingers. On examination there was severe weakness of the muscles innervated by the posterior interosseous nerve. Because of the weakness of finger extension there was doubt about the strength in spreading the fingers, but two weeks after the onset of weakness needle EMG showed abnormalities not only in the muscles innervated by the interosseous posterior nerve but also in the abductor digiti quinti muscle. During the slow recovery of the finger extensors, over the course of a few months, it became unequivocally evident that there was also weakness of the interossei and abductor digiti quinti muscles of the right hand, in the territory of the ulnar nerve.

It has been proposed that in such cases the lesion is still within the corresponding fascicle of the brachial plexus rather than in the separate trunk of the nerve in question (Rennels and Ochoa, 1980). As a general explanation that view is not only far-fetched but also is contradicted by the occasional involvement of nerves outside the brachial plexus: the phrenic nerve (Schwind and Solcher, 1958; Cape and Fincham, 1965; Dinsmore *et al.*, 1985; Leys *et al.*, 1989; Mulvey *et al.*, 1993), and lower cranial nerves such as the facial nerve (Byrne, 1987), the vagus nerve (Dinsmore *et al.*, 1985), the recurrent laryngeal nerve (Sanders *et al.*, 1988), the accessory nerve (Byrne, 1987), or even the four last cranial nerves together (Pierre *et al.*, 1990).

Bilateral involvement does occur, in as many as one-third of the patients in the large series reported from the Mayo Clinic (Tsairis *et al.*, 1972); from our personal experience we estimate that the proportion of bilateral cases is, at most, 10%.

Rarely, the lumbosacral plexus may be affected (Evans *et al.*, 1981; Sander and Sharp, 1981; Marra, 1987; Refisch and van Laack, 1989; van Alfen and van Engelen, 1997).

A 71-year-old man received an influenza vaccination in his right buttock. Two days later he experienced, with abrupt onset, severe pain in the ventral part of the right thigh, radiating laterally and anteriorly to the knee. Two hours later he was no longer able to walk because of the pain. Coughing or straining did not increase the pain. Ten days after the onset of the pain he noted weakness of his right leg. Examination on that same day showed moderate weakness of the right iliopsoas, quadriceps and adductor muscles. The right knee jerk and right adductor jerk were absent. Sensation was entirely normal. The mobility of the lumbar spine was unimpaired. When the right leg was passively extended in the hip the pain increased.

The following investigations were normal or negative: erythrocyte sedimentation rate, fasting blood sugar, antibodies against *Treponema pallidum* and *Borrelia burgdorferi*, cerebrospinal fluid (including immunoglobin G index), plain radiographs of the pelvis and lumbar spine, CT of the pelvis, retroperitoneal space, and lumbar spine, and contrast myelography (this was in 1988). Three weeks after the onset of weakness, needle EMG showed signs of denervation in the right quadriceps and adductor muscles, without involvement of the paraspinal muscles.

Four weeks after the onset of the first symptoms the pain started to decrease spontaneously. Three months after onset the pain had completely disappeared, and after six months muscle strength in the right leg had returned to normal.

Normally episodes of neuralgic amyotrophy do not recur, but inevitably there are exceptions (Bradley *et al.*, 1975; Dinsmore *et al.*, 1985; Michotte *et al.*, 1988).

Familial neuralgic amyotrophy is inherited as an autosomal dominant trait. In these cases the attacks tend to recur, but otherwise follow the usual pattern of episodes, with pain, followed by weakness and atrophy predominantly involving the shoulder and arm, and less commonly the recurrent laryngeal nerve (vocal cords), other cranial nerves, the leg, or axial musculature. Congenital anomalies, particularly hypotelorism and syndactyly, are common in affected members of these families. Attacks may start in childhood (Dunn *et al.*, 1978). The episodes may be precipitated by pregnancy or non-specific illness (Geiger *et al.*, 1974; Arts *et al.*, 1983). At autopsy the peripheral and central nervous system shows only non-specific changes (Arts *et al.*, 1983). In one family, only the long thoracic nerve was involved (Phillips, 1986). The disorder is associated with a mutation on distal chromosome 17q (Pellegrino *et al.*, 1996; Stögbauer *et al.*, 1997; Wehnert *et al.*, 1997), and is genetically distinct from hereditary neuropathy with liability to pressure palsies (Chance *et al.*, 1994; Gouider *et al.*, 1994). A case report of a woman with relapsing bilateral brachial plexopathy during pregnancy, without a family history, may well have represented a new mutation (Redmond *et al.*, 1989).

Differential diagnosis

The typical history and the clinical findings mentioned above usually leave little doubt about the diagnosis of the idiopathic form of amyotrophic neuralgia. If a painful disorder of the brachial plexus develops after the wearing of a heavy backpack (rucksack paralysis), the distinction from direct mechanical injury to the brachial plexus is difficult, especially since physical exercise is thought to be one of the many factors that may precipitate neuralgic amyotrophy (Tsairis *et al.*, 1972). The line of division becomes even more vague when the weakness is confined to the serratus anterior muscle, as isolated lesions of the long thoracic nerve may form part of the clinical spectrum of neuralgic amyotrophy (Foo and Swann, 1983; England and Sumner, 1987). Compression during sleep is unlikely if the patient has severe pain. Guillain–Barré disease almost invariably involves the legs first, while pain is only rarely a prominent feature. Multifocal motor neuropathy is bilateral (although asymmetrical), painless, and slower in onset. Lead poisoning may also cause (bilateral) painless brachial neuropathy (Antonini *et al.*, 1989). Painful lesions of the brachial plexus may result from radiation therapy (Malow and Dawson, 1991).

The spinal fluid is normal, but in some cases the total protein content is slightly elevated. This may help to exclude poliomyelitis, if the clinical and geographical features make this necessary. Radiological investigations are rarely necessary.

Needle EMG often provides evidence of multifocal axonal lesions within the brachial plexus or its branches, but may also be suggestive of an individual peripheral nerve lesion (England and Sumner, 1987; Wertsch, 1992). Examinations of the paraspinal muscles are usually normal. There may be some slowing of motor conduction to proximal muscles and sensory nerve action potential amplitudes may be reduced (Flaggman and Kelly, 1980).

Prognosis

The painful episode seldom lasts longer than one or two weeks. In contrast, the weakness may not recover until after many months, or sometimes even years. In one study, 32 of 44 patients still showed some degree of motor deficit after 1–17 years of follow-up (Huffmann, 1973). In another series of 99 patients, functional recovery had occurred in 36% within one year, in 75% within two years, and 89% had recovered by the end of the third year (Tsairis *et al.*, 1972). In this same series weakness of the shoulder muscles had recovered in 60% by the end of the first year, whereas no patient with predominantly lower plexus involvement had reached normal function. Paralysis of the diaphragm may persist up to 30 years later (Leys *et al.*, 1989).

Treatment

No effective treatment is known for this disorder. Given the reasonably good prognosis success can be claimed for almost any intervention, given it is started before the onset of spontaneous recovery. Of course corticosteroids have been tried, but no convincing evidence about their efficacy has been reported. If the shoulder muscles are involved to such an extent that elevation of the shoulder has become impaired, it is important to order passive (and later active) exercises of the shoulder joint to prevent a 'frozen shoulder' syndrome.

Chapter 25
Hereditary neuropathy with liability to pressure palsies

This disorder is characterized by the familial occurrence of recurrent deficits in the territory of single or multiple peripheral nerves, after slight compression or traction (de Jong, 1947; Davies, 1954; Earl *et al.*, 1964; Staal *et al.*, 1965). Its precise incidence is unknown, but most neurologists will have encountered at least one family with this condition.

Clinical features

A characteristic example is a Dutch family in which 13 members, spanning four generations, were affected (Staal *et al.*, 1965). Many of them were employed as farmhands in digging flower bulbs; this required much squatting and kneeling, resulting in multiple episodes of peroneal palsy. In the family the disorder was therefore known as 'bulb digger's palsy'. The age of onset varied between 14 and 30 years. Peroneal palsies also occurred after sitting with crossed legs for as short a time as 15 minutes, or even without apparent cause. Many other focal neuropathies also occurred in this family, involving the radial, median, ulnar, suprascapular and supraorbital nerves.

The episodes are always painless. Sometimes not a single peripheral nerve but the entire brachial plexus is involved (Bosch *et al.*, 1980; Martinelli *et al.*, 1989). A few years after the report about the family referred to above (Staal *et al.*, 1965), one of us saw a young man from the fourth generation with a severe but transient lesion of one brachial plexus after he had carried his little brother's small and lightweight bicycle on his shoulder for only 10 minutes. Recovery is the rule with all variants. Only after repeated episodes may some degree of deficit remain, for example a drop foot with muscle atrophy. Also, tendon reflexes may become negative. In a clinical variant of this neuropathy, reported in five siblings, the palsies were painful and associated with episodes of abdominal colic (Trockel *et al.*, 1983); genetic mapping was not possible at the time.

Genetics

The pattern of inheritance is autosomal dominant. In some families the disorder predominates in males (Staal *et al.*, 1965), which may be explained by a difference in everyday activities, as no evidence has since emerged to support the notion of incomplete expression in females (Meier and Moll, 1982). The underlying chromosomal abnormality is a large interstitial deletion at chromosome 17p11.2–12 (Chance *et al.*, 1993). The deleted region appears uniform in unrelated pedigrees (Chance *et al.*, 1993; Ohnishi *et al.*, 1995). It includes the gene for peripheral myelin protein 22 (PMP-22) and in fact all markers that are known to map with the duplication in type 1A of hereditary motor and sensory neuropathy

(HMSN 1A); also, the breakpoints appear to be similar (Chance *et al.*, 1993). This suggests that the two disorders may be reciprocal products of unequal crossover during meiosis: hereditary neuropathy with liability to pressure palsies with a single allele (monosomy, through deletion) and HMSN IA with three alleles (trisomy, through reduplication). *De novo* mutations have been reported (Reisecker *et al.*, 1994; Gonnaud *et al.*, 1995). The genetic relationship between the two diseases may explain why some patients show the phenotype of a symmetrical demyelinating sensorimotor neuropathy, after a series of pressure palsies (Staal *et al.*, 1965), or sometimes as the presenting feature, without previous history (Mancardi *et al.*, 1995). Recurrent episodes of acute, ascending, symmetrical sensorimotor polyneuropathy have also been associated with tomaculous neuropathy, in a single patient, but at that time presence of the mutation could not yet be verified (Joy and Oh, 1989).

Morphology

The morphological characteristics of this disorder are focal, large, sausage-shaped thickenings ('tomacula') of the myelin sheath after teasing and staining of individual nerve fibres in biopsy specimens of the sural or another cutaneous nerve (Behse *et al.*, 1972; Bradley *et al.*, 1975). These abnormalities are also found in carriers in whom pressure palsies have not yet occurred (Verhagen *et al.*, 1993). On electron microscopic study, the tomacula correspond to regions of uncompacted myelin lamellae, folded back longitudinally or circumferentially (Yoshikawa and Dyck, 1991).

Electrophysiological studies

At the site of nerve compression, findings are not different from those found with non-inherited compression palsies: local slowing and conduction block. In severe cases secondary signs of denervation will be found. The crucial finding is the co-existence of mild to moderate slowing of nerve conduction in clinically unaffected nerves (Earl *et al.*, 1964; Staal *et al.*, 1965; Behse *et al.*, 1972; Bradley *et al.*, 1975; Verhagen *et al.*, 1993). Most conduction blocks are found at classical sites such as the ulnar groove or the fibular head. These blocks may last for weeks, months, or even several years, and may be recurrent (Magistris and Roth, 1985). Hereditary neuropathy with liability to pressure palsies is the only hereditary neuropathy in which conduction blocks occur. With regard to the distinction from hereditary brachial plexus neuropathy, it is important that the latter is a focal axonal disorder (Dunn *et al.* 1978).

Differential diagnosis

The only condition that may be confused with hereditary neuropathy with liability to pressure palsies is the hereditary form of neuralgic amyotrophy. The locus for this disorder is unknown, but it is genetically distinct from hereditary neuralgic amyotrophy (Chance *et al.*, 1994; Gouider *et al.*, 1994). Although the brachial plexus may be involved in hereditary neuropathy with liability to pressure palsies, this is always painless and other mononeuropathies are bound to occur (Bosch *et al.*, 1980).

Management

Although there is no effective treatment it is important that patients and their siblings should know about the practical implications of the diagnosis. Genetic counselling is possible to identify children who are possibly affected (Mandich *et al.*, 1995; Gonnaud *et al.*, 1995). They should avoid sitting with crossed legs, wearing rucksacks or choosing certain professions, for example work where frequent kneeling is necessary. In the case of operations, anaesthetists need to be informed that limbs should be positioned even more carefully than usual. Obviously, decompressive operations for acute peripheral nerve deficits are superfluous, as are injections with corticosteroids.

Chapter 26
Infectious neuropathies

Mononeuropathies as a result of infectious diseases ('neuritis' in its true sense) occur mostly with leprosy, more rarely with the acquired immune deficiency syndrome (Fuller *et al.*, 1993) and, exceptionally, with bacterial infections (Banerjee *et al.*, 1993). Herpes zoster and borreliosis will be briefly discussed, although these infections tend to affect nerve roots rather than limb nerves; we shall also refer to diphtheria, in which cranial nerves may be involved.

Leprosy

This infection occurs in many parts of the world, mostly in tropical regions but also in the cooler areas of China, Japan and Korea (Sabin *et al.*, 1993). In some areas the prevalence is as high as 1% or more; the total prevalence is now estimated at 5.5 million, which is about half of the number between the mid-1960s and mid-1980s, thanks to the introduction of multi-drug therapy by the World Health Organization (Noordeen *et al.*, 1992). The world annual case detection rate remains at around 600 000 new patients, many being at an early stage of the disease (Waters and Jacobs, 1996). It is unknown why it has disappeared in Europe. The disease should still be suspected in immigrants, and also in Europeans who return home after having lived in an endemic area for years (see case history on page 130). The incubation period is at least three years, and often longer (Shepard, 1982).

Clinical features

Sensory loss is the leading symptom; it precedes paralysis in all types of leprosy (Sabin *et al.*, 1993). The first symptoms are non-specific and consist of paraesthesia, pruritus and pain. *Mycobacterium leprae* is the only microorganism that selectively enters the small sensory intracutaneous nerve endings, leading to granulomatous inflammation with thickening of the affected nerve or nerves. In the tuberculoid (localized) form of the disease the bacteria slowly proliferate and often involve only a single nerve; the lepromatous form is extensive and diffuse, with many bacilli present and a high infectivity. At an early stage the infection often causes patchy hypopigmentation of the skin, with analgesia. However, depigmentation is not always present, and in such cases the delay in the correct diagnosis may be extensive, especially in Europe.

In the tuberculoid form the bacilli slowly spread from the intracutaneous nerve endings in a centripetal direction to thicker parts of the nerve. Eventually, motor branches are also affected. The most frequently affected nerves are the posterior tibial nerve (sensory), the ulnar and median nerves, and the common peroneal nerve (Schmutzhard *et al.*, 1984;

Van Brakel and Khawas, 1994; Richardus *et al.*, 1996). The superficial branch of the radial nerve is involved only later in the disease, but in one of our own patients it was the second nerve to be infected, after the posterior tibial nerve (see case history on page 130). Even if the disease is clinically arrested, acid-fast bacilli can still be demonstrated many years later (Job *et al.*, 1997).

If nerves are infected at well-known entrapment points (the carpal tunnel, the ulnar groove, or the tarsal tunnel), swelling of the nerve may cause secondary compression and dysfunction.

Diagnosis

Often one or more peripheral nerves in superficial locations are thickened over part of their course. Careful palpation, by brushing the skin with a fingertip, may disclose the characteristic enlargements, which are fusiform and tender. It is perhaps unnecessary to add that one needs to have palpated normal nerves regularly enough to recognize thickening of nerves. Special attention should be given to the ulnar nerve at the elbow, the peroneal nerve at the head of the fibula, and the greater auricular nerve in the neck. When, clinically, only a single nerve seems affected, nerve conduction studies may demonstrate involvement of other nerves. The presence of hypopigmented areas greatly increases the probability of leprosy; obviously this is relatively difficult to ascertain in whites. Perception of pain is lost early in affected areas, whereas distinction between blunt and sharp objects may still be intact; position sense and vibration sense are similarly preserved modalities. The skin lesions are often anhidrotic. If fingers and toes are involved these may show painless ulcerations.

For a definitive diagnosis acid-fast bacilli must be demonstrated. If skin biopsy is uninformative, biopsy of a sensory nerve is often necessary. If more diffuse involvement is suspected, stained smears of nasal swabs may be worthwhile, since bacilli are often transmitted via nasal secretions (Padma and Bhatia, 1983). A modern approach is DNA amplification by means of the polymerase chain reaction (Warndorff *et al.*, 1996).

Differential diagnosis

Thickening of nerves may also occur with hypertrophic forms of hereditary neuropathies, von Recklinghausen's disease, Refsum's disease (phytanic acid deficiency), or amyloidosis. With the first two disorders other members of the family will often be affected, as these disorders are inherited with an autosomal dominant pattern; Refsum's disease (autosomal recessive) and amyloidosis (various patterns) may occur in only a single member of a family.

Treatment

The World Health Organization recommended a multidrug therapy regimen for multibacillary leprosy patients in 1982 which was to be administered for a minimum period of two years or until a skin smear was negative for acid-fast bacilli, whichever was later. This regimen contains rifampin, dapsone and clofazimine (Shepard, 1982).

Human immunodeficiency virus infection

Peripheral neuropathies with HIV-1 infection occur especially in late stages of the disease (Barohn *et al.*, 1993; Ghika Schmid *et al.*, 1994); not infrequently the central nervous system is also involved (Hall *et al.*, 1991). The most common patterns involve several rather than single nerves. Six subtypes of peripheral neuropathy can be distinguished: acute inflammatory demyelinating polyneuropathy; chronic inflammatory demyelinating polyneuropathy;

mononeuritis multiplex; an axonal, predominantly sensory, painful polyneuropathy; a sensory ataxic neuropathy due to ganglioneuronitis; and an inflammatory polyradiculoneuropathy presenting as cauda equina syndrome (Dalakas and Pezeshkpour, 1988). To differentiate between these various types of nerve involvement, electromyographic and nerve conduction studies are helpful (Lange, 1994). Demyelination in sural nerve specimens can be found even in asymptomatic patients, during life (de la Monte *et al.*, 1988) or at autopsy (Mah *et al.*, 1988).

The symmetrical inflammatory forms of neuropathy may be caused by necrotizing arteritis of the vasa nervorum, secondary to perivascular replication of virus in infiltrating mononuclear cells (Gherardi *et al.*, 1989a). Widespread multiple mononeuropathy may occur in patients with AIDS with CD4 counts less than 50 and it is then usually caused by cytomegalovirus (CMV) infection; these neuropathies are usually progressive unless antiviral treatment is given. Progressive polyradiculopathy usually also occurs in patients with AIDS and low CD4 counts. If the cerebrospinal fluid has a polymorphonuclear pleocytosis, CMV infection is almost always present, and progression is expected unless ganciclovir therapy is started promptly (de Gans *et al.*, 1990; Simpson and Olney, 1992; Roullet *et al.*, 1994).

Isolated *mononeuropathies* without apparent local compression have been reported in the lateral cutaneous nerve of the thigh, the common peroneal nerve, the median nerve and the facial nerve (Fuller *et al.*, 1993; Mumenthaler and Schliack, 1993); bilateral radial nerve palsy may be a manifestation of multiple mononeuropathy (Sturzenegger and Rutz, 1990).

Herpes zoster

Varicella-zoster virus is a ubiquitous infectious agent. Over 90% of the adult population in the western world is infected with the virus, against approximately 50% in tropical countries. Transmission is largely through inhalation of infectious aerosols; direct contact with active varicella or zoster lesions less often leads to infection (Straus, 1994). The incubation period is 10–21 days. The primary infection in the non-immune host is chickenpox (shingles). After the acute, often trivial, primary infection in childhood, the virus becomes latent in nerve cells.

In the 'immune' host, reactivation of the virus results in zoster, a predominantly dermatomal infection. The annual incidence of herpes zoster is between 150 and 225 per 100 000 general population (Glynn *et al.*, 1990; Donahue *et al.*, 1995; Paul and Thiel, 1996). Only 5% of cases occur in children under 15 years of age; the chance of acquiring zoster rises with age. Overall, at least 20% of all adults suffer from zoster at some time. The risk of zoster is greatly enhanced by immunosuppression or in patients infected with HIV (Balfour *et al.*, 1983; Guiloff, 1989).

Clinical features

Herpes zoster involves truncal roots in more than 50% of patients, followed by cervical (17%), lumbar (10%) and sacral dermatomes (5%); the trigeminal nerve is infected in 12% (Glynn *et al.*, 1990). Pain and sometimes paraesthesia may be present for up to three weeks before skin eruptions become manifest. Subtle skin lesions may be hidden in skin folds and can be missed on superficial inspection. The disease may be accompanied by low-grade fever, general malaise, headache, sometimes neck stiffness, or regional swelling of lymph nodes. The pain usually abates after the skin has healed, but 10–20% of patients develop the dreaded complication of post-herpetic neuralgia.

Apart from pain and sensory loss in affected dermatomes, other neurological complications infrequently supervene. Limb weakness through concomitant infection of ventral roots ('segmental zoster paresis') is uncommon, occurring in 3–5% of patients with cutaneous zoster (Thomas and Howard, 1972; Merchut and Gruener, 1996). In many more patients, however, EMG studies of paraspinal muscles show evidence of motor denervation (Greenberg *et al.*, 1992). Recovery occurs in 75%, but may take as long as two years. Much more rare complications are brachial plexus neuropathy (Fabian *et al.*, 1997), myelitis, encephalitis, acute ascending polyradiculopathy, and cerebral infarction via infiltration of major vessels (Elliott, 1994). Some degree of aseptic meningitis is often, although not always, present, at least in the early stages. *Mononeuropathies* are definitely rare and may affect the median, ulnar, long thoracic, recurrent laryngeal or phrenic nerves (Merchut and Gruener, 1996).

Treatment

Acyclovir (800 mg five times a day) and related drugs are the drugs of choice for herpes zoster, especially in immunocompromised patients in whom they are given intravenously rather than orally (Balfour *et al.*, 1983). Acyclovir shortens the period with pain and skin lesions, and a meta-analysis of five adequate trials has suggested this treatment also halves the incidence of post-herpetic neuralgia (Jackson *et al.*, 1997). Recently, valaciclovir and famciclovir have become available; because of their better bioavailability, the dosing schedule with these drugs can be reduced to three times daily (Gnann, 1994). Combining acyclovir with oral prednisolone does not prevent the occurrence of post-herpetic neuralgia (Esmann *et al.*, 1987; Wood, 1994).

The pain of postherpetic neuralgia can be decreased by application of a 5% lidocaine gel, as shown in a controlled study (Rowbotham *et al.*, 1995). A solution of acetylsalicylic acid has also been recommended, although with less solid evidence (King, 1993); chlorophorm is a potentially toxic solvent, and alcohol is the preferred medium (van Horssen, 1995).

Lyme borreliosis

Lyme borreliosis is a complex multi-system infection with worldwide distribution (Steere, 1989). The disorder is caused by the spirochaete, *Borrelia burgdorferi*, which is transmitted by ticks of the *Ixodes ricinus* complex. Certain species of mice are critical in the life cycle of the spirochaete, and deer or sheep appear to be crucial to the tick; infected ticks are found especially in forested areas. Lyme disease commonly begins in summer with a characteristic skin lesion, erythema migrans, accompanied by flu-like or meningitis-like symptoms. Weeks or months later, the patient may have neurologic or cardiac abnormalities, migratory musculoskeletal pain, or arthritis, and more than a year after onset some patients have chronic joint, skin or neurologic abnormalities. Diagnosis in these late stages is not straightforward, if only because about half of the patients do not remember a tick bite. Also, skin manifestations may have been lacking or unobtrusive (Reik, *et al.*, 1986).

The two most common patterns of neuropathy are symmetrical distal, non-painful paraesthesia, and asymmetric radicular pain, with plexopathy or multiple mononeuritis in only a minority (Pachner and Steere, 1985; Halperin *et al.*, 1990; Logigian and Steere, 1992). Mononeuropathies in the limbs are definitely infrequent, with the exception of carpal tunnel syndrome (Halperin *et al.*, 1989). In contrast, cranial neuropathies are often seen, especially facial palsy on one or both sides (Kindstrand, 1995). In all these neuropathies the pattern of electrophysiological abnormalities is indicative of axonal damage (Halperin *et al.*, 1990).

After the first several weeks of infection, almost all patients have a positive antibody response to the spirochaete. However, the seroconversion may have taken place in the distant past, and the diagnosis of active neuroborreliosis should always be supported by the demonstration of pleiocytosis in the cerebrospinal fluid (Finkel and Halperin, 1992).

For the treatment of neuroborreliosis ceftriaxone is more efficacious than high-dose penicillin (Dattwyler *et al.*, 1988).

Diphtheria

Although rigorous vaccination programmes have nearly eradicated diphtheria in many western countries, outbreaks do occur, not only in developing countries but also in Eastern Europe (Sasse *et al.*, 1994), and adult travellers who are no longer fully immune may import the disease after a visit to these regions (Lumio *et al.*, 1993).

Two to three weeks after the primary throat infection, multiple cranial nerves may be affected; in these cases cranial nerve involvement is inevitably followed after 8–12 weeks by a motor and sensory polyneuropathy (Scheid, 1952; Fisher and Adams, 1956). Exceptionally, the clinical picture is that of acute inflammatory demyelinating polyneuropathy (Creange *et al.*, 1995).

Chapter 27

Multiple mononeuropathy

Multiple mononeuropathy (mononeuritis multiplex) occurs with many systemic diseases. It may be the presenting feature of the underlying disease, which is often a form of vasculitis (Moore and Fauci, 1981; Kissel *et al.*, 1985; Said *et al.*, 1988; Chalk *et al.*, 1993). Vasculitis affecting the peripheral nervous system may also give rise to symmetric polyneuropathy (Davies *et al.*, 1996); in polyarteritis nodosa and Wegener's granulomatosis this pattern is as common as multiple mononeuropathy (Moore and Cupps, 1983).

Clinical features

Several peripheral or cranial nerves become involved one after another, within days or weeks. The main symptoms are paraesthesia, pain, sensory loss and weakness. The more nerves become involved, the more the clinical deficits resemble those of polyneuropathy. Signs and symptoms of the underlying systemic disease may or may not accompany those of the neurological deficits.

Electrophysiological studies

In most cases electrophysiological studies in vasculitic neuropathy show typical changes of an axonal neuropathy. Needle EMG of the involved muscles will demonstrate signs of denervation and reinnervation. Nerve conduction velocities are normal or mildly decreased; the amplitudes of the sensory potentials and compound muscle action potentials may be reduced. In a minority of cases conduction blocks may be found (Ropert and Metral, 1990; Jamieson *et al.*, 1991).

Causes

Vasculitis is the most frequent condition underlying mononeuritis multiplex, but blood diseases or inflammatory conditions should be considered as well (Table 27.1). If the affected nerves lie close together, of course imaging studies are necessary to exclude local mass lesions. A few common (vasculitic) causes are considered separately below (Moore and Cupps, 1983; Lockwood, 1996). In all these forms the mainstay of treatment consists of corticosteroids, although this notion is not backed up by evidence from controlled clinical trials.

Vasculitis

Polyarteritis nodosa

Polyarteritis nodosa is a vasculitis of medium-sized arteries. The clinical manifestations reflect the size of vessel involved: the gastrointestinal, renal or cerebral vasculature may be involved. Peripheral neuropathy is seen in

Table 27.1
Causes of multiple mononeuropathy

Vasculitis
- Polyarteritis nodosa (Walker, 1978)
- Allergic granulomatosis and angiitis (Churg-Strauss syndrome) (Moore *et al.*, 1985; Marazzi *et al.*, 1992; Kurita *et al.*, 1994; Shintani *et al.*, 1995)
- Connective tissue disorders
  - Rheumatoid arthritis (Chang *et al.*, 1984; Schneider *et al.*, 1985; Puechal *et al.*, 1995)
  - Sjögren syndrome (Andonopoulos *et al.*, 1990; Hebbar *et al.*, 1995)
  - Systemic lupus erythematosus (Hughes *et al.*, 1982)
- Wegener's granulomatosis (Baker and Robinson, 1978; Nishino *et al.*, 1993a,b; Finkelman *et al.*, 1993; Sheldon, 1994)
- Vasculitis associated with cryoglobulinaemia (Konishi *et al.*, 1982; Peppard *et al.*, 1986; Vital *et al.*, 1988; Thomas *et al.*, 1992; Murai *et al.*, 1995), sometimes in association with HIV infection (Stricker *et al.*, 1992)
- Giant cell arteritis (Feigal *et al.*, 1985; Golbus and McCune, 1987; McAlindon and Ferguson, 1989)
- Behçet's disease (Takeuchi *et al.*, 1989)
- Non-systemic vasculitis of peripheral nerves (Dyck *et al.*, 1987)
- Angiitis associated with amphetamine use (Stafford *et al.*, 1975)
- Paraneoplastic vasculitis (Johnson, P.C. *et al.*, 1979)

Haematological disorders
- Acute myeloid leukaemia (Lekos *et al.*, 1994)
- Myelodysplastic syndrome (Shiozawa *et al.*, 1991)
- Plasmocytoma (Gherardi *et al.*, 1989b)
- Paraproteinaemia (Yee *et al.*, 1989)
- Waldenstrom's macroglobulinaemia (Fraser *et al.*, 1976; Tassin *et al.*, 1980)
- Lymphoma (Roux *et al.*, 1995), angioimmunoblastic lymphadenopathy (Ferrer *et al.*, 1988)

Infections or other inflammatory disorders
- Meningococcal septicaemia (Roig *et al.*, 1985)
- Infective endocarditis (Lazzarino *et al.*, 1994)
- Cutaneous polyarthritis, in children (Draaisma *et al.*, 1992)
- Non-vasculitic, steroid-responsive form (Logigian *et al.*, 1993)
- Sarcoidosis (Kompf *et al.*, 1976; Vital *et al.*, 1982; Zuniga *et al.*, 1991)

Miscellaneous conditions
- Diabetes (see Chapter 28)
- Neurofibromatosis (see Chapter 30)
- Jellyfish stings (Filling-Katz, 1984)

approximately 50% of patients, mostly in the form of multiple mononeuritis or a symmetrical polyneuropathy (Walker, 1978). Moderate to severe hypertension is common. Circulating anti-neutrophil cytoplasmic antibodies (cANCA) are rarely found, and when present may indicate the coincident development of the smaller vessel vasculitis. In the same patients lupus anticoagulant may be found (Cohney *et al.*, 1995), or an associated α-1-antitrypsin deficiency (Fortin *et al.*, 1991).

The disease may present at any age and is more common in men (men/women 2 : 1). General malaise, with tachycardia, fever and weight loss is frequent; these symptoms may be accompanied by striking clinical signs such as an acute abdomen, myocardial infarction, stroke or severe hypertension. Biopsy of affected tissue helps to establish the diagnosis; in the case of mononeuritis multiplex, the biopsy is of muscle or the sural nerve.

The prognosis in untreated patients is poor. With corticosteroid therapy, partial to complete recovery of neurological function occurs in about half the patients, over months or a few years (Chalk *et al.*, 1993).

Churg–Strauss syndrome

This vasculitic syndrome is characterized by granulomatous necrotizing vasculitis, which predominantly affects the lungs and, to a lesser extent, other organs. Typically, patients present with a prodromal phase with asthma and eosinophilia before the onset of systemic vasculitis, which may include neurological deficits corresponding to single or multiple peripheral nerves. Fulminant forms may resemble Guillain–Barré syndrome (Ng *et al.*, 1997). In a large series of 30 patients, peripheral nerves were involved in 19 (Chumbley *et al.*, 1977).

A 26-year-old woman one day felt paraesthesia of the lateral part of the lower leg. Two days later this was followed by a drop foot, while paraesthesia changed to pain; within two or three weeks the pain moved to the region of first and second toe. During this entire period she suffered from malaise, night sweats and some loss of weight. During that same summer, one or two months before, she had a brief spell of red spots on both her legs. Her previous history included severe asthmatic bronchitis, with a recent exacerbation for which she was treated with prednisone (120 mg/day) and bronchodilating agents. On examination there was weakness of the left tibialis anterior, extensor hallucis longus and peroneus muscles, but also of the tibialis posterior muscle. Skin sensation was impaired over the lateral part of the lower leg and the dorsum of the foot. The left ankle jerk was absent. She was admitted for a series of investigations: erythrocyte sedimentation rate 55 mm; leukocytes 12.7×10^9/l, with 11% eosinophilic cells; cerebrospinal fluid normal; MRI scan of lumbosacral area normal. Within one week after admission her asthmatic symptoms deteriorated and she developed a dark-red rash over both legs, with large and confluent lesions. The proportion of eosinophilic cells had increased to 43%, and a skin biopsy showed extensive perivascular infiltrates with eosinophilic cells and granulocytic cells. Steroid treatment was increased to massive doses of dexamethasone; despite this she suddenly died four days later. Autopsy showed severe, predominantly eosinophilic, infiltration of the myocardium, pericardium, lungs, pleural cavity, spleen and lymph nodes.

Confirmation comes from demonstration of vasculitis on biopsy, in which the affected tissues frequently show eosinophilic infiltrates.

Rheumatoid arthritis

Polyneuropathy and, especially, multiple mononeuritis is a rare complication of rheumatoid arthritis (Chang *et al.*, 1984; Schneider *et al.*, 1985; Puechal *et al.*, 1995). Vasculitis secondary to rheumatoid arthritis is associated with long-standing disease, seropositivity and florid subcutaneous nodule formation. It may affect small arteries, arterioles, capillaries and venules, and often causes little in the way of symptoms. At the time of death one-quarter of patients show evidence of systemic vasculitis (Peyronnard *et al.*, 1982; Endtz *et al.*, 1983). One should keep in mind that joint deformities and synovial swelling may lead to entrapment neuropathies (Pallis and Scott, 1965); of course such deficits should not be attributed to vasculitis. If multiple mononeuritis does occur with rheumatoid arthritis, the outcome is not necessarily poor (Chang *et al.*, 1984; Vollertsen *et al.*, 1986).

Systemic lupus erythematosus

Neurological complications are common in this non-organ-specific autoimmune disorder, especially effects on the brain and spinal cord (Feinglass *et al.*, 1976; Wong *et al.*, 1991). Yet involvement of the peripheral nervous system is occasionally the presenting feature (Bloch *et al.*, 1979; Hughes *et al.*, 1982; Millette *et al.* 1986; Tola *et al.*, 1992). Peripheral neuropathy may show the pattern of multiple mononeuritis or of chronic inflammatory polyneuropathy, with a tendency to spontaneous recovery (McCombe *et al.*, 1987).

Giant-cell arteritis

Giant-cell (cranial, senile or temporal) arteritis is rare before the age of 50 years and chiefly affects those aged 65–75 years with a male/female ratio of 1 : 2. The malaise, fever and anaemia are similar to those in polymyalgia rheumatica; the differences are in the vascular symptoms. The majority of patients have temporal features, with headache, scalp sensitivity and tender thickened arteries.

Overwhelming generalized headache and the feared complication of irreversible loss of vision are more readily recognized. If the peripheral nervous system is involved, not only may multiple mononeuritis accompany the disorder (Feigal *et al.*, 1985; Golbus and McCune, 1987; McAlindon and Ferguson, 1989), but also mononeuropathy (Caselli *et al.*, 1988) or polyneuropathy (Golbus and McCune, 1987; Caselli *et al.*, 1988). Corticosteroids quickly lead to impressive recovery of the systemic as well as of the neurological complications. This treatment should often be continued for many months, or even years; the ESR is a useful measure for titration of dosage.

Wegener's granulomatosis

Wegener's granulomatosis is a systemic necrotizing vasculitis characterized by granulomatous vasculitis of the respiratory tract, with or without glomerulonephritis or arthralgia. Peripheral neuropathy may accompany this disorder in a symmetric form (Baker and Robinson, 1978; Nishino *et al.*, 1993a) as well as in the form of multiple mononeuropathy (Baker and Robinson, 1978; Finkelman *et al.*, 1993; Sheldon, 1994). Other patterns of neurological involvement are cranial neuropathy, external ophthalmoplegia, cerebrovascular events, seizures, cerebritis, aseptic meningitis, myelitis and diabetes insipidus (Drachman, 1963; Anderson *et al.*, 1975; Nishino *et al.*, 1993a). Both cranial and peripheral neuropathies may occur transiently, resolving over a period of hours (Moore and Cupps, 1983).

Behçet's disease

Behçet's disease is characterized by relapsing ocular lesions and recurrent oral and genital ulcers. Small-vessel vasculitis with mononuclear cell infiltrate is common and can be demonstrated in the skin, in gastrointestinal ulcers, and occasionally in the central nervous system. Neurological abnormalities include meningoencephalitis, corticospinal tract involvement, pseudo-tumour, cerebellar ataxia, pseudo-bulbar palsy, paraplegia, sensory disturbances and seizures (Wolf *et al.*, 1965; Serdaroglu *et al.*, 1989); the brainstem is the most frequent site of focal disease. Peripheral neuropathy is rare; if it does occur it is in the form of multiple mononeuritis (Takeuchi *et al.*, 1989).

Sarcoidosis

Sarcoidosis is a chronic multisystem disorder histologically characterized by infiltration of affected tissues (most often the lung) by T lymphocytes and mononuclear phagocytes, with formation of non-caseating epitheloid granulomas. The causes are unknown. The nervous system is involved in approximately 5% of patients with sarcoidosis (Stern *et al.*, 1985), and the peripheral nervous system in 3% (Matthews, 1993). Cranial neuropathy is the most frequent problem, mostly involving the facial nerve, and sometimes has a fluctuating course (as may also occur in Wegener's granulomatosis).

Involvement of peripheral nerves most often takes the form of mononeuritis multiplex (Kompf *et al.*, 1976; Vital *et al.*, 1982; Zuniga *et al.*, 1991). The following combinations have been observed, for example: weakness of the serratus anterior muscle with peroneal nerve involvement, bilateral radial and median nerve palsies, slight weakness of limbs in a radicular fashion, or asymmetrically absent tendon reflexes, not parallel to motor or sensory deficit (Matthews, 1993). Mononeuritis multiplex may be accompanied by cranial nerve lesions or lesions in the central nervous system. Other patterns of peripheral nerve disorders are a symmetrical polyneuropathy (Scott *et al.*, 1993), compression of the median nerve secondary to synovitis (Bleton *et al.*, 1991), or sensory loss over large areas of the trunk (Matthews, 1993).

Sural nerve biopsy may confirm the diagnosis by showing epineurial and endoneurial granulomas, with secondary demyelination (Brochet *et al.*, 1988; Gainsborough *et al.*, 1991). Corticosteroids are again the preferred treatment, but the response is extremely variable.

Chapter 28
Mononeuropathies due to metabolic and endocrine disorders

Diabetes mellitus

The most frequent types of diabetic neuropathy are cranial neuropathies and a distal sensory and motor neuropathy, followed by *isolated peripheral nerve lesions*. These are often located at the well-known entrapment points (Johnson, 1993). Not infrequently, these are superimposed on a polyneuropathy, which may be symptomatic or clinically silent (evident only from nerve conduction studies). Often it is difficult to know whether the mononeuropathy is induced by external pressure to the nerve or whether it is purely intrinsic; that is, caused by focal ischaemia or infarction secondary to occlusion of small blood vessels supplying the nerve (Raff and Asbury, 1968). Entrapment is presumably not an important factor in femoral neuropathy, one of the commonest mononeuropathies in diabetes (mostly involving other nerves as well, see below under diabetic amyotrophy). The probability of diabetes in a patient with an unexplained femoral nerve palsy is so high that relevant tests will uncover diabetes in a large proportion of patients in whom no obvious cause is present; for example, 15 of 23 patients in a series of 44 patients with femoral neuropathy, against 11 already known to have diabetes (Lazzarino *et al.*, 1991).

Entrapment neuropathies in diabetes mostly involve ulnar, median, radial and peroneal nerves, as in patients without diabetes. Also, entrapment of the superficial branch of the radial nerve (cheiralgia paraesthetica) has been associated with diabetes mellitus (Massey and O'Brian, 1978). The onset of diabetic mononeuropathy may be acute or insidious. The gradual types are the majority and mostly concern the median nerve at the wrist or the ulnar nerve at the elbow (Fraser *et al.*, 1979). Symptomatic carpal tunnel syndrome is found in approximately 11% of patients with diabetes mellitus (Dyck *et al.*, 1993). A co-existent polyneuropathy is found in 80% of diabetic patients with an ulnar nerve palsy, versus only 20% of patients with carpal tunnel syndrome and diabetes mellitus (Fraser *et al.*, 1979).

Acute peroneal neuropathy

It is rare to see acute, painless peroneal palsy in a diabetic patient without some degree of compression. We saw two patients who, during a phase of renewed regulation of poorly controlled diabetes, within a few hours developed a subtotal deficit of the common peroneal nerve, followed by the same deficit in the other leg two days later; in both, recovery occurred in a few weeks.

A 56-year-old housewife was admitted to hospital for adjustment of her severe insulin-dependent diabetes from which she had been suffering for 25 years. One day her right foot became weak, with numbness of the lower leg, and the next day the same symptoms occurred in the other foot. Examination showed on both sides a severe but slightly asymmetrical weakness of the foot and toe extensors, and diminished skin sensation at the dorsum of the feet and the lateral part of the lower legs; tendon jerks were normal. In the course of about three weeks both peroneal nerve palsies recovered.

Brachial plexus neuropathy

A form of brachial plexus neuropathy (unilateral or bilateral) has been described in four diabetic patients with a typical radiculo-plexopathy of the legs (symmetrical or asymmetrical, see below), against the background of a generalized sensorimotor polyneuropathy (Riley and Shields, 1984). The onset was subacute in two patients and much more gradual in the others; in the subacute cases the causal relationship with diabetes is uncertain, as the pathogenesis may have been similar to that of neuralgic amyotrophy in patients without diabetes. Similarly, phrenic neuropathy in diabetic patients may be part of an otherwise asymptomatic episode of neuralgic amyotrophy, although subclinical forms of phrenic neuropathy are common in diabetics (Wolf *et al.*, 1983).

Diabetic amyotrophy

Unilateral or asymmetrical proximal neuropathy in the lower limbs is fairly typical of diabetes (Barohn *et al.*, 1991; Said *et al.*, 1994). It may occur against the background of a chronic, symmetrical polyneuropathy. Often, the femoral nerve bears the brunt of the motor deficit, but

other nerves may be affected as well. Although small infarcts are found in peripheral nerve trunks, the lumbosacral plexus may be similarly affected (Raff and Asbury, 1968), and electrophysiological studies suggest involvement of spinal roots (Bastron and Thomas, 1981). For this reason the term 'diabetic radiculo-plexopathy' has been proposed; others prefer the descriptive term 'proximal diabetic neuropathy' (Asbury, 1977) or 'lower limb asymmetric motor neuropathy' (Thomas and Tomlinson, 1993).

The syndrome mainly occurs in middle-aged or elderly diabetics. It may be the first manifestation of diabetes, but in previously diagnosed patients the diabetes may be mild and well controlled. At onset there may be severe pain at the anterior side of the thigh. The quadriceps and iliopsoas muscles are most commonly involved, with an absent knee jerk, but the adductor muscles (obturator nerve) may be weak as well. Sensory deficits are rare. There is a strong tendency towards at least some degree of recovery, beginning within weeks of onset, and the diagnosis should be in doubt if no improvement at all has occurred after several months. Enhancement of lumbar nerve roots on MRI scanning may sometimes identify autoimmune vasculitis rather than diabetes as the cause (O'Neill *et al.*, 1997). The recovery is incomplete in almost half of patients (Coppack and Watkins, 1991; Donaghy, 1991).

Truncal neuropathy

Thoracic radiculopathy (truncal neuropathy, thoracoabdominal neuropathy) is a relatively uncommon form of diabetic neuropathy (Ellenberg, 1978; Kikta *et al.*, 1982; Streib and Sun, 1984) which presents with severe pain in the chest or abdomen, often not typically radicular in character, and bilateral in about half of cases. It may be confused with an abdominal hernia or acute intra-abdominal disorders (Longstreth and Newcomer, 1977; Parry and Floberg, 1989). Often there is associated weight loss. The muscles of the abdominal wall may bulge, because the motor fibres are involved. Sensory deficits are highly variable: unilateral or bilateral, mostly involving several adjacent dermatomes, corresponding to entire spinal nerves, or to dorsal rami or ventral branches only (Stewart, 1989). The prognosis for recovery is good.

Hypothyroidism

Carpal tunnel syndrome is the most common neuropathy associated with hypothyroidism; it is often bilateral (Gelberman *et al.*, 1980). It is probably caused by myxoedematous deposits in the connective tissue of tendon sheaths and synovial membranes. Most patients improve following hormone substitution therapy; surgical section of the transverse carpal ligament is usually unnecessary (Frymoyer and Bland, 1973). Deep peroneal palsy is the only other mononeuropathy described in association with hypothyroidism (Yasuoka *et al.*, 1993).

A predominantly sensory and sometimes painful polyneuropathy may occasionally complicate hypothyroidism (Meier and Bischoff, 1977; Pollard *et al.*, 1982).

Hyperthyroidism

Mononeuropathies of the common peroneal nerve and of the lateral cutaneous nerve of the thigh have been reported in association with hyperthyroidism (Ijichi *et al.*, 1990). Thyrotoxic polyneuropathy is equally uncommon (Feibel and Campa, 1976; Florin and Walls, 1984).

Acromegaly

Carpal tunnel syndrome is a well-recognized complication of acromegaly (O'Duffy *et al.*, 1973). It occurs in about half of patients and tends to recover after pituitary surgery (Pickett *et al.*, 1975). In one of our patients, a 40-year-old nurse, the carpal tunnel syndrome preceded the other manifestations of acromegaly by several years. Other neuromuscular complications of acromegaly are myopathy (Pickett *et al.*, 1975) and a subclinical polyneuropathy, independent of the presence of diabetes (Low *et al.*, 1974).

Chapter 29
Ischaemic neuropathy

For peripheral nerve tissue to be damaged by ischaemia requires extensive compromise of blood flow to the region, in view of the richness of anastomotic connections within the nutrient arterial supply as well as in the vasa nervorum themselves (Lundborg, 1975). Extensive ligation is needed to produce experimental ischaemia (Hess *et al.*, 1979).

Sudden occlusion of a major limb artery may complicate arterial disease, often influenced by risk factors such as diabetes, hypertension and cigarette smoking, or by heart disease, most commonly atrial fibrillation, myocardial infarction or rheumatic heart disease. Embolic mononeuropathy has also been reported with bacterial endocarditis (Jones and Siekert, 1968). After the initial phase of paleness and coldness, reperfusion (for example by embolectomy) may restore the pulse, colour and temperature of the limb. Yet a distal neuropathy may remain, often with burning pain and sensory loss. This may involve a single nerve, such as peroneal neuropathy with occlusion of the femoral or popliteal arteries (Ferguson and Liversedge, 1954; Welti *et al.*, 1961) or several nerves in a single limb (ischaemic monomelic neuropathy) (Wilbourn *et al.*, 1983). A correlation exists between the level of the vascular lesion (aortic, aortoiliac or distally) and the type of peripheral nerve deficit (D'Amour *et al.*, 1987). Iatrogenic sciatic nerve lesions may result from occlusion of the femoral artery, after bypass surgery (Boontje and Haaxma, 1987), or in patients undergoing prolonged periods of intra-aortic balloon pump therapy with a catheter placed through the femoral artery ipsilateral to the sciatic nerve lesion (McManis, 1994). Improvement often takes months and may be incomplete. Haemodialysis shunts placed between the brachial artery and the antecubital vein may cause multiple brachial neuropathies (Bolton *et al.*, 1979).

Neuropathy from chronic vascular insufficiency is much less clearly defined. Atherosclerosis severe enough to produce intermittent claudication and ischaemic skin ulceration may cause mild neuropathy (Eames and Lange, 1967).

Chapter 30
Peripheral nerve tumours

Every nerve may become involved by all sorts of tumours, from metastases to lymphomas (Roncaroli *et al.*, 1997), but in this chapter we deal only with tumours originating in peripheral nerves. Table 30.1 lists the most common types. The majority of peripheral nerve tumours originate from the nerve sheath.

Clinical features

In general there is a slowly progressive mononeuropathy. Typically, an initial phase with paraesthesia is followed by motor or sensory deficits, or both. The tumour itself may be seen or felt. Signs and symptoms occur relatively early if the tumour is located in a confined space such as the carpal tunnel. With benign schwannomas the tumour is mobile from side to side but not in the vertical axis of the limb (Birch, 1993). Tomographic neuroimaging techniques may be helpful in detecting nerve tumours in deep parts

of a limb (Kchouk *et al.*, 1993; Zingale *et al.*, 1993), or even to identify fatty components as a characteristic of fibrolipoma (De Maeseneer *et al.*, 1997). Nerve conduction studies may be helpful in localizing a nerve tumour. However, the diagnostic possibilities are limited with deeply seated tumours and with tumours that cause little compression of the nerve fibres, which is usually the case with schwannomas.

Malignant transformation of nerve sheath tumours is uncommon, but if this occurs pain can be a prominent symptom. Pain and paraesthesia may be exacerbated by local pressure, such as by sitting with tumours of the sciatic nerve in the buttock, or by walking if the nerve tumour is in the foot. In addition, patients with malignant nerve sheath tumours may show general symptoms such as loss of weight or anaemia. The prognosis is generally poor because radical excision is only rarely possible. Radiation and

Table 30.1
Classification of peripheral nerve tumours (after Birch, 1993)

	Benign	Malignant
Nerve sheath tumours	Schwannoma (neurilemmoma) Solitary neurofibroma Plexiform neurofibroma Fibrolipoma	Malignant schwannoma Neurofibrosarcoma Neuroepithelioma
Neuronal tumours	Ganglioneuroma	Ganglioneuroblastoma Neuroblastoma

chemotherapy are not helpful (Birch, 1993).

Schwannomas

Schwannomas (neurilemmomas, neurinomas) arise from Schwann cells only and form encapsulated nerve sheath tumours. It is possible to extirpate these tumours without damaging the nerve. They may occur as isolated forms or associated with type 1 neurofibromatosis. In 3–5% of patients with neurofibromatosis malignant transformation of schwannomas will occur in the limbs, trunk or head (Ducatman *et al.*, 1986). In exceptional instances a neurinoma may be associated with hyperprolactinaemia (Katsuren *et al.*, 1997).

Neurofibromas

This type of tumour is made up of all cell types in perineurial tissue. Multiple benign neurofibromas occur in type 1 neurofibromatosis, in which case the tumours originate from cutaneous nerve branches. The clinical manifestations range from the asymptomatic stage to malignant transformation with dedifferentiation to neurofibrosarcoma or metastatic angiosarcoma (Macaulay, 1978). If the tumours originate from large nerves they may give rise to mononeuropathies, either single or multiple. Enucleation without sacrificing the nerve is impossible even with histologically benign tumours, because the tumour is intermingled with normal nerve fibres.

Localized hypertrophic mononeuropathy

Localized hypertrophic mononeuropathy is characterized clinically by slowly progressive motor mononeuropathy with little or no pain or numbness.

A 53-year-old man reported gradually increasing weakness of the left hand over the course of two years. He had no sensory symptoms. On examination there was severe weakness of finger extension and wrist extension (MRC grade 2). There was no atrophy, sensation was normal, and the tendon jerks were symmetrical. Percutaneous stimulation of the radial nerve halfway up the upper arm did not result in a motor response in the extensor muscles or the brachioradialis. The most proximal site where a motor response could be evoked was about 5 cm above the lateral epicondyle. In contrast, radial sensory conduction in the arm was completely normal. Needle electromyography showed no fibrillations in the weak muscles of the forearm, but much spontaneous activity in the form of fasciculations and rhythmic motor unit discharges. On maximal volition a single pattern of polyphasic motor unit potentials was obtained. Radiological studies of the left arm were unremarkable.

On surgical exploration a waxy, gray swelling of the radial nerve was found, extending from 6 to 12 cm proximally to the lateral epicondyle. At this level the nerve had not yet divided in its motor and sensory branches. The neurosurgeon refrained from attempts to extirpate the tumour completely. The biopsy specimen showed concentric onion bulb structures, mainly around smaller nerve fibres. There were no signs of inflammation. Several large fibres showed signs of myelin degeneration, and there was an increased amount of endoneural collagen.

The condition may occur with type 1 neurofibromatosis but also in an isolated form. Morphological changes consist of primary perineurial cell hyperplasia (Hawkes *et al.*, 1974; Mitsumoto *et al.*,

1980); superficially these resemble onion bulbs, as in generalized hypertrophic neuropathy, but other than in that condition the whorls are separated from each other by cells identical to those forming the whorls, and not by loose endoneurial collagen (Mitsumoto *et al.*, 1980). Almost any peripheral nerve may be affected, and even spinal roots (Yassini *et al.*, 1993). Surgical resection may be followed by some improvement (Phillips *et al.*, 1991; Taras and Melone, 1995).

Chapter 31
Injury by physical agents

Vibration

Daily work with vibrating tools such as pneumatic hammers may damage the median and ulnar nerves distal to the wrist (Farkkila *et al.*, 1985; Farkkila *et al.*, 1988). Other possible complications of pneumatic tools are the Raynaud phenomenon (Palmer and Collin, 1994) and, more controversial, spinal muscular atrophy (Gallagher and Sanders, 1983).

Lightning and electric injury

It is well known that lightning injuries may kill instantaneously, but less well known that survivors may show neurological sequelae, including peripheral nerve damage. One or more nerves in a limb may be injured directly (Savitsky and Gerson, 1942; DiVicenti *et al.*, 1969), or occasionally multiple points of entry can result in a pattern of acute polyneuropathy (Hawkes and Thorpe, 1992). Damage to the central nervous system by lightning is more common, with cerebral oedema, intracerebral haematoma (Hanson and McIlwraith, 1973; Cwinn and Cantrill, 1985) or delayed myelopathy (Davidson and Deck, 1988).

High voltage injury from other sources may lead to similar injuries to peripheral nerves (Engrav *et al.*, 1990) or the central nervous system (Grube *et al.*, 1990).

Burns and heat

Burning may cause focal neuropathy by vascular occlusion of the vasa nervorum, direct thermal injury or secondarily by scar formation (Salisbury and Dingeldein, 1982; Marquez *et al.*, 1993). In a large series of 800 patients with burns, 19 had signs and symptoms of neuropathy. Mononeuritis multiplex was the most common finding in these patients, occurring in 11; three patients (19%) had an isolated mononeuropathy, one a radiculopathy and one a generalized axonal polyneuropathy, which may have been caused by a disseminated neurotoxin (Marquez *et al.*, 1993). Mononeuritis multiplex was also the most common pattern of neuropathy in another series (Dagum *et al.*, 1993); nerves can be affected in burned and unburned areas.

Heat injury of hand nerves, either single or multiple, may follow injudicious use of microwave ovens (Dickason and Barutt, 1984; Marchiori *et al.*, 1995). An iatrogenic thermal lesion of the sciatic nerve may be caused during operations, by overheating of an electrode placed on the dorsal side of the thigh (Mumenthaler and Schliack, 1993).

Cold

Exposure to cold may lead to sensory symptoms and, subsequently, to permanent nerve damage in the limbs, with motor and sensory deficits. This occurs not only with frost-bite but also after prolonged chilling short of freezing. Examples are: the so-called 'trench foot' in the First World War, from prolonged exposure to water, cold and mud in the trenches; and 'immersion foot' in the Second World War, in shipwreck survivors in northern seas. The affected limbs are numb and weak, with swollen tissues that may eventually become necrotic. The motor and sensory deficits occur distally, in the territory of several and not single nerves (Ungley *et al.*, 1945). An iatrogenic form of nerve damage by cold is phrenic nerve injury in heart surgery, by the use of iced slush for topical hypothermia (Rousou *et al.*, 1985; Efthimiou *et al.*, 1991).

Abnormal sensitivity to cold may occur in a syndrome of cold hyperalgesia associated with cold hypaesthesia, in patients with peripheral polyneuropathy or mononeuropathy of various causes (Ochoa and Yarnitsky, 1994). The presumed explanation is sensory disinhibition, where diminished input from cold-specific A-δ fibres releases cold pain input carried by C nociceptors.

Radiation

Therapeutic X-rays, cobalt therapy and radioisotopes may all lead to nerve injuries, depending not only on the total dose but also on the fractionation of doses. A well-known form is damage of the brachial plexus after radiation for breast cancer, or less commonly of the lumbosacral plexus in the case of pelvic cancer. The interval may be as short as 1 year or as long as 30 years.

A 64-year-old widow came to see one of us in 1997 because of a left drop foot which had gradually started to appear in 1992, with progression over one or two years. Extensive investigations, including MRI scans of the leg and pelvis, had failed to show a cause. On examination the weakness was not confined to the dorsiflexors of the foot and toes (MRC 4, with atrophy), but it was even more marked on inversion of the foot against resistance (MRC 3). Also, the left ankle jerk was absent. Other than the motor deficit, the sensory deficit more or less corresponded with the territory of the common peroneal nerve, involving the lateral part of the leg and the dorsum of the foot. Electrophysiological studies had shown signs of denervation in the left tibialis anterior and calf muscles. Apart from a marginally increased soleus H-reflex, nerve conduction studies in the left leg were normal. The solution emerged after renewed enquiry into her previous history: in 1962 she had undergone a hysterectomy for recurrent hypermenorrhagia. Her questions about the diagnosis had never been answered, but subsequently she had been treated 40 times with radiotherapy.

Almost invariably the plexus rather than an individual nerve is involved, but isolated lesions of the long thoracic nerve have been reported, after radiation for breast cancer (Pugliese *et al.*, 1987). Other variants are transient paraesthesia (Salner *et al.*, 1981) and an exclusively motor deficit ('monomelic amyotrophy') of the arm (Jackson, 1992) or the leg (Lamy *et al.*, 1991). Factors predisposing to radiation plexopathy of the arm are concomitant chemotherapy, relatively young age, and fractions exceeding 2 Gy (Olsen *et al.*, 1993).

An important diagnostic question in a patient with involvement of the brachial plexus after radiation for breast cancer is the exclusion of tumour recurrence as a cause for the deficits. Involvement of the lower plexus and lymphoedema favour radiation neuropathy, whereas severe pain as the presenting symptom and upper plexus involvement occur relatively often with tumour regrowth

(Kori *et al.*, 1981; Lederman and Wilbourn, 1984; Harper *et al.*, 1989). A mass lesion seen on CT scanning is also strongly suggestive of tumour infiltration, although it is not definite proof (Cascino *et al.*, 1983; Harper *et al.*, 1989). MRI scanning is probably even more sensitive (Thyagarajan *et al.*, 1995). EMG studies may also be helpful in the differentiation between radiation-induced and neoplastic plexopathy. The occurrence of repetitive series of spontaneous motor unit potentials (myokymic discharges) is highly suggestive of a radiation lesion (Aho and Sainio, 1983; Lederman and Wilbourn, 1984; Thomas *et al.*, 1985; Harper *et al.*, 1989). In addition, with radiation injury needle EMG shows signs of partial denervation and reinnervation.

Rarely, a brachial plexopathy complicating breast cancer is not caused not by radiation or local tumour but by a paraneoplastic inflammatory process (Lachance *et al.*, 1991).

Treatment with anticoagulants for radiation injury of the brain, spinal cord or nerve plexus has been advocated on the basis of an uncontrolled study, in which neurological deficits were arrested or reversed in a few patients (Glantz *et al.*, 1994). The rationale is that anticoagulation may arrest and reverse small-vessel endothelial injury and proliferation, which is the underlying process in radiation necrosis. Obviously this claim needs to be substantiated in a controlled study, despite encouraging experiences elsewhere (Koehler *et al.*, 1995).

Injury by physical agents

References

Abdel Salam, A., Eyres, K.S. and Cleary, J. (1991) Drivers' elbow: a cause of ulnar neuropathy. *J. Hand Surg. Br.* **16**, 436–437.

Abel, J.G. and Ali, J. (1992) Thoracostomy. In: Hall, J.R., Schmidt, G.A. and Wood, L.D.H. (eds), *Principles of Critical Care*, pp. 224–229. New York: McGraw Hill.

Abram, L.J. and Froimson, A.I. (1991) Saphenous nerve injury. An unusual arthroscopic complication. *Am. J. Sports Med.* **19**, 668–669.

Achauer, B.M., Braly, P., Berman, M.L. and DiSaia, P.J. (1984) Immediate vaginal reconstruction following resection for malignancy using the gluteal thigh flap. *Gynecol. Oncol.* **19**, 79–89.

Adamson, J.E., Srouji, S.J., Horton, C.E. and Mladick, R.A. (1971) The acute carpal tunnel syndrome. *Plast. Reconstr. Surg.* **47**, 332–336.

Adornato, B.T. and Carlini, W.G. (1992) 'Pushing palsy': a case of self-induced bilateral peroneal palsy during natural childbirth. *Neurology* **42**, 936–937.

Agnesi, R., Dal Vecchio, L., Todros, A., Sparta, S. and Valentini, F. (1993) Neuropatia del nervo ulnare a livello del gomito in addette all'uso di macchine per cucire a colonna: casistica e follow-up. [Ulnar neuropathy at the elbow in workers using column sewing machines: case reports and follow-up] *Med. Lav.* **84**, 147–161.

Aguayo, A., Nair, C.P. and Midgley, R. (1971) Experimental progressive compression neuropathy in the rabbit. Histologic and electrophysiologic studies. *Arch. Neurol.* **24**, 358–364.

Aho, K. and Sainio, K. (1983) Late irradiation-induced lesions of the lumbosacral plexus. *Neurology* **33**, 953–955.

Aiello, I., Serra, G., Traina, G.C. and Tugnoli, V. (1982) Entrapment of the suprascapular nerve at the spinoglenoid notch. *Ann. Neurol.* **12**, 314–316.

Aita, J.F. (1984) An unusual compressive neuropathy. *Arch. Neurol.* **41**, 341.

Akizuki, S. and Matsui, T. (1984) Entrapment neuropathy caused by tophaceous gout. *J. Hand Surg. Br.* **9**, 331–332.

Alevizon, S.J. and Finan, M.A. (1996) Sacrospinous colpopexy: management of postoperative pudendal nerve entrapment. *Obstet. Gynecol.* **88**, 713–715.

Alfonsi, E., Moglia, A., Sandrini, G., Pisoni, M.R. and Arrigo, A. (1986) Electrophysiological study of long thoracic nerve conduction in normal subjects. *Electromyogr. Clin. Neurophysiol.* **26**, 63–67.

Alhadeff, J. and Lee, C.K. (1995) Gastrocnemius muscle herniation at the knee causing peroneal nerve compression resembling sciatica. *Spine* **20**, 612–614.

al Hakim, M. and Katirji, B. (1993) Femoral mononeuropathy induced by the lithotomy position: a report of 5 cases with a review of literature. *Muscle Nerve* **16**, 891–895.

Aljure, J., Eltorai, I., Bradley, W.E., Lin, J.E. and Johnson, B. (1985) Carpal tunnel syndrome in paraplegic patients. *Paraplegia* **23**, 182–186.

Allen, I.M. (1931) The neurological complications of serum treatment. *Lancet* **ii**, 1128–1131.

Allen, R.E., Hosker, G.L., Smith, A.R. and Warrell, D.W. (1990) Pelvic floor damage and childbirth: a neurophysiological study. *Br. J. Obstet. Gynaecol.* **97**, 770–779.

al Naib, I. (1994) Humeral supracondylar spur and Struthers' ligament. A rare cause of neurovascular entrapment in the upper limb. *Int. Orthop.* **18**, 393–394.

al Qattan, M.M. and Duerksen, F. (1992) A variant of flexor carpi ulnaris causing ulnar nerve compression. *J. Anat.* **180**, 189–190.

al Qattan, M.M. and Husband, J.B. (1991) Median nerve compression by the supracondylar process: a case report. *J. Hand Surg. Br.* **16**, 101–103.

Alter, M. (1973) The digiti quinti sign of mild hemiparesis. *Neurology* **23**, 503–505.

Altissimi, M., Antenucci, R., Fiacca, C. and Mancini, G.B. (1986) Long-term results of conservative treatment of fractures of the distal radius. *Clin. Orthop.* 202–210.

Ames, P.A., Lenet, M.D. and Sherman, M. (1980) Joplin's neuroma. *J. Am. Podiatr. Assoc.* **70**, 99–101.

Amoiridis, G. (1992) Median–ulnar nerve communications and anomalous innervation of the intrinsic hand muscles: an electrophysiological study. *Muscle Nerve* **15**, 576–597.

Amoiridis, G., Wohrle, J., Grunwald, I. and Przuntek, H. (1993) Malignant tumour of the psoas: another cause of meralgia paraesthetica. *Electromyogr. Clin. Neurophysiol.* **33**, 109–112.

Anderson, J.M., Jamieson, D.G. and Jefferson, J.M. (1975) Non-healing granuloma and the nervous system. *Q. J. Med.* **44**, 309–323.

Andonopoulos, A.P., Lagos, G., Drosos, A.A. and Moutsopoulos, H.M. (1990) The spectrum of neurological involvement in Sjogren's syndrome. *Br. J. Rheumatol.* **29**, 21–23.

Antoniadis, G., Braun, V., Rath, S., Moese, G. and Richter, H.P. (1995) Die Meralgia paraesthetica und ihre operative Behandlung. [Meralgia paraesthetica and its surgical treatment.] *Nervenarzt* **66**, 614–617.

Antoniadis, G., Richter, H.P., Rath, S., Braun, V. and Moese, G. (1996) Suprascapular nerve entrapment: experience with 28 cases. *J. Neurosurg.* **85**, 1020–1025.

Antonini, G., Palmieri, G., Spagnoli, L.G. and Millefiorini, M. (1989) Lead brachial neuropathy in heroin addiction. A case report. *Clin. Neurol. Neurosurg.* **91**, 167–170.

Appel, H. (1991) Handcuff neuropathy. *Neurology* **41**, 955.

Arancio, O., Bongiovanni, L.G. and De Grandis, D. (1985) Acute peroneal compartmental

syndrome. Report of a case. *Eur. Neurol.* **24**, 69–72.

Aranoff, S.M., Levy, H.B., Tuchman, A.J. and Daras, M. (1985) Alopecia in meralgia paresthetica. *J. Am. Acad. Dermatol.* **12**, 176–178.

Arboleya, L. and Garcia, A. (1993) Suprascapular nerve entrapment of occupational etiology: clinical and electrophysiological characteristics. *Clin. Exp. Rheumatol.* **11**, 665–668.

Arnoldussen, W.J. and Korten, J.J. (1980) Pressure neuropathy of the posterior femoral cutaneous nerve. *Clin. Neurol. Neurosurg.* **82**, 57–60.

Aro, H., Koivunen, T., Katevuo, K., Nieminen, S. and Aho, A.J. (1988) Late compression neuropathies after Colles' fractures. *Clin. Orthop.* 217–225.

Arts, W.F.M., Busch, H.F.M., Van den Brand, H.J., Jennekens, F.G.I., Frants, R.R. and Stefanko, S.Z. (1983) Hereditary neuralgic amyotrophy. Clinical, genetic, electrophysiological and histopathological studies. *J. Neurol. Sci.* **62**, 261–279.

Asbury, A.K. (1977) Proximal diabetic neuropathy. *Ann. Neurol.* **2**, 179–180.

Asbury, A.K. and Fields, H.L. (1984) Pain due to peripheral nerve damage: an hypothesis. *Neurology* **34**, 1587–1590.

Ashleigh, R.J. and Marcuson, R.W. (1993) False aortic aneurysm presenting as sciatic nerve root pain. *Eur. J. Vasc. Surg.* **7**, 214–216.

Assmus, H. (1994) Die einfache Dekompression des N. ulnaris beim Kubitaltunnelsyndrom mit und ohne morphologische Veranderungen. Erfahrungsbericht anhand von 523 Fallen. [Simple decompression of the ulnar nerve in cubital tunnel syndrome with and without morphologic changes. Report of experiences based on 523 cases.] *Nervenarzt* **65**, 846–853.

Azuma, H. and Taneda, H. (1989) Rotational acetabular osteotomy in congenital dysplasia of the hip. *Int. Orthop.* **13**, 21–28.

Babins, D.M. and Lubahn, J.D. (1994) Palmar lipomas associated with compression of the median nerve. *J. Bone Joint Surg. [Am.]* **76**, 1360–1362.

Bacourt, F., Mercier, F. and Benoist, M. (1994) Anevrysme rompu de l'artère hypogastrique revelé par une paralysie sciatique. Un cas et revue de la litterature. [Ruptured hypogastric aneurysm presenting as a sciatic paralysis. Case report and review of the literature.] *J. Mal. Vasc.* **19**, 147–150.

Bademosi, O., Osuntokun, B.O., Van de Werd, H.J., Bademosi, A.K. and Ojo, O.A. (1980) Obstetric neuropraxia in the Nigerian African. *Int. J. Gynaecol. Obstet.* **17**, 611–614.

Baker, G.S., Parsons, W.R. and Welch, J.S. (1966) Endometriosis within the sheath of the sciatic nerve. Report of two patients with progressive paralysis. *J. Neurosurg.* **25**, 652–655.

Baker, S.B. and Robinson, D.R. (1978) Unusual renal manifestations of Wegener's granulomatosis. Report of two cases. *Am. J. Med.* **64**, 883–889.

Balfour, H.H., Jr., Bean, B., Laskin, O.L., Ambinder, R.F., Meyers, J.D., Wade, J.C., Zaia, J.A., Aeppli, D., Kirk, L.E., Segreti, A.C. and Keeney, R.E. (1983) Acyclovir halts progression of herpes zoster in immunocompromised patients. *N. Engl. J. Med.* **308**, 1448–1453.

Ball, N.A., Stempien, L.M., Pasupuleti, D.V. and Wertsch, J.J. (1989) Radial nerve palsy: a complication of walker usage. *Arch. Phys. Med. Rehabil.* **70**, 236–238.

Banerjee, T. and Koons, D.D. (1981) Superficial peroneal nerve entrapment. Report of two cases. *J. Neurosurg.* **55**, 991–992.

Banerjee, T.K., Grubb, W., Otero, C., McKee, M., Brady, R.O. and Barton, N.W. (1993) Musculocutaneous mononeuropathy complicating *Capnocytophaga canimorsus* infection. *Neurology* **43**, 2411–2412.

Barker, B., Bloch, T., Vakili, S.T. and Waller, B.F. (1986) One pathologist went to mow, went to mow a meadow . . . [letter]. *JAMA* **255**, 200.

Barohn, R.J., Sahenk, Z., Warmolts, J.R. and Mendell, J.R. (1991) The Bruns–Garland syndrome (diabetic amyotrophy) revisited 100 years later. *Arch. Neurol.* **48**, 1130–1135.

Barohn, R.J., Gronseth, G.S., Le Force, B.R., McVey, A.L., McGuire, S.A., Butzin, C.A. and King, R.B. (1993) Peripheral nervous system involvement in a large cohort of human immunodeficiency virus-infected individuals. *Arch. Neurol.* **50**, 167–171.

Barontini, F. and Macucci, M. (1986) Simultaneous femoral nerve palsy due to hemorrhage in both iliac muscles. *Ital. J. Neurol. Sci.* **7**, 463–465.

Bartosh, R.A., Dugdale, T.W. and Nielsen, R. (1992) Isolated musculocutaneous nerve injury complicating closed fracture of the clavicle. A case report. *Am. J. Sports Med.* **20**, 356–359.

Bassett, F.H.3rd. and Nunley, J.A. (1982) Compression of the musculocutaneous nerve at the elbow. *J. Bone Joint Surg. [Am.]* **64**, 1050–1052.

Bastron, J.A. and Thomas, J.E. (1981) Diabetic polyradiculopathy: clinical and electromyographic findings in 105 patients. *Mayo Clin. Proc.* **56**, 725–732.

Beard, L., Kumar, A. and Estep, H.L. (1985) Bilateral carpal tunnel syndrome caused by Graves' disease. *Arch. Intern. Med.* **145**, 345–346.

Beaudry, Y., Stewart, J.D. and Errett, L. (1989) Distal sciatic nerve compression by a popliteal artery aneurysm. *Can. J. Neurol. Sci.* **16**, 352–353.

Beghi, E., Kurland, L.T., Mulder, D.W. and Nicolosi, A. (1985) Brachial plexus neuropathy in the population of Rochester, Minnesota, 1970–1981. *Ann. Neurol.* **18**, 320–323.

Behse, F. and Buchthal, F. (1971) Normal sensory conduction in the nerves of the leg in man. *J. Neurol. Neurosurg. Psychiatry* **34**, 404–414.

Behse, F., Buchthal, F., Carlsen, F. and Knappeis, G.G. (1972) Hereditary neuropathy with liability to pressure palsies. Electrophysiological and histopathological aspects. *Brain* **95**, 777–794.

Belsh, J.M. (1991) Anterior femoral cutaneous nerve injury following femoral artery reconstructive surgery. *Arch. Neurol.* **48**, 230–232.

Benini, A. (1992) Die Ilioinguinalis- und Genitofemoralisneuralgie. Ursachen, Klinik, Therapie. [Ilio-inguinal and genito-femoral neuralgia. Causes, clinical aspects, therapy.] *Schweiz. Rundsch. Med. Prax.* **81**, 1114–1120.

Benini, A. and Di Martino, E. (1976) Die Schadigung des Ramus profundus nervi radialis (Supinatorsyndrom). [Lesion of the ramus profundus of the radial nerve (supinator syndrome). Dissociated radial paralysis of the proximal underarm type.] *Schweiz. Med. Wochenschr.* **106**, 639–643.

Beresford, H.R. (1971) Meralgia paresthetica after seat-belt trauma. *J. Trauma.* **11**, 629–630.

Bergqvist, A., Bergqvist, D., Lindholm, K. and Linell, F. (1987) Endometriosis in the uterosacral ligament giving orthopedic symptoms through compression of the sciatic nerve and surgically treated via an extraperitoneal approach keeping the pelvic organs intact. *Acta Obstet. Gynecol. Scand.* **66**, 93–94.

Berkowitz, A.R., Melone, C.P., Jr. and Belsky, M.R. (1992) Pisiform–hamate coalition with ulnar neuropathy. *J. Hand Surg. Am.* **17**, 657–662.

Berlemann, U. and Dunkerton, M.C. (1994) Compression of the radial digital nerve of the thumb. *J. Hand Surg. Br.* **19**, 288.

Berlit, P. (1993) Car toll neuropathy [letter]. *J. Neurol. Neurosurg. Psychiatry* **56**, 1329.

Berlusconi, M. and Capitani, D. (1991) Post-traumatic hematoma of the iliopsoas muscle with femoral nerve entrapment: description of a rare occurrence in a professional cyclist. *Ital. J. Orthop. Traumatol.* **17**, 563–566.

Bernard, F., Perdrix, J.P., Lepape, A., Grozel, J.M. and Caillot, J.L. (1991) Ischemie intestinale aigue dans les suites d'une intoxication medicamenteuse volontaire. [Acute intestinal ischemia after voluntary drug poisoning.] *Ann. Fr. Anesth. Reanim.* **10**, 158–160.

Bernhardt, M. (1895) Ueber isolirt im Gebiete des N. cutaneus femoris externus vorkommende Parästhesien. [About isolated paraesthesia in the distribution of the lateral cutaneous nerve.] *Neurol. Centralbl.* **14**, 242–244.

Berry, H. and Bril, V. (1982) Axillary nerve palsy following blunt trauma to the shoulder region: a clinical and electrophysiological review. *J. Neurol. Neurosurg. Psychiatry* **45**, 1027–1032.

Berry, H. and Richardson, P.M. (1976) Common peroneal nerve palsy: a clinical and electrophysiological review. *J Neurol. Neurosurg. Psychiatry* **39**, 1162–1171.

Berry, P.R. and Wallis, W.E. (1977) Venepuncture nerve injuries. *Lancet* **i**, 1236–1237.

Bieber, E.J., Moore, J.R. and Weiland, A.J. (1986) Lipomas compressing the radial nerve at the elbow. *J. Hand Surg. [Am.]* **11**, 533–535.

Bierman, H.R. (1959) Nerve compression due to a tight watchband. *N. Engl. J. Med.* **261**, 237–238.

Bilge, T., Kaya, A., Alatli, M., Bilge, S. and Alatli, C. (1989) Hemangioma of the peroneal nerve: case report and review of the literature. *Neurosurgery* **25**, 649–652.

Billings, R. and Grahame, R. (1975) Neuralgic amyotrophy with hemidiaphragmatic paralysis. *Rheumatol. Rehabil.* **14**, 260–261.

Bimmler, D., von Wartburg, U., Frick, T.W. and Meyer, V.E. (1993) Ergebnisse der operativen Therapie des Sulcus-ulnaris-Syndroms. Submuskulare Vorverlagerung versus einfache Dekompression des N. ulnaris. [Results of surgical therapy of ulnar sulcus syndrome. Submuscular anterior transposition versus simple decompression of the ulnar nerve.] *Helv. Chir. Acta* **59**, 697–700.

Binder, A., Snaith, M.L. and Isenberg, D. (1988) Sjogren's syndrome: a study of its neurological complications. *Br. J. Rheumatol.* **27**, 275–280.

Bindra, R.R., Evanoff, B.A., Chough, L.Y., Cole, R.J., Chow, J.C.Y. and Gelberman, R.H. (1997) The use of routine wrist radiography in the evaluation of patients with carpal tunnel syndrome. *J. Hand Surg. [Am.]* **22**, 115–119.

Birch, R. (1993) Peripheral nerve tumours. In: Dyck, P.J., Thomas, P.K., Griffin, J.W., Low, P.A. and Poduslo, J.F. (eds), *Peripheral Neuropathy*, 3rd edn, pp. 1623–1640. Philadelphia: W.B. Saunders.

Bischoff, C. and Schonle, P.W. (1991) Obturator nerve injuries during intra-abdominal surgery. *Clin. Neurol. Neurosurg.* **93**, 73–76.

Bjork, K.J., Mucha, P. and Cahill, D.R. (1988) Obturator hernia. *Surg. Gynecol. Obstet.* **167**, 217–222.

Black, P.R.M., Flowers, M.J. and Saleh, M. (1997) Acute carpal tunnel syndrome as a complication of oral anticoagulant therapy. *J. Hand Surg. [Br.]* **22**, 50–51.

Blankenship, J.C. (1991) Median and ulnar neuropathy after streptokinase infusion. *Heart Lung* **20**, 221–223.

Bleecker, M.L., Bohlman, M., Moreland, R. and Tipton, A. (1985) Carpal tunnel syndrome: role of carpal canal size. *Neurology* **35**, 1599–1604.

Blennow, G., Bekassy, A.N., Eriksson, M. and Rosendahl, R. (1982) Transient carpal tunnel syndrome accompanying rubella infection. *Acta Paediatr. Scand.* **71**, 1025–1028.

Bleton, R., Alnot, J.Y., Kahn, M.F. and Bocquet, L. (1991) Synovite sarcoidosique. A propos d'un cas de localization au niveau des tendons flechisseurs des doigts. [Sarcoid synovitis. A case report of localization at the level of the flexor tendons of the fingers.] *Ann. Chir. Main. Memb. Super.* **10**, 360–363.

Blexrud, M.D., Windebank, A.J. and Daube, J.R. (1993) Long-term follow-up of 121 patients with benign fasciculations. *Ann. Neurol.* **34**, 622–625.

Bloch, S.L., Jarrett, M.P., Swerdlow, M. and Grayzel, A.I. (1979) Brachial plexus neuropathy as the initial presentation of systemic lupus erythematosus. *Neurology* **29**, 1633–1634.

Blom, S. and Dahlback, L.O. (1970) Nerve injuries in dislocations of the shoulder joint and fractures of the neck of the humerus. A clinical and electromyographical study. *Acta Chir. Scand.* **136**, 461–466.

Boc, S.F. and Kushner, S. (1994) Plantar fibromatosis causing entrapment syndrome of the medial plantar nerve. *J. Am. Podiatr. Med. Assoc.* **84**, 420–422.

Boden, S.D., Davis, D.O., Dina, T.S., Patronas, N.J. and Wiesel, S.W. (1990) Abnormal magnetic-resonance scans of the lumbar spine in asymptomatic subjects – a prospective investigation. *J. Bone Joint Surg. [Am.]* **72**, 403–408.

Boe, S. and Holst Nielsen, F. (1987) Intra-articular entrapment of the median nerve after dislocation of the elbow. *J. Hand Surg. [Br.]* **12**, 356–358.

Bolton, C.F. and McFarlane, R.M. (1978) Human pneumatic tourniquet paralysis. *Neurology* **28**, 787–793.

Bolton, C.F., Driedger, A.A. and Lindsay, R.M. (1979) Ischaemic neuropathy in uraemic patients caused by bovine arteriovenous shunt. *J. Neurol. Neurosurg. Psychiatry* **42**, 810–814.

Boontje, A.H. and Haaxma, R. (1987) Femoral neuropathy as a complication of aortic surgery. *J. Cardiovasc. Surg. (Torino.)* **28**, 286–289.

Bors, E.J. and Blinn, K.A. (1959) Bulbocavernosus reflex. *J. Urol.* **82**, 128.

Bosch, E.P., Chui, H.C., Martin, M.A. and Cancilla, P.A. (1980) Brachial plexus involvement in familial pressure-sensitive neuropathy: electrophysiological and morphological findings. *Ann. Neurol.* **8**, 620–624.

Both, R., Mühlau, G. and Wieckszorek, V. (1983) Schlaflähmung – eine spezielle Form der akuten Drucklähmung. [Sleep paralysis – a special form of acute pressure neuropathy.] *Wiss. Z. Ernst-Moritz-Arndt Univ. Greifsw. Med.* **32**, 44–45.

Bowen, T.L. and Stone, K.H. (1966) Posterior interosseous nerve paralysis caused by a ganglion at the elbow. *J. Bone Joint Surg. [Br.]* **48**, 774–776.

Boyce, J.R. (1984) Meralgia paresthetica and tight trousers [letter]. *JAMA* **251**, 1553.

Braddom, R.L. and Wolfe, C. (1978) Musculocutaneous nerve injury after heavy exercise. *Arch. Phys. Med. Rehabil.* **59**, 290–293.

Bradley, W.G., Madrid, R., Thrush, D.C. and Campbell, M.J. (1975) Recurrent brachial plexus neuropathy. *Brain* **98**, 381–398.

Brady, K.A., McCarron, J.P., Jr, Vaughan, E.D., Jr and Javidian, P. (1993) Benign schwannoma of the retroperitoneal space: case report. *J. Urol.* **150**, 179–181.

Brain, W.R., Wright, A.D. and Wilkinson, M. (1947) Spontaneous compression of both median nerves in the carpal tunnel. *Lancet* **i**, 277–282.

Braithwaite, I.J. (1992) Bilateral median nerve palsy in a cyclist. *Br. J. Sports Med.* **26**, 27–28.

Brand, M.G. and Gelberman, R.H. (1988) Lipoma of the flexor digitorum superficialis causing triggering at the carpal canal and median nerve compression. *J. Hand Surg. Am.* **13**, 342–344.

Brandenberger, A.W., Hauser, R. and Bronz, L.B. (1992) Postpartum periarticular hip abscess with later coxitis caused by group B streptococcus. *Eur. J. Obstet. Gynecol. Reprod. Biol.* **47**, 255–257.

Brasch, R.C., Bufo, A.J., Kreienberg, P.F. and Johnson, G.P. (1995) Femoral neuropathy secondary to the use of a self-retaining retractor. Report of three cases and review of the literature. *Dis. Colon Rectum* **38**, 1115–1118.

Brenninkmeyer, R. (1979) The carpal tunnel syndrome and the antidrome sensory latencies to the first and fourth finger [abstract]. *Acta Neurol. Scand.* **60**(Suppl. 73), 119.

Britt, B.A. and Gordon, R.A. (1964) Peripheral nerve injuries associated with anaesthesia. *Can. Anaesth. Soc. J.* **2**, 515–535.

Britton, J.M. and Dunkerley, D.R. (1990) Closed nailing of a femoral fracture followed by sciatic nerve palsy. *J. Bone Joint Surg. [Br.]* **72**, 318.

Brochet, B., Louiset, P., Lagueny, A., Coquet, M., Vital, C. and Loiseau, P. (1988) Neuropathie peripherique revelatrice d'une sarcoidose. [Peripheral neuropathies disclosing sarcoidosis.] *Rev. Neurol. (Paris)* **144**, 590–595.

Broin, E.O., Horner, C., Mealy, K., Kerin, M.J., Gillen, P., O'Brien, M. and Tanner, W.A. (1995) Meralgia paraesthetica following laparoscopic inguinal hernia repair. An anatomical analysis. *Surg. Endosc.* **9**, 76–78.

Bronisch, F.W. (1960) Die Ulnarisschädigung im Handbereich. [Damage to the ulnar nerve in the region of the hand.] *Dtsch. Zschr. Nervenheilk.* **181**, 1–14.

Bronisch, F.W. (1971) Zur Pathogenese und Therapie der nichttraumatischen Lahmung des Ramus profundus n. radialis. [Pathogenesis and therapy of non-traumatic paralysis of ramus profundus nervi radialis.] *Nervenarzt* **42**, 32–35.

Brooke, M.M., Heard, D.L., de Lateur, B.J., Moeller, D.A. and Alquist, A.D. (1991) Heterotopic ossification and peripheral nerve entrapment: early diagnosis and excision. *Arch. Phys. Med. Rehabil.* **72**, 425–429.

Brooks, D.M. (1952) Nerve compression by simple ganglia. A review of thirteen collected cases. *J. Bone Joint Surg. [Br.]* **34**, 391–401.

Brooks, J.P. and Pascal, R.R. (1984) Malignant giant cell tumour of bone: ultrastructural and immunohistologic evidence of histiocytic origin. *Hum. Pathol.* **15**, 1098–1100.

Brown, R.A., Gelberman, R.H., Seiler, J.G., Abrahamsson, S.O., Weiland, A.J., Urbaniak, J.R., Schoenfeld, D.A. and Furcolo, D. (1993) Carpal tunnel release. A prospective, randomized assessment of open and endoscopic methods. *J. Bone Joint Surg. [Am.]* **75**, 1265–1275.

Brown, R.E. and Storm, B.W. (1994) 'Congenital' common peroneal nerve compression. *Ann. Plast. Surg.* **33**, 326–329.

Brown, W.F. and Watson, B.V. (1991) Quantitation of axon loss and conduction block in peroneal nerve palsies. *Muscle Nerve* **14**, 237–244.

Brown, W.F., Yates, S.K. and Ferguson, G.G. (1980) Cubital tunnel syndrome and ulnar neuropathy. *Ann. Neurol.* **7**, 289–290.

Bruijn, J.D. and Koning, J. (1992) Compression of the ulnar nerve by an aneurysm. A case of late complication after a supracondylar fracture. *Acta Orthop. Scand.* **63**, 223–224.

Bruyn, R.P.M. (1994) Occupational neuropathy of the sural nerve. *Ital. J. Neurol. Sci.* **15**, 119–120.

Buch, K.A. and Campbell, J. (1993) Acute onset meralgia paraesthetica after fracture of the anterior superior iliac spine. *Injury* **24**, 569–570.

Buchberger, W., Judmaier, W., Birbamer, G., Hasenohrl, K. and Schmidauer, C. (1993) Der Stellenwert von Sonographie und MR-Tomographie in Diagnose und Therapiekontrolle des Karpaltunnelsyndroms. [The role of sonography and MR tomography in the diagnosis and therapeutic control of the carpal tunnel syndrome.] *Rofo. Fortschr. Geb. Rontgenstr. Neuen. Bildgeb. Verfahr.* **159**, 138–143.

Buckmiller, J.F. and Rickard, T.A. (1987) Isolated compression neuropathy of the palmar cutaneous branch of the median nerve. *J. Hand Surg. [Am.]* **12**, 97–99.

Budny, P.G., Regan, P.J. and Roberts, A.H. (1992) Localized nodular synovitis: a rare cause of ulnar nerve compression in Guyon's canal. *J. Hand Surg. [Am.]* **17**, 663–664.

Burczak, J.R. (1994) Median nerve palsy after operative treatment of intraarticular distal humerus fracture with intact supracondylar process. *J. Orthop. Trauma* **8**, 252–254.

Burke, D., Skuse, N.F. and Lethlean, A.K. (1974) Sensory conduction of the sural nerve in polyneuropathy. *J. Neurol. Neurosurg. Psychiatry* **37**, 647–652.

Burney, T.L., Campbell, E.C., Jr, Naslund, M.J. and Jacobs, S.C. (1993) Complications of staging laparoscopic pelvic lymphadenectomy. *Surg. Laparosc. Endosc.* **3**, 184–190.

Bush, D.C. and Schneider, L.H. (1984) Tuberculosis of the hand and wrist. *J. Hand Surg. Am.* **9**, 391–398.

Butler, E.T., Johnson, E.W. and Kaye, Z.A. (1974) Normal conduction velocity in the lateral femoral cutaneous nerve. *Arch. Phys. Med. Rehabil.* **55**, 31–32.

Byrne, E. (1987) Extended neuralgic amyotrophy syndrome. *Aust. N.Z. J. Med.* **17**, 34–38.

Cahill, B.R. and Palmer, R.E. (1983) Quadrilateral space syndrome. *J. Hand Surg. [Am.]* **8**, 65–69.

Caldwell, J.W., Crane, C.R. and Boland, G.L. (1968) Determinations of intercostal motor conduction time in diagnosis of nerve root compression. *Arch. Phys. Med. Rehabil.* **49**, 515–518.

Callahan, J.D., Scully, T.B., Shapiro, S.A. and Worth, R.M. (1991) Suprascapular nerve entrapment. A series of 27 cases. *J. Neurosurg.* **74**, 893–896.

Campbell, W.W. (1989) AAEE case report 18: Ulnar neuropathy in the distal forearm. *Muscle Nerve* **12**, 347–352.

Campbell, W.W., Pridgeon, R.M. and Sahni, S.K. (1988) Entrapment neuropathy of the ulnar nerve at its point of exit from the flexor carpi ulnaris muscle. *Muscle Nerve* **11**, 467–470.

Campbell, W.W., Sahni, S.K., Pridgeon, R.M., Riaz, G. and Leshner, R.T. (1988a) Intraoperative electroneurography: management of ulnar neuropathy at the elbow. *Muscle Nerve* **11**, 75–81.

Campbell, W.W., Pridgeon, R.M. and Sahni, K.S. (1992) Short segment incremental studies in the evaluation of ulnar neuropathy at the elbow. *Muscle Nerve* **15**, 1050–1054.

Cape, C.A. and Fincham, R.W. (1965) Paralytic brachial neuritis with diaphragmatic paralysis. *Neurology* **15**, 191–193.

Capener, N. (1966) The vulnerability of the posterior interosseous nerve of the forearm. A case report and an anatomical study. *J. Bone Joint Surg. [Br.]* **48**, 770–773.

Caplan, L., Corbett, J., Goodwin, J., Thomas, C., Shenker, D. and Schatz, N. (1983) Neuro-ophthalmologic signs in the angiitic form of neurosarcoidosis. *Neurology* **33**, 1130–1135.

Carayon, A., Giordano, C., Colomar, R. and Courbil, L.J. (1966) Nerf cubital à ressaut. [Leaping ulnar nerve]. *Bull. Soc. Med. Afr. Noire. Lang. Fr.* **11**, 66–69.

Cardelia, J.M., Dormans, J.P., Drummond, D.S., Davidson, R.S., Duhaime, C. and Sutton, L. (1995) Proximal fibular osteochondroma with associated peroneal nerve palsy: a review of six cases. *J. Pediatr. Orthop.* **15**, 574–577.

Carfi, J. and Dong, M. (1985) Posterior interosseous nerve syndrome revisited. *Muscle Nerve* **8**, 499–502.

Carlson, D.A., Dobozi, W.R. and Rabin, S. (1995) Peroneal nerve palsy and compartment syndrome in bilateral femoral fractures. *Clin.Orthop.* 115–118.

Carney, L.R. (1967) The dimple sign in peroneal palsy. *Neurology* **17**, 922.

Carroll, R.E. and Green, D.P. (1972) The significance of the palmar cutaneous nerve at the wrist. *Clin. Orthop.* 24–28.

Carrozzella, J., Stern, P.J. and Von Kuster, L.C. (1989) Transection of radial digital nerve of the thumb during trigger release. *J. Hand Surg. [Am.]* **14**, 198–200.

Casagrande, P.A. and Danahy, P.R. (1971) Delayed sciatic-nerve entrapment following the use of self-curing acrylic. A case report. *J. Bone Joint Surg. [Am.]* **53**, 167–169.

Cascino, T.L., Kori, S., Krol, G. and Foley, K.M. (1983) CT of the brachial plexus in patients with cancer. *Neurology* **33**, 1553–1557.

Case, D.B. (1967) An acute carpal tunnel syndrome in a haemophiliac. *Br. J. Clin. Pract.* **21**, 254–255.

Caselli, R.J., Daube, J.R., Hunder, G.G. and Whisnant, J.P. (1988) Peripheral neuropathic syndromes in giant cell (temporal) arteritis. *Neurology* **38**, 685–689.

Caspi, I., Ezra, E., Nerubay, J. and Horoszovski, H. (1987) Musculocutaneous nerve injury after coracoid process transfer for clavicle instability. Report of three cases. *Acta Orthop. Scand.* **58**, 294–295.

Casscells, C.D., Lindsey, R.W., Ebersole, J. and Li, B. (1993) Ulnar neuropathy after median sternotomy. *Clin. Orthop.* 259–265.

Cavanagh, N.P., Yates, D.A. and Sutcliffe, J. (1979) Thenar hypoplasia with associated radiologic abnormalities. *Muscle Nerve* **2**, 431–436.

Chaise, F. and Boucher, P. (1987) Les resultats eloignes de la decompression chirurgicale du nerf tibial posterieur dans les neuropathies de la maladie de Hansen. [Remote results of the surgical decompression of the posterior tibial nerve in the neuropathies of Hansen's disease.] *J. Chir. Paris.* **124**, 315–318.

Chaise, F. and Sedel, L. (1984) Les compressions isolées de la branche motrice du nerf cubital. [Isolated compression of the motor branch of the ulnar nerve.] *Sem. Hop.* **60**, 694–697.

Chalk, C.H., Dyck, P.J. and Conn, D.L. (1993) Vasculitic neuropathy. In: Dyck, P.J., Thomas, P.K., Griffin, J.W., Low, P.A. and Poduslo, J.F. (eds), *Peripheral Neuropathy*, 3rd edn, pp. 1424–1436. Philadelphia: W.B. Saunders.

Chammas, M., Reckendorf, G.M.Z. and Allieu, Y. (1995) Compression of the ulnar nerve in Guyon's canal by pseudotumoural calcinosis in systemic scleroderma. *J. Hand Surg. [Br.]* **20**, 794–796.

Chance, P.F., Alderson, M.K., Leppig, K.A., Lensch, M.W., Matsunami, N., Smith, B., Swanson, P.D., Odelberg, S.J., Disteche, C.M. and Bird, T.D. (1993) DNA deletion associated with hereditary neuropathy with liability to pressure palsies. *Cell* **72**, 143–151.

Chance, P.F., Lensch, M.W., Lipe, H., Brown, R.H., Sr, Brown, R.H., Jr and Bird, T.D. (1994) Hereditary neuralgic amyotrophy and hereditary neuropathy with liability to pressure palsies: two distinct genetic disorders. *Neurology* **44**, 2253–2257.

Chang, C.W. and Oh, S.J. (1988) Medial antebrachial cutaneous neuropathy: case report. *Electromyogr. Clin. Neurophysiol.* **28**, 3–5.

Chang, C.W. and Oh, S.J. (1990) Sensory nerve conduction study in forearm on superficial radial nerve: standardization of technique. *EMG Clin. Neurophysiol.* **30**, 349–351.

Chang, R.W., Bell, C.L. and Hallett, M. (1984) Clinical characteristics and prognosis of vasculitic mononeuropathy multiplex. *Arch. Neurol.* **41**, 618–621.

Chantraine, A. (1973) EMG examination of the anal and urethral sphincters. In: Desmedt, J.E. (ed.), *New Developments in Electromyography and Clinical Neurophysiology.* pp. 421–432. Basel: Karger.

Chapman, D.R., Bennett, J.B., Bryan, W.J. and Tullos, H.S. (1982) Complications of distal radial fractures: pins and plaster treatment. *J. Hand Surg. [Am.]* **7**, 509–512.

Charles, N., Vial, C., Chauplannaz, G. and Bady, B. (1990) Clinical validation of antidromic stimulation of the ring finger in early electrodiagnosis of mild carpal tunnel syndrome. *Electroencephalogr. Clin. Neurophysiol.* **76**, 142–147.

Chen, W.S. (1992) Lipome a l'origine d'un syndrome du tunnel tarsien. A propos de 2 cas.

[Lipoma responsible for tarsal tunnel syndrome. Apropos of 2 cases.] *Rev. Chir. Orthop. Reparatrice. Appar. Mot.* **78**, 251–254.

Chen, W.S. (1994) Bipartite piriformis muscle: an unusual cause of sciatic nerve entrapment. *Pain* **58**, 269–272.

Cherington, M. (1977) Anterior interosseous nerve syndrome straight thumb sign [letter]. *Neurology* **27**, 800–801.

Chiao, H.C., Marks, K.E., Bauer, T.W. and Pflanze, W. (1987) Intraneural lipoma of the sciatic nerve. *Clin. Orthop.* 267–271.

Chokroverty, S., Deutsch, A., Guha, C., Gonzalez, A., Kwan, P., Burger, R. and Goldberg, J. (1995) Thoracic spinal nerve and root conduction: a magnetic stimulation study. *Muscle Nerve* **18**, 987–991.

Chopra, J.S., Khanna, S.K. and Murthy, J.M. (1979) Congenital arteriovenous fistula producing carpal tunnel syndrome. *J. Neurol. Neurosurg. Psychiatry* **42**, 815–817.

Chumbley, L.C., Harrison, E.G.J. and DeRemee, R.A. (1977) Allergic granulomatosis and angiitis (Churg–Strauss syndrome). Report and analysis of 30 cases. *Mayo Clin. Proc.* **52**, 477–484.

Chutkow, J.G. (1988) Posterior femoral cutaneous neuralgia. *Muscle Nerve* **11**, 1146–1148.

Ciulla, T.A., Frederick, A.R., Jr, Kelly, C. and Amrein, R. (1996) Postvitrectomy positioning complicated by ulnar nerve palsy. *Am. J. Ophthalmol.* **122**, 739–740.

Cobb, T.K., Amadio, P.C., Leatherwood, D.F., Schleck, C.D. and Ilstrup, D.M. (1996) Outcome of reoperation for carpal tunnel syndrome. *J. Hand Surg. [Am.]* **21A**, 347–356.

Coccurollo, G.D.G. and Galvagno, S. (1984) Paralisi del nervo ulnare: rara complicanza della frature del polso. Analisi di cinque casi. [Ulnar nerve palsy: a rare complication of wrist fracture. Analysis of five cases.] *Minerva Ortop.* **35**, 421–426.

Cohney, S., Savige, J. and Stewart, M.R. (1995) Lupus anticoagulant in anti-neutrophil cytoplasmic antibody-associated polyarteritis. *Am. J. Nephrol.* **15**, 157–160.

Colbert, D.S., Cunningham, F. and Mackey, D. (1975) Sural nerve entrapment – case report. *Ir. Med. J.* **68**, 544.

Cole, J.D. and Bolhofner, B.R. (1994) Acetabular fracture fixation via a modified Stoppa limited intrapelvic approach. Description of operative technique and preliminary treatment results. *Clin. Orthop.* 112–123.

Collier, F.C. (1985) Acute monetary sciatica [letter]. *Lancet* **ii**, 1079.

Copeland, J., Wells-HG, J. and Puckett, C.L. (1989) Acute carpal tunnel syndrome in a patient taking coumadin. *J. Trauma* **29**, 131–132.

Coppack, S.W. and Watkins, P.J. (1991) The natural history of diabetic femoral neuropathy. *Q. J. Med.* **79**, 307–313.

Corner, N.B., Milner, S.M., MacDonald, R. and Jubb, M. (1990) Isolated musculocutaneous nerve lesion after shoulder dislocation. *J. R. Army Med. Corps* **136**, 107–108.

Costigan, D., Tindall, S.C. and Lexow, S. (1991) Tibial nerve entrapment by the tendinous arch of the origin of the soleus muscle: diagnostic difficulties. *Muscle Nerve* **14**, 880.

Cravens, G. and Kline, D.G. (1990) Posterior interosseous nerve palsies. *Neurosurgery* **27**, 397–402.

Creange, A., Meyrignac, C., Roualdes, B., Degos, J.D. and Gherardi, R.K. (1995) Diphtheritic neuropathy. *Muscle Nerve* **18**, 1460–1463.

Cremer, G.M., Goldstein, N.P. and Paris, J. (1969) Myxedema and ataxia. *Neurology* **19**, 37–46.

Creton, D. (1991) Resultat des strippings saphène interne sous anesthésie locale en ambulatoire (700 cas). [The results of internal saphenous vein stripping under local anesthesia in outpatient care (700 cases).] *Phlebologie* **44**, 303–311.

Crow, R.S. (1960) Treatment of the carpal tunnel syndrome. *Br. Med. J.* **i**, 1611–1615.

Cruz Martinez, A. (1987) Slimmer's paralysis: electrophysiological evidence of compressive lesion. *Eur. Neurol.* **26**, 189–192.

Cruz Martinez, A., Gonzalez, P., Garza, E., Bescansa, E. and Anciones, B. (1987) Electrophysiologic follow-up in Whipple's disease. *Muscle Nerve* **10**, 616–620.

Cumming, W.J., Thrush, D.C. and Kenward, D.H. (1978) Bilateral neuralgic amyotrophy complicating Weil's disease. *Postgrad. Med. J.* **54**, 680–681.

Currie, S. and Henson, R.A. (1971) Neurological syndromes in the reticuloses. *Brain* **94**, 307–320.

Cusimano, M.D., Bilbao, J.M. and Cohen, S.M. (1988) Hypertrophic brachial plexus neuritis: a pathological study of two cases. *Ann. Neurol.* **24**, 615–622.

Cwinn, A.A. and Cantrill, S.V. (1985) Lightning injuries. *J. Emerg. Med.* **2**, 379–388.

Dagum, A.B., Peters, W.J., Neligan, P.C. and Douglas, L.G. (1993) Severe multiple mononeuropathy in patients with major thermal burns. *J. Burn. Care Rehabil.* **14**, 440–445.

Dalakas, M.C. and Pezeshkpour, G.H. (1988) Neuromuscular diseases associated with human immunodeficiency virus infection. *Ann. Neurol.* **23**(Suppl.), S38–S48.

Daly, K.E., Chow, J.W. and Vickers, R.H. (1993) Excision of the hamate for an unusual hand tumour. *J. Hand Surg. [Br.]* **18**, 606–608.

D'Amour, M.L., Lebrun, L.H., Rabbat, A., Trudel, J. and Daneault, N. (1987) Peripheral neurological complications of aortoiliac vascular disease. *Can. J. Neurol. Sci.* **14**, 127–130.

Danner, R. (1983) Unilateral thenar hypoplasia. *Clin. Neurol. Neurosurg.* **85**, 123–128.

Dap, F., Dautel, G., Bour, C., Marin Braun, F. and Merle, M. (1992) Lipofibrome du nerf median. A propos d'un cas. [Lipofibroma of the median nerve. Apropos of a case.] *Ann. Chir. Main. Memb. Super.* **11**, 51–55.

Darzi, A., Paraskeva, P.A., Quereshi, A., Menzies Gow, N., Guillou, P.J. and Monson, J.R. (1994) Laparoscopic herniorrhaphy: initial experience in 126 patients. *J. Laparoendosc. Surg.* **4**, 179–183.

Dattwyler, R.J., Halperin, J.J., Volkman, D.J. and Luft, B.J. (1988) Treatment of late Lyme borreliosis–randomized comparison of ceftriaxone and penicillin. *Lancet* **i**, 1191–1194.

Daupleix, D. and Dreyfus, P. (1984) (letter) Meralgie paresthesique compliquant le prelevement d'un greffon iliaque. A propos de 3 observations. [Meralgia paresthetica complicating iliac bone graft removal. Apropos of 3 cases.] *Presse Méd.* **13**, 681–682.

Davidson, G.S. and Deck, J.H. (1988) Delayed myelopathy following lightning strike: a demyelinating process. *Acta Neuropathol. (Berl.)* **77**, 104–108.

Davies, D.M. (1954) Recurrent peripheral nerve palsies in a family. *Lancet* **ii**, 266–268.

Davies, L., Spies, J.M., Pollard, J.D. and McLeod, J.G. (1996) Vasculitis confined to peripheral nerves. *Brain* **119**, 1441–1448.

Davies, M.A., Vonau, M., Blum, P.W., Kwok, B.C., Matheson, J.M. and Stening, W.A. (1991) Results of ulnar neuropathy at the elbow treated by decompression or anterior transposition. *Aust. N.Z. J. Surg.* **61**, 929–934.

Dawson, D.M. and Krarup, C. (1989) Perioperative nerve lesions. *Arch. Neurol.* **46**, 1355–1360.

Dawson, D.M., Hallett, M. and Millender, L.H. (1990) *Entrapment Neuropathies*, 2nd edn. Boston: Little, Brown and Co.

de Coninck, A., Helou, S. and Bins Ely, J. (1983) Le mal perforant plantaire. Neurolyse interfasciculaire du nerf tibial postérieur. [Perforating plantar ulcer. Interfascicular neurolysis of the posterior tibial nerve.] *Sem. Hop.* **59**, 1823–1826.

de Gans, J., Portegies, P., Tiessens, G., Troost, D., Danner, S.A. and Lange, J.M. (1990) Therapy for cytomegalovirus polyradiculomyelitis in patients with AIDS: treatment with ganciclovir. *AIDS* **4**, 421–425.

DeHertogh, D., Ritland, D. and Green, R. (1988) Carpal tunnel syndrome due to gonococcal tenosynovitis. *Orthopedics* **11**, 199–200.

de Jong, J.G.Y. (1947) Over families met hereditaire dispositie tot het optreden van neuritiden, gecombineerd met migraine. [On families with hereditary predisposition for the development of neuritis, associated with migraine.] *Psychiatr. Neurol. Bl.* **50**, 60–76.

de Jong, P.J. and van Weerden, T.W. (1983) Inferior and superior gluteal nerve paresis and femur neck fracture after spondylolisthesis and lysis: a case report. *J. Neurol.* **230**, 267–270.

Dekel, S., Papaioannou, T., Rushworth, G. and Coates, R. (1980) Idiopathic carpal tunnel syndrome caused by carpal stenosis. *Br. Med. J.* **280**, 1297–1299.

de Krom, M.C., Kester, A.D., Knipschild, P.G. and Spaans, F. (1990a) Risk factors for carpal tunnel syndrome. *Am. J. Epidemiol.* **132**, 1102–1110.

de Krom, M.C., Knipschild, P.G., Kester, A.D. and Spaans, F. (1990b) Efficacy of provocative tests for diagnosis of carpal tunnel syndrome. *Lancet* **335**, 393–395.

de Krom, M.C., Knipschild, P.G., Kester, A.D., Thijs, C.T., Boekkooi, P.F. and Spaans, F. (1992) Carpal tunnel syndrome: prevalence in the general population. *J. Clin. Epidemiol.* **45**, 373–376.

de Laat, E.A., Visser, C.P., Coene, L.N., Pahlplatz, P.V. and Tavy, D.L. (1994) Nerve lesions in primary shoulder dislocations and humeral neck fractures. A prospective clinical and EMG study. *J. Bone Joint Surg. [Br.]* **76**, 381–383.

de la Monte, S.M., Gabuzda, D.H., Ho, D.D., Brown, R.H., Jr, Hedley-Whyte, E.T., Schooley, R.T., Hirsch, M.S. and Bhan, A.K. (1988) Peripheral neuropathy in the acquired immunodeficiency syndrome. *Ann. Neurol.* **23**, 485–492.

Deleu, D. (1992) Mouse-directed computers and ulnar sensory neuropathy [letter]. *J. Neurol. Neurosurg. Psychiatry* **55**, 232.

DeLisa, J.A. and Saeed, M.A. (1983) The tarsal tunnel syndrome. *Muscle Nerve* **6**, 664–670.

dell'Omo, M., Muzi, G., Cantisani, T.A., Ercolani, S., Accattoli, M.P. and Abbritti, G. (1995) Bilateral median and ulnar neuropathy at the wrist in a parquet floorer. *Occup. Environ. Med.* **52**, 211–213.

Dellon, A.L. (1990) Deep peroneal nerve entrapment on the dorsum of the foot. *Foot Ankle* **11**, 73–80.

Dellon, A.L. (1992) Treatment of Morton's neuroma as a nerve compression. The role for neurolysis. *J. Am. Podiatr. Med. Assoc.* **82**, 399–402.

Dellon, A.L. and Mackinnon, S.E. (1986) Radial sensory nerve entrapment. *Arch. Neurol.* **43**, 833–835.

Dellon, A.L., Hament, W. and Gittelshon, A. (1993) Nonoperative management of cubital tunnel syndrome: an 8-year prospective study. *Neurology* **43**, 1673–1677.

Del Pino, J.G., Delgado-Martínez, A.D., González, I.G. and Lovic, A. (1997) Value of the carpal compression test in the diagnosis of carpal tunnel syndrome. *J. Hand Surg. [Br.]* **22**, 38–41.

Del Sasso, L., Mondini, A., Brambilla, S. (1988) A case of isolated paralysis of serratus anterior. *Ital. J. Orthop. Traumatol.* **14**, 533–537.

De Maeseneer, M., Jaovisidha, S., Lenchik, L., Witte, D., Schweitzer, M.E., Sartoris, D.J. and Resnick, D. (1997) Fibrolipomatous hamartoma: MR imaging findings. *Skeletal Radiol.* **26**, 155–160.

Denislic, M. and Bajec, J. (1994) Bilateral tarsal tunnel syndrome [letter]. *J. Neurol. Neurosurg. Psychiatry* **57**, 239.

De Smet, L., Bande, S. and Fabry, G. (1994) Giant lipoma of the deep palmar space, mimicking persistent carpal tunnel syndrome. *Acta Orthop. Belg.* **60**, 334–335.

Desta, K., O'Shaughnessy, M. and Milling, M.A. (1994) Non-Hodgkin's lymphoma presenting as median nerve compression in the arm. *J. Hand Surg. [Br.]* **19**, 289–291.

De Stoop, N., Suykens, S., Goossens, M., Coppens, M., Badile, N. and Dewitte, A. (1989) Tarsal tunnel syndrome: clinical and pathological results. *Acta Orthop. Belg.* **55**, 461–466.

Deutinger, M., Kuzbari, R., Paternostro Sluga, T., Quittan, M., Zauner Dungl, A., Worseg, A.,

Todoroff, B. and Holle, J. (1995) Donor-site morbidity of the gracilis flap. *Plast. Reconstr. Surg.* **95**, 1240–1244.

Dharapak, C. and Nimberg, G.A. (1974) Posterior interosseous nerve compression. Report of a case caused by traumatic aneurysm. *Clin. Orthop.* 225–228.

Dhillon, M.S. and Nagi, O.N. (1992) Sciatic nerve palsy associated with total hip arthroplasty. *Ital. J. Orthop. Traumatol.* **18**, 521–526.

Dhôte, R., Tudoret, L., Bachmeyer, C., Legmann, P. and Christoforov, B. (1996) Cyclic sciatica – a manifestation of compression of the sciatic nerve by endometriosis. A case report. *Spine* **21**, 2277–2279.

Dickason, W.L. and Barutt, J.P. (1984) Investigation of an acute microwave-oven hand injury. *J. Hand Surg. [Am.]* **9**, 132–135.

Dieck, G.S. and Kelsey, J.L. (1985) An epidemiologic study of the carpal tunnel syndrome in an adult female population. *Prev.Med.* **14**, 63–69.

Di Guglielmo, G., Torrieri, F., Repaci, M. and Uncini, A. (1997) Conduction block and segmental velocities in carpal tunnel syndrome. *Electroenceph. Clin. Neurophysiol.* **105**, 321–327.

Dimitri, W.R., West, I.E. and Williams, B.T. (1987) A quick and atraumatic method of autologous vein harvesting using the subcutaneous extraluminal dissector. *J. Cardiovasc. Surg. Torino* **28**, 103–111.

Dinsmore, W.W., Irvine, A.K. and Callender, M.E. (1985) Recurrent neuralgic amyotrophy with vagus and phrenic nerve involvement. *Clin. Neurol. Neurosurg.* **87**, 39–40.

DiRisio, D., Lazaro, R. and Popp, A.J. (1994) Nerve entrapment and calf atrophy caused by a Baker's cyst: case report. *Neurosurgery* **35**, 333–334.

Distefano, S. (1989) Neuropathy due to entrapment of the long thoracic nerve. A case report. *Ital. J. Orthop. Traumatol.* **15**, 259–262.

DiVicenti, F.C., Moncrief, J.A. and Pruitt, B.A. (1969) Electrical injuries: a review of 65 cases. *J. Trauma* **9**, 497–507.

Dobyns, J.H., O'Brien, E.T., Linscheid, R.L. and Farrow, G.M. (1972) Bowler's thumb: diagnosis and treatment. A review of seventeen cases. *J. Bone Joint Surg. [Am.]* **54**, 751–755.

Docks, G.W. and Salter, M.S. (1979) Sural nerve entrapment: an unusual case report. *J. Foot Surg.* **18**, 42–43.

Donaghy, M. (1991) Diabetic proximal neuropathy: therapy and prognosis. *Q. J. Med.* **79**, 287–288.

Donahue, F., Turkel, D.H., Mnaymneh, W. and Mnaymneh, L.G. (1996) Intraosseous ganglion cyst associated with neuropathy. *Skeletal Radiol.* **25**, 675–678.

Donahue, J.G., Choo, P.W., Manson, J.E. and Platt, R. (1995) The incidence of herpes zoster. *Arch. Intern. Med.* **155**, 1605–1609.

Dormans, J.P., Squillante, R. and Sharf, H. (1995) Acute neurovascular complications with supracondylar humerus fractures in children. *J. Hand Surg. [Am.]* **20**, 1–4.

Doublet, J.D., Gattegno, B. and Thibault, P. (1994) Laparoscopic pelvic lymph node dissection for staging of prostatic cancer. *Eur. Urol.* **25**, 194–198.

Draaisma, J.M., Fiselier, T.J. and Mullaart, R.A. (1992) Mononeuritis multiplex in a child with cutaneous polyarteritis. *Neuropediatrics* **23**, 28–29.

Drachman, D.A. (1963) Neurological complications of Wegener's granulomatosis. *Arch. Neurol.* **8**, 145–154.

Ducatman, B.S., Scheithauer, B.W., Piepgras, D.G., Reiman, H.M. and Ilstrup, D.M. (1986) Malignant peripheral nerve sheath tumours. A clinicopathologic study of 120 cases. *Cancer* **57**, 2006–2021.

Dumitru, D. and Nelson, M.R. (1990) Posterior femoral cutaneous nerve conduction. *Arch. Phys. Med. Rehabil.* **71**, 979–982.

Dumitru, D., Walsh, N. and Visser, B. (1988) Congenital hemihypertrophy associated with posterior interosseous nerve entrapment. *Arch. Phys. Med. Rehabil.* **69**, 696–698.

Duncan, M.A., Lotze, M.T., Gerber, L.H. and Rosenberg, S.A. (1983) Incidence, recovery, and management of serratus anterior muscle palsy after axillary node dissection. *Phys. Ther.* **63**, 1243–1247.

Dunn, H.G., Daube, J.R. and Gomez, M.R. (1978) Heredofamilial brachial plexus neuropathy (hereditary neuralgic amyotrophy with brachial predilection) in childhood. *Dev. Med. Child Neurol.* **20**, 28–46.

Dupont, C., Cloutier, G.E., Prévost, Y. and Dion, M.A. (1965) Ulnar tunnel syndrome at the wrist. *J. Bone Joint Surg. [Br.]* **47**, 757–761.

Durrani, Z. and Winnie, A.P. (1991) Piriformis muscle syndrome: an underdiagnosed cause of sciatica. *J. Pain Symptom Manage.* **6**, 374–379.

Dyck, P.J., Benstead, T.J., Conn, D.L., Stevens, J.C., Windebank, A.J. and Low, P.A. (1987) Nonsystemic vasculitic neuropathy. *Brain* **110**, 843–853.

Dyck, P.J., Kratz, K.M., Karnes, J.L., Litchy, W.J., Klein, R., Pach, J.M., Wilson, D.M., O'Brien, P.C., Melton, L.J.,III and Service, F.J. (1993) The prevalence by staged severity of various types of diabetic neuropathy, retinopathy, and nephropathy in a population-based cohort: the Rochester diabetic neuropathy study. *Neurology* **43**, 817–824.

Eames, R.A. and Lange, L.S. (1967) Clinical and pathological study of ischaemic neuropathy. *J. Neurol. Neurosurg. Psychiatry* **30**, 215–226.

Earl, C.J., Fullerton, P.M., Wakefield, G.S. and Schutta, H.S. (1964) Hereditary neuropathy with liability to pressure palsies – a clinical and electrophysiological study of four families. *Q. J. Med.* **132**, 481–498.

Eaton, L.M. (1937) Paralysis of the peroneal nerve caused by crossing the legs: report of a case. *Mayo Clin. Proc.* **12**, 206–208.

Ebeling, P., Gilliatt, R.W. and Thomas, P.K. (1960) A clinical and electrical study of ulnar nerve lesions in the hand. *J. Neurol. Neurosurg. Psychiatry* **23**, 1–10.

Ecker, A.D. and Woltman, H.W. (1938) Meralgia paresthetica: a report of one hundred and fifty cases. *JAMA* **110**, 1650–1652.

Edelson, R. and Stevens, P. (1994) Meralgia paresthetica in children. *J. Bone Joint Surg. [Am.]* **76**, 993–999.

Edlich, H.S., Fariss, B.L., Phillips, V.A., Chang, D.E., Smith, J.F., Hartigan, C. and Edlich, R.F. (1987) Talotibial exostoses with entrapment of the deep peroneal nerve. *J. Emerg. Med.* **5**, 109–113.

Edwards, J.C., Green, C.T. and Riefel, E. (1989) Neurilemoma of the saphenous nerve presenting as pain in the knee. A case report. *J. Bone Joint Surg. [Am.]* **71**, 1410–1411.

Edwards, M.S.D., Hirigoyen, M. and Burge, P.D. (1995) Compression of the common peroneal nerve by a cyst of the lateral meniscus. A case report. *Clin. Orthop.* 131–133.

Edwards, P. and Kurth, L. (1992) Postoperative radial nerve paralysis caused by fracture callus. *J. Orthop. Trauma* **6**, 234–236.

Edwards, P. and Nilsson, B.E. (1969) The time of disability following fracture of the shaft of the tibia. *Acta Orthop. Scand.* **40**, 501–506.

Efthimiou, J., Butler, J., Woodham, C., Benson, M.K. and Westaby, S. (1991) Diaphragm paralysis following cardiac surgery: role of phrenic nerve cold injury. *Ann. Thorac. Surg.* **52**, 1005–1008.

Ehrmann, L., Lechner, K., Mamoli, B., Novotny, C. and Kos, K. (1981) Peripheral nerve lesions in haemophilia. *J. Neurol.* **225**, 175–182.

Eiras, J. and Garcia Cosamalon, P.J. (1979) Intraneural ganglion of the common peroneal nerve. *Neurochirurgia. Stuttg.* **22**, 145–150.

Ekelund, A.L. (1990) Bilateral nerve entrapment in the popliteal space. *Am. J. Sports Med.* **18**, 108.

Ekman, O.G., Salgeback, S. and Ordeberg, G. (1987) Carpal tunnel syndrome in pregnancy. A prospective study. *Acta Obstet. Gynecol. Scand.* **66**, 233–235.

Ellenberg, M. (1978) Diabetic truncal mononeuropathy – a new clinical syndrome. *Diabetes Care* **1**, 10–13.

Elliott, K.J. (1994) Other neurological complications of herpes zoster and their management. *Ann. Neurol.* **35**(Suppl.), S57–S61.

Ellis, R.J., Geisse, H., Holub, B.A. and Swenson, M.R. (1992) Ilioinguinal nerve conduction [abstract]. *Muscle Nerve* **15**, 1194.

Endtz, L.J., Frenay, J. and Goor, C. (1983) Vasculitic neuropathy in RA [letter]. *Neurology* **33**, 1635–1636.

England, J.D. and Sumner, A.J. (1987) Neuralgic amyotrophy: an increasingly diverse entity. *Muscle Nerve* **10**, 60–68.

Engrav, L.H., Gottlieb, J.R., Walkinshaw, M.D., Heimbach, D.M., Trumble, T.E. and Grube, B.J. (1990) Outcome and treatment of electrical injury with immediate median and ulnar nerve palsy at the wrist: a retrospective review and a survey of members of the American Burn Association. *Ann. Plast. Surg.* **25**, 166–168.

Engstrom, J.W., Layzer, R.B., Olney, R.K. and Edwards, M.B. (1993) Idiopathic, progressive mononeuropathy in young people. *Arch. Neurol.* **50**, 20–23.

Enzenauer, R.J. and Nordstrom, D.M. (1991) Anterior interosseous nerve syndrome associated with forearm band treatment of lateral epicondylitis. *Orthopedics* **14**, 788–790.

Erickson, S.J., Quinn, S.F., Kneeland, J.B., Smith, J.W., Johnson, J.E., Carrera, G.F., Shereff, M.J., Hyde, J.S. and Jesmanowicz, A. (1990) MR imaging of the tarsal tunnel and related spaces: normal and abnormal findings with anatomic correlation. *Am. J. Roentgenol.* **155**, 323–328.

Esmann, V., Geil, J.P., Kroon, S., Fogh, H., Peterslund, N.A., Petersen, C.S., Ronne-Rasmussen, J.O. and Danielsen, L. (1987) Prednisolone does not prevent post-herpetic neuralgia. *Lancet* **ii**, 126–129.

Esselman, P.C., Tomski, M.A., Robinson, L.R., Zisfein, J. and Marks, S.J. (1993) Selective deep peroneal nerve injury associated with arthroscopic knee surgery. *Muscle Nerve* **16**, 11–92.

Etienne, G., Constantin, J.M. and Hevia, M. (1995) Le cryo-eveinage: une avancee dans le traitement de la maladie variqueuse. 3811 membres opérés. [Cryo-stripping: an advance in the treatment of varicose veins. 3811 operated limbs.] *Presse Méd.* **24**, 1017–1020.

Eustace, S., McCarthy, C., O'Byrne, J., Breatnach, E. and Fitzgerald, E. (1994) Computed tomography of the retroperitoneum in patients with femoral neuropathy. *Can. Assoc. Radiol. J.* **45**, 277–282.

Evans, B.A., Stevens, J.C. and Dyck, P.J. (1981) Lumbosacral plexus neuropathy. *Neurology* **31**, 1327–1330.

Evans, J.D., Neumann, L. and Frostick, S.P. (1994) Compression neuropathy of the common peroneal nerve caused by a ganglion. *Microsurgery.* **15**, 193–195.

Fabian, R.H., Norcross, K.A. and Hancock, M.B. (1987) Surfer's neuropathy [letter]. *N. Engl. J. Med.* **316**, 555.

Fabian, V.A., Wood, B., Crowley, P. and Kakulas, B.A. (1997) Herpes zoster brachial plexus neuritis. *Clin. Neuropathol.* **16**, 61–64.

Fabra, M., Frieling, A., Porst, H. and Schneider, E. (1993) Schwerpunktneuropathie des N. pudendus bei Alkoholikern mit erektiler Dysfunction? [Pressure neuropathy of the pudendal nerve in alcoholics with erectile dysfunction?] *Z. EEG-EMG* **24**, 274–279.

Falck, B. and Alaranta, H. (1983) Fibrillation potentials, positive sharp waves and fasciculation in the intrinsic muscles of the foot in healthy subjects. *J. Neurol. Neurosurg. Psychiatry* **46**, 681–683.

Falck, B., Hurme, M., Hakkarainen, S. and Aarnio, P. (1984) Sensory conduction velocity of plantar digital nerves in Morton's metatarsalgia. *Neurology* **34**, 698–701.

Farber, J.S. and Bryan, R.S. (1968) The anterior interosseous nerve syndrome. *J. Bone Joint Surg. [Am.]* **50**, 521–523.

Farkkila, M., Aatola, S., Starck, J., Pyykko, I. and Korhonen, O. (1985) Vibration-induced neuropathy among forestry workers. *Acta Neurol. Scand.* **71**, 221–225.

Farkkila, M., Pyykko, I., Jantti, V., Aatola, S., Starck, J. and Korhonen, O. (1988) Forestry workers exposed to vibration: a neurological study. *Br. J. Ind. Med.* **45**, 188–192.

Favero, K.J., Hawkins, R.H. and Jones, M.W. (1987) Neuralgic amyotrophy. *J. Bone Joint Surg. [Br.]* **69**, 195–198.

Feibel, J.H. and Campa, J.F. (1976) Thyrotoxic neuropathy (Basedow's paraplegia). *J. Neurol. Neurosurg.Psychiatry* **39**, 491–497.

Feigal, D.W., Robbins, D.L. and Leek, J.C. (1985) Giant cell arteritis associated with mononeuritis multiplex and complement-activating 19S IgM rheumatoid factor. *Am. J. Med.* **79**, 495–500.

Feinglass, E.J., Arnett, F.C., Dorsch, C.A., Zizic, T.M. and Stevens, M.B. (1976) Neuropsychiatric manifestations of systemic lupus erythematosus: diagnosis, clinical spectrum, and relationship to other features of the disease. *Medicine (Baltimore)* **55**, 323–339.

Feinstein, B., Pattle, R.E. and Weddell, C.T. (1945) Metabolic factors affecting fibrillations in denervated muscle. *J. Neurol. Neurosurg. Psychiatry* **8**, 1–16.

Feldman, M.D., Rotman, M.B. and Manske, P.R. (1995) Compression of the deep motor branch of the ulnar nerve by a midpalmar ganglion. *Orthopedics* **18**, 65–67.

Felsenthal, G. (1983) Bedrail palsy: the etiology of bilateral footdrop. *Md. State. Med. J.* **32**, 173–174.

Felsenthal, G., Mondell, D.L., Reischer, M.A. and Mack, R.H. (1984) Forearm pain secondary to compression syndrome of the lateral cutaneous nerve of the forearm. *Arch. Phys. Med. Rehabil.* **65**, 139–141.

Felsenthal, G., Butler, D.H. and Shear, M.S. (1992) Across-tarsal-tunnel motor-nerve conduction technique. *Arch. Phys. Med. Rehabil.* **73**, 64–69.

Fenichel, G.M. (1982) Neurological complications of immunization. *Ann. Neurol.* **12**, 119–128.

Ferguson, F.R. and Liversedge, L.A. (1954) Ischaemic lateral popliteal nerve palsy. *Br. Med. J.* **2**, 333–335.

Ferlic, D.C. and Ries, M.D. (1990) Epineural ganglion of the ulnar nerve at the elbow. *J. Hand Surg. [Am.]* **15**, 996–998.

Fernandez, A.M. and Tiku, M.L. (1994) Posterior interosseous nerve entrapment in rheumatoid arthritis. *Semin. Arthritis Rheum.* **24**, 57–60.

Fernandez, E., Pallini, R. and Talamonti, G. (1987) Sleep palsy (Saturday-night palsy) of the deep radial nerve. Case report. *J. Neurosurg.* **66**, 460–461.

Fernandez Garcia, S., Pi Folguera, J. and Estallo Matino, F. (1994) Bifid median nerve compression due to a musculotendinous anomaly of FDS to the middle finger. *J. Hand Surg. [Br.]* **19**, 616–617.

Ferrer, I., Vidaller, A., Fernandez de Sevilla, A., Martinez Matos, J.A., Montero, J. and Romagosa, V. (1988) Peripheral neuropathy associated with angioimmunoblastic lymphadenopathy. *Clin. Neurol. Neurosurg.* **90**, 159–162.

Fettweis, E. (1966) Kniegelenks-und Huftgelenkskontrakturen bei narbiger Irritation des sensiblen Astes des Nervus obturatoius. [Contractures of the knee and hip joint in scarry irritation of the sensory branch of nervus obturatorius.] *Dtsch. Med. Wochenschr.* **91**, 313–314.

Filler, A.G., Kliot, M., Howe, F.A., Hayes, C.E., Saunders, D.E., Goodkin, R., Bell, B.A., Winn, H.R., Griffiths, J.R. and Tsuruda, J.S. (1996) Application of magnetic resonance neurography in the evaluation of patients with peripheral nerve pathology. *J. Neurosurg.* **85**, 299–309.

Filling-Katz, M.R. (1984) Mononeuritis multiplex following jellyfish stings [letter]. *Ann. Neurol.* **15**, 213.

Finelli, P.F. (1977) Anterior interosseous nerve syndrome following cutdown catheterization. *Ann. Neurol.* **1**, 205–206.

Finkel, M.J. and Halperin, J.J. (1992) Nervous system Lyme borreliosis – revisited. *Arch. Neurol.* **49**, 102–107.

Finkelman, R., Munsat, T., Mandell, H., Adelman, L. and Logigian, E. (1993) Neuromuscular manifestations of Wegener's granulomatosis: a case report. *Neurology* **43**, 617–618.

Fisher, A.P. and Hanna, M. (1987) Transcutaneous electrical nerve stimulation in meralgia paraesthetica of pregnancy. *Br. J. Obstet. Gynaecol.* **94**, 603–604.

Fisher, C.M. and Adams, R.D. (1956) Diphtheritic polyneuritis, a pathological study. *J. Neuropathol. Exp. Neurol.* **15**, 243–268.

Fishman, J.R., Moran, M.E. and Carey, R.W. (1993) Obturator neuropathy after laparoscopic pelvic lymphadenectomy. *Urology* **42**, 198–200.

Fitzsimmons, A.S., O'Dell, M.W., Guiffra, L.J. and Sandel, M.E. (1993) Radial nerve injury associated with traumatic myositis ossificans in a brain injured patient. *Arch. Phys. Med. Rehabil.* **74**, 770–773.

Flaggman, P.D. and Kelly, J.J.J. (1980) Brachial plexus neuropathy. An electrophysiologic evaluation. *Arch. Neurol.* **37**, 160–164.

Fletcher, H.S. and Frankel, J. (1976) Ruptured abdominal aneurysms presenting with unilateral peripheral neuropathy. *Surgery* **79**, 120–121.

Florin, T. and Walls, R.S. (1984) Neurological complications of thyrotoxicosis in the elderly [letter]. *Ann.Neurol.* **15**, 608.

Floros, C. and Davis, P.K. (1991) Complications and long-term results following abdominoplasty: a retrospective study. *Br. J. Plast. Surg.* **44**, 190–194.

Flügel, K.A., Sturm, U. and Skiba, N. (1984) Somatosensibel evozierte Potentiale nach Stimulation des N. cutaneus femoris lateralis bei Normalpersonen und Patienten mit Meralgia paraesthetica. [Somatosensory evoked potentials following stimulation of the lateral femoral cutaneous nerve in normal persons and in patients with meralgia paraesthetica.] *EEG EMG Z. Elektroenzephalogr. Verwandte. Geb.* **15**, 88–93.

Foo, C.L. and Swann, M. (1983) Isolated paralysis of the serratus anterior. A report of 20 cases. *J. Bone Joint Surg. [Br.]* **65**, 552–556.

Fortin, P.R., Fraser, R.S., Watts, C.S. and Esdaile, J.M. (1991) Alpha-1 antitrypsin deficiency and systemic necrotizing vasculitis. *J. Rheumatol.* **18**, 1613–1616.

Fortuna, R., Grisostomi, E. and Grisostomi, C. (1989) La sindrome del tunnel carpale nelle orlatrici calzaturiere. [Carpal tunnel syndrome in shoe hemmers.] *Chir. Organi. Mov.* **74**, 79–82.

Fosse, E. and Fjeld, N.B. (1991) Kirurgisk pleurodese ved spontanpneumothorax. [Surgical pleurodesis in spontaneous pneumothorax.] *Tidsskr. Nor. Laegeforen.* **111**, 196–197.

Foucher, G., Berard, V., Snider, G., Lenoble, E. and Constantinesco, A. (1993) Distal ulnar nerve entrapment due to tumours of Guyon's canal. A series of ten cases. *Handchir. Mikrochir. Plast. Chir.* **25**, 61–65.

Foxworthy, M. and Kinninmonth, A.W. (1992) Median nerve compression in the proximal forearm as a complication of partial rupture of the distal biceps brachii tendon. *J. Hand Surg. Br.* **17**, 515–517.

Francel, T.J., Dellon, A.L. and Campbell, J.N. (1991) Quadrilateral space syndrome: diagnosis and operative decompression technique. *Plast. Reconstr. Surg.* **87**, 911–916.

Francis, H., March, L., Terenty, T. and Webb, J. (1987) Benign joint hypermobility with neuropathy: documentation and mechanism of tarsal tunnel syndrome. *J. Rheumatol.* **14**, 577–581.

Franzini, A., Scaioli, V., Leocata, F., Palazzini, E. and Broggi, G. (1995) Pain syndrome and focal myokymia due to anterior interosseous neurovascular relationships: report of a case and neurophysiological considerations. *J. Neurosurg.* **82**, 578–580.

Fraser, D.M., Parker, A.C., Amer, S. and Campbell, I.W. (1976) Mononeuritis multiplex in a patient with macroglobulinaemia. *J. Neurol. Neurosurg. Psychiatry* **39**, 711–715.

Fraser, D.M., Campbell, I.W., Ewing, D.J. and Clarke, B.F. (1979) Mononeuropathy in diabetes mellitus. *Diabetes* **28**, 96–101.

Fricker, R.M., Troeger, H. and Pfeiffer, K.M. (1997) Obturator nerve palsy due to fixation of an acetabular reinforcement ring with transacetabular screws – A case report. *J. Bone Joint Surg. [Am.]* **79A**, 444–446.

Fritz, R.C., Helms, C.A., Steinbach, L.S. and Genant, H.K. (1992) Suprascapular nerve entrapment: evaluation with MR imaging. *Radiology* **182**, 437–444.

Frymoyer, J.W. and Bland, J. (1973) Carpal-tunnel syndrome in patients with myxedematous arthropathy. *J. Bone Joint Surg. [Am.]* **55**, 78–82.

Fu, R., DeLisa, J.A. and Kraft, G.H. (1980) Motor nerve latencies through the tarsal tunnel in normal adult subjects: standard determinations corrected for temperature and distance. *Arch. Phys. Med. Rehabil.* **61**, 243–248.

Fuller, G.N., Jacobs, J.M. and Guiloff, R.J. (1993) Nature and incidence of peripheral nerve syndromes in HIV infection. *J. Neurol. Neurosurg. Psychiatry* **56**, 372–381.

Fullerton, P.M. (1963) The effect of ischaemia on nerve conduction in the carpal tunnel. *J. Neurol. Neurosurg. Psychiatry* **26**, 385–397.

Gabel, G.T. and Amadio, P.C. (1990) Reoperation for failed decompression of the ulnar nerve in the region of the elbow. *J. Bone Joint Surg. [Am.]* **72**, 213–219.

Gadelrab, R.R. (1990) Sciatic nerve entrapment in an osseous tunnel as a late complication of fracture dislocation of the hip. *Orthopedics* **13**, 1262–1264.

Gainsborough, N., Hall, S.M., Hughes, R.A. and Leibowitz, S. (1991) Sarcoid neuropathy. *J. Neurol.* **238**, 177–180.

Gallagher, J.P. and Sanders, M. (1983) Apparent motor neuron disease following the use of pneumatic tools [letter]. *Ann. Neurol.* **14**, 694–695.

Galzio, R.J., Magliani, V., Lucantoni, D. and D'Arrigo, C. (1987) Bilateral anomalous course of the ulnar nerve at the wrist causing ulnar and median nerve compression syndrome. Case report. *J. Neurosurg.* **67**, 754–756.

Ganglani, R.D., Turk, A.A., Mehra, M.R., Beaver, W.L. and Lach, R.D. (1991) Contralateral femoral neuropathy: an unusual complication of anticoagulation following PTCA. *Cathet. Cardiovasc. Diagn.* **24**, 176–178.

Gardner Thorpe, C. (1974) Anterior interosseous nerve palsy: spontaneous recovery in two patients. *J. Neurol. Neurosurg. Psychiatry* **37**, 1146–1150.

Garland, H. and Moorhouse, D. (1952) Compressive lesions of the external popliteal (common peroneal) nerve. *Br. Med. J.* **2**, 1373–1378.

Garlipp, M. (1979) Spongiosaentnahme am Beckenkamm und Meralgia paraesthetica. [Meralgia paraesthetica [author's transl].] *Zentralbl. Chir.* **104**, 658–660.

Gasecki, A.P., Ebers, G.C., Vellet, A.D. and Buchan, A. (1992) Sciatic neuropathy associated with persistent sciatic artery. *Arch. Neurol.* **49**, 967–968.

Gauthier, G. (1979) Thomas Morton's disease: a nerve entrapment syndrome. A new surgical technique. *Clin. Orthop.* 90–92.

Gaynor, R., Hake, D., Spinner, S.M. and Tomczak, R.L. (1989) A comparative analysis of conservative versus surgical treatment of Morton's neuroma. *J. Am. Podiatr. Med. Assoc.* **79**, 27–30.

Geelen, J.A., de Graaff, R., Biemans, R.G., Prevo, R.L. and Koch, P.W. (1985) Sciatic nerve compression by an aneurysm of the internal iliac artery. *Clin. Neurol. Neurosurg.* **87**, 219–222.

Geiger, L.R., Mancall, E.L., Penn, A.S. and Tucker, S.H. (1974) Familial neuralgic amyotrophy. Report of three families with review of the literature. *Brain* **97**, 87–102.

Geissler, W.B., Corso, S.R. and Caspari, R.B. (1992) Isolated rupture of the popliteus with posterior tibial nerve palsy. *J. Bone Joint Surg. [Br.]* **74**, 811–813.

Gelberman, R.H., Aronson, D. and Weisman, M.H. (1980) Carpal-tunnel syndrome. Results of a prospective trial of steroid injection and splinting. *J. Bone Joint Surg. Am.* **62**, 1181–1184.

Gellman, H., Gelberman, R.H., Tan, A.M. and Botte, M.J. (1986) Carpal tunnel syndrome. An evaluation of the provocative diagnostic tests. *J. Bone Joint Surg. Am.* **68**, 735–737.

Gerardi, J.A., Mack, G.R. and Lutz, R.B. (1989) Acute carpal tunnel syndrome secondary to septic arthritis of the wrist. *J. Am. Osteopath. Assoc.* **89**, 933–934.

Gersbach, P. and Waridel, D. (1976) Paralysie après prévention antitétanique. *Schweiz. Med. Wochenschr.* **106**, 150–153.

Gherardi, R., Lebargy, F., Gaulard, P., Mhiri, C., Bernaudin, J.F. and Gray, F. (1989a) Necrotizing vasculitis and HIV replication in peripheral nerves [letter]. *N. Engl. J. Med.* **321**, 685–686.

Gherardi, R.K., Amiel, H., Martin Mondiere, C., Viard, J.P., Salama, J. and Delaporte, P. (1989b) Solitary plasmacytoma of the skull revealed by a mononeuritis multiplex associated with immune complex vasculitis. *Arthritis Rheum.* **32**, 1470–1473.

Ghika Schmid, F., Kuntzer, T., Chave, J.P., Miklossy, J. and Regli, F. (1994) Diversité de l'atteinte neuromusculaire de 47 patients infectés par le virus de l'immunodéficience humaine. [Range of neuromuscular involvement in 47 patients infected with the human immunodeficiency virus.] *Schweiz. Med. Wochenschr.* **124**, 791–800.

Giannestras, N.J. and Bronson, J.L. (1975) Malignant schwannoma of the medial plantar branch of the posterior tibial nerve (unassociated with von Recklinghausen's disease). A case report. *J. Bone Joint Surg. [Am.]* **57**, 701–703.

Gilliatt, R.W. and Wilson, T.G. (1953) A pneumatic tourniquet test in the carpal tunnel syndrome. *Lancet* **ii**, 595–597.

Gilliatt, R.W., Willison, R.G., Dietz, V. and Williams, I.R. (1978) Peripheral nerve conduction in patients with a cervical rib and band. *Ann. Neurol.* **4**, 124–129.

Giuliani, G., Poppi, M., Pozzati, E. and Forti, A. (1990) Ulnar neuropathy due to a carpal ganglion: the diagnostic contribution of. *Neurology* **40**, 1001–1002.

Glantz, M.J., Burger, P.C., Friedman, A.H., Radtke, R.A., Massey, E.W. and Schold, S.C., Jr (1994) Treatment of radiation-induced nervous system injury with heparin and warfarin. *Neurology* **44**, 2020–2027.

Glover, M.G. and Convery, F.R. (1989) Migration of fractured greater trochanteric osteotomy wire with resultant sciatica. A report of two cases. *Orthopedics* **12**, 743–744.

Glynn, C., Crockford, G., Gavaghan, D., Cardno, P., Price, D. and Miller, J. (1990) Epidemiology of shingles. *J. R. Soc. Med.* **83**, 617–619.

Gnann, J.W., Jr (1994) New antivirals with activity against varicella-zoster virus. *Ann. Neurol.* **35**(suppl.), S69–S72.

Golbus, J. and McCune, W.J. (1987) Giant cell arteritis and peripheral neuropathy: a report of 2 cases and review of the literature. *J. Rheumatol.* **14**, 129–134.

Goldberg, V.M. and Jacobs, B. (1975) Osteoid osteoma of the hip in children. *Clin. Orthop.* 41–47.

Golding, D.N. (1970) Hypothyroidism presenting with musculoskeletal symptoms. *Ann. Rheum. Dis.* **29**, 10–14.

Goldman, S., Honet, J.C., Sobel, R. and Goldstein, A.S. (1969) Posterior interosseous nervepalsy in the absence of trauma. *Arch. Neurol.* **21**, 435–441.

Gonnaud, P.M., Sturtz, F., Fourbil, Y. *et al.* (1995) DNA analysis as a tool to confirm the diagnosis of asymptomatic hereditary neuropathy with liability to pressure palsies (HNPP) with further evidence for the occurrence of *de novo* mutations. *Acta Neurol. Scand.* **92**, 313–318.

Goodfellow, J., Fearn, C.B. and Matthews, J.M. (1967) Iliacus haematoma. A common complication of haemophilia. *J. Bone Joint Surg. [Br.]* **49**, 748–756.

Goodgold, J., Kopell, H.P. and Spielholz, N.I. (1965) The tarsal tunnel syndrome: objective diagnostic criteria. *N. Engl. J. Med.* **273**, 742–745.

Goodwin, D.R. and Arbel, R. (1985) Pseudogout of the wrist presenting as acute median nerve compression. *J. Hand Surg. [Br.]* **10**, 261–262.

Gore, D.R. (1971) Carpometacarpal dislocation producing compression of the deep branch of the ulnar nerve. *J. Bone Joint Surg. [Am.]* **53**, 1387–1390.

Gottlieb, N.L. and Riskin, W.G. (1980) Complications of local corticosteroid injections. *JAMA* **243**, 1547–1548.

Gouet, P., Castets, M., Touchard, G., Payen, J. and Alcalay, M. (1984) Bilateral carpal tunnel syndrome due to tuberculosis tenosynovitis: a case report [letter]. *J. Rheumatol.* **11**, 721–722.

Gouider, R., LeGuern, E., Emile, J., Tardieu, S., Cabon, F., Samid, M., Weissenbach, J., Agid, Y., Bouche, P. and Brice, A. (1994) Hereditary neuralgic amyotrophy and hereditary neuropathy with liability to pressure palsies: two distinct clinical, electrophysiologic, and genetic entities. *Neurology* **44**, 2250–2252.

Gould, N. and Trevino, S. (1981) Sural nerve entrapment by avulsion fracture of the base of the fifth metatarsal bone. *Foot Ankle* **2**, 153–155.

Goulding, P.J. and Schady, W. (1993) Favourable outcome in non-traumatic anterior interosseous nerve lesions. *J. Neurol.* **240**, 83–86.

Gousheh, J. and Razian, M. (1991) Les blessures de guerre du nerf crural. A propos d'une série de vingt-sept cas. [War injuries of the femoral nerve. Apropos of a series of 27 cases.] *Ann. Chir. Plast. Esthet.* **36**, 527–531.

Grabois, M., Puentes, J. and Lidsky, M. (1981) Tarsal tunnel syndrome in rheumatoid arthritis. *Arch. Phys. Med. Rehabil.* **62**, 401–403.

Grace, D.M. (1987) Meralgia paresthetica after gastroplasty for morbid obesity. *Can. J. Surg.* **30**, 64–65.

Greco, R.J. and Curtsinger, L.J. (1993) Carpal tunnel release complicated by necrotizing fasciitis. *Ann. Plast. Surg.* **30**, 545–548.

Greenberg, M.K., McVey, A.L. and Hayes, T. (1992) Segmental motor involvement in herpes zoster: an EMG study. *Neurology* **42**, 1122–1123.

Greenfield, J., Rea, J. and Ilfeld, F.W. (1984) Morton's interdigital neuroma. Indications for treatment by local injections versus surgery. *Clin. Orthop.* **185**, 142–144.

Gross, J.A., Hamilton, W.J. and Swift, T.R. (1980) Isolated mechanical lesions of the sural nerve. *Muscle Nerve* **3**, 248–249.

Gross, P.T. and Jones, H.R., Jr (1992) Proximal median neuropathies: electromyographic and clinical correlation. *Muscle Nerve* **15**, 390–395.

Groulier, P., Benaim, J.L., Curvale, G. and Guillermet, R. (1987) Un cas de compression du nerf tibial postérieur par un kyste synovial developpé aux dépens de l'articulation péroneo-tibiale supérieure. [A case of compression of the posterior tibial nerve by a synovial cyst with impact on the superior tibiofibular joint.] *Rev. Chir. Orthop.* **73**, 67–69.

Grube, B.J., Heimbach, D.M., Engrav, L.H. and Copass, M.K. (1990) Neurologic consequences of electrical burns. *J. Trauma* **30**, 254–258.

Guillain, G., Bourguignon, G. and Corre, L. (1940) Les paralysies du nerf cubital chez les cyclistes. [Ulnar nerve palsies in cyclists.] *Bull. Soc. Méd. Hôp.* **56**, 489–492.

Guillemin, F., Czorny, A. and Pourel, J. (1991) Sciatic nerve compression by hematoma. Case report of a late complication of Harrington's operation. *Spine* **16**, 237–239.

Guiloff, R.J. (1979) Carbamazepine in Morton's neuralgia. *Br. Med. J.* **2**, 904.

Guiloff, R.J. (1989) AIDS: neurological opportunist infections in central London. *J. R. Soc. Med.* **82**, 278–280.

Guiloff, R.J. and Sherratt, R.M. (1977) Sensory conduction in medial plantar nerve: normal values, clinical applications, and a comparison with the sural and upper limb sensory nerve action potentials in peripheral neuropathy. *J. Neurol. Neurosurg. Psychiatry* **40**, 1168–1181.

Guiloff, R.J., Scadding, J.W. and Klenerman, L. (1984) Morton's metatarsalgia. Clinical, electrophysiological and histological observations. *J. Bone Joint Surg. [Br.]* **66**, 586–591.

Haddad, F.S., Jones, D.H., Vellodi, A., Kane, N. and Pitt, M.C. (1997) Carpal tunnel syndrome in the mucopolysaccharidoses and mucolipidoses. *J. Bone Joint Surg. [Br.]* **79**, 576–582.

Hadley, M.N., Sonntag, V.K. and Pittman, H.W. (1986) Suprascapular nerve entrapment. A summary of seven cases. *J. Neurosurg.* **64**, 843–848.

Hah, J.S., Kim, D.E. and Oh, S.J. (1992) Lateral plantar neuropathy: a heretofore unrecognized neuropathy. *Muscle Nerve* **15**, 1175.

Hahn, L. (1989) Clinical findings and results of operative treatment in ilioinguinal nerve entrapment syndrome. *Br. J. Obstet. Gynaecol.* **96**, 1080–1083.

Haldeman, S., Bradley, W.E., Bhatia, N.N. and *et al* (1982) Neurologic evaluation of bladder, bowel and sexual disturbances in diabetic man. In: Goto, Y., Hiriuchi, A. and Kogure, K. (eds), *Diabetic Neuropathy*, pp. 298–307. Amsterdam: Excerpta Medica.

Hale, B.R. (1976) Handbag paraesthesia [letter]. *Lancet* **ii**, 470.

Hall, C.D., Snyder, C.R., Messenheimer, J.A., Wilkins, J.W., Robertson, W.T., Whaley, R.A. and Robertson, K.R. (1991) Peripheral neuropathy in a cohort of human immunodeficiency virus-infected patients. Incidence and relationship to other nervous system dysfunction. *Arch. Neurol.* **48**, 1273–1274.

Hall, M.C., Koch, M.O. and Smith, J.A., Jr (1995) Femoral neuropathy complicating urologic abdominopelvic procedures. *Urology.* **45**, 146–149.

Halperin, J.J., Volkman, D.J., Luft, B.J. and Dattwyler, R.J. (1989) Carpal tunnel syndrome in Lyme borreliosis. *Muscle Nerve* **12**, 397–400.

Halperin, J.J., Luft, B.J., Volkman, D.J. and Dattwyler, R.J. (1990) Lyme neuroborreliosis. Peripheral nervous system manifestations. *Brain* **113**, 1207–1221.

Hankey, G.J. (1988) Median nerve compression in the palm of the hand by an anomalously enlarged ulnar artery. *Aust. N.Z. J. Surg.* **58**, 511–513.

Hankey, G.J. and Gubbay, S.S. (1988) Compressive mononeuropathy of the deep palmar branch of the ulnar nerve in cyclists. *J. Neurol. Neurosurg. Psychiatry* **51**, 1588–1590.

Hannington-Kiff, J.G. (1980) Absent thigh adductor reflex in obturator hernia. *Lancet* **i**, 180.

Hanson, G.C. and McIlwraith, G.R. (1973) Lightning injury: two case histories and a review of management. *Br. Med. J.* **4**, 271–274.

Hardegger, F. and Segmuller, G. (1982) Ischamische Nekrose der tiefen Vorderarmstrecker: ein seltenes Compartment-Syndrom. [Ischemic necrosis of the deep extensors of the forearm: a rare compartment syndrome.] *Schweiz. Med. Wochenschr.* **112**, 1549–1556.

Harding, A.E. and Le, F.J. (1977) Carpal tunnel syndrome related to antebrachial Cimino-Brescia fistula. *J. Neurol. Neurosurg. Psychiatry* **40**, 511–513.

Harness, D. and Sekeles, E. (1971) The double anastomotic innervation of thenar muscles. *J. Anat.* **109**, 461–466.

Harper, C.M., Jr, Thomas, J.E., Cascino, T.L. and Litchy, W.J. (1989) Distinction between neoplastic and radiation-induced brachial plexopathy, with emphasis on the role of EMG. *Neurology* **39**, 502–506.

Harrison, M.J., Leis, H.T., Johnson, B.A., MacDonald, W.D. and Goldman, C.D. (1995) Hemangiopericytoma of the sciatic notch presenting as sciatica in a young healthy man: case report. *Neurosurgery* **37**, 1208–1211.

Hartz, C.R., Linscheid, R.L., Gramse, R.R. and Daube, J.R. (1981) The pronator teres syndrome: compressive neuropathy of the median nerve. *J. Bone Joint Surg. [Am.]* **63**, 885–890.

Haskard, D.O. and Panayi, G.S. (1988) Multiple peripheral nerve entrapment in Forestier's disease (diffuse idiopathic skeletal hyperostosis). *Br. J. Rheumatol.* **27**, 407–408.

Haskin, J.S., Jr (1994) Ganglion-related compression neuropathy of the palmar cutaneous branch of the median nerve: a report of two cases. *J. Hand Surg. [Am.]* **19**, 827–828.

Hawkes, C.H. and Thorpe, J.W. (1992) Acute polyneuropathy due to lightning injury. *J. Neurol. Neurosurg. Psychiatry* **55**, 388–390.

Hawkes, C.H., Jefferson, J.M., Jones, E.L. and Thomas, S.W. (1974) Hypertrophic mononeuropathy. *J. Neurol. Neurosurg. Psychiatry* **37**, 76–81.

Hayashi, Y., Kojima, T. and Kohno, T. (1984) A case of cubital tunnel syndrome caused by the snapping of the medial head of the triceps brachii muscle. *J. Hand Surg. [Am.]* **9**, 96–99.

Hayes, J.M. and Zehr, D.J. (1981) Traumatic muscle avulsion causing winging of the scapula. A case report. *J. Bone Joint Surg. [Am.]* **63**, 495–497.

Healy, C., Watson, J.D., Longstaff, A. and Campbell, M.J. (1990) Magnetic resonance imaging of the carpal tunnel. *J. Hand Surg. [Br.]* **15**, 243–248.

Hebbar, M., Hebbar Savean, K., Hachulla, E., Brouillard, M., Hatron, P.Y. and Devulder, B. (1995) Participation of cryoglobulinaemia in the severe peripheral neuropathies of primary Sjogren's syndrome. *Ann. Med. Intern. Paris.* **146**, 235–238.

Heidenreich, W. and Lorenzoni, E. (1983) Lasion des Nervus cutaneus femoris lateralis. Eine seltene Komplikation nach gynakologischen Eingriffen. [Injury of the lateral cutaneous nerve of the thigh. A rare complication following gynecologic surgery.] *Geburtshilfe. Frauenheilkd.* **43**, 766–768.

Helbling, F., Wyss, P. and Maroni, E. (1994) Einseitige, sensomotorische Femoralisparese nach einer abdominalen gynakologischen Operation. [Unilateral, sensorimotor femoral nerve paralysis following abdominal gynecological operation.] *Geburtshilfe. Frauenheilkd.* **54**, 250–252.

Hemler, D.E., Ward, W.K., Karstetter, K.W. and Bryant, P.M. (1991) Saphenous nerve entrapment caused by pes anserine bursitis mimicking stress fracture of the tibia. *Arch. Phys. Med. Rehabil.* **72**, 336–337.

Henlin, J.L., Rousselot, J.P., Monnier, G., Sevrin, P. and Bady, B. (1992) Syndrome canalaire du nerf sus-scapulaire dans le défilé spino-glénoidien. [Suprascapular nerve entrapment at the spinoglenoid notch.] *Rev. Neurol. (Paris)* **148**, 362–367.

Henricson, A.S. and Westlin, N.E. (1984) Chronic calcaneal pain in athletes: entrapment of the calcaneal nerve? *Am. J. Sports Med.* **12**, 152–154.

Herndon, J.H., Eaton, R.G. and Littler, J.W. (1974) Carpal-tunnel syndrome. An unusual presentation of osteoid-osteoma of the capitate. *J. Bone Joint Surg. Am.* **56**, 1715–1718.

Herrera, B., Sanmarti, R., Ponce, A., Lopez-Soto, A. and Muñoz-Gómez, J. (1997) Carpal tunnel syndrome heralding polymyalgia rheumatica. *Scand. J. Rheumatol.* **26**, 222–224.

Hershlag, A., Loy, R.A., Lavy, G. and DeCherney, A.H. (1990) Femoral neuropathy after laparoscopy. A case report. *J. Reprod. Med.* **35**, 575–576.

Herskovitz, S., Berger, A.R. and Lipton, R.B. (1995) Low-dose, short-term oral prednisone in the treatment of carpal tunnel syndrome. *Neurology* **45**, 1923–1925.

Hess, K., Eames, R.A., Darveniza, P. and Gilliatt, R.W. (1979) Acute ischaemic neuropathy in the rabbit. *J. Neurol. Sci.* **44**, 19–43.

Heuck, A., Hochholzer, T. and Keinath, C. (1992) Die MRT von Hand und Handgelenk bei Sportkletterern. Darstellung von Verletzungen und Uberlastungsfolgen. [MRT of the hand and wrist of sport climbers. Imaging of injuries and consequences of stress overload.] *Radiologe.* **32**, 248–254.

Heuser, M. (1982) Das exogene Kompressionssyndrom des N. suralis. 'Kamerad- Schnurschuh-Syndrom'. [Suralis compression syndrome from tightly laced boots.] *Nervenarzt* **53**, 223–224.

Highet, W.B. (1943) Innervation and function of thenar muscles. *Lancet* **i**, 227–230.

Ho, V.W., Peterfy, C. and Helms, C.A. (1993) Tarsal tunnel syndrome caused by strain of an anomalous muscle: an MRI-specific diagnosis. *J. Comput. Assist. Tomogr.* **17**, 822–823.

Hodgkinson, P.D. and McLean, N.R. (1994) Ulnar nerve entrapment due to epitrochleo-anconeus muscle. *J. Hand Surg. [Br.]* **19**, 706–708.

Hoefnagels, W.A., Vielvoye, G.J., de Jonge, F.A., Peetermans, W.E., Wondergem, J.H. and Roos, R.A.C. (1991) Sciatic neuritis as initial symptom of spontaneous clostridial myonecrosis. *Clin. Neurol. Neurosurg.* **93**, 149–150.

Hofmann, A., Jones, R.E. and Schoenvogel, R. (1982) Pudendal-nerve neurapraxia as a result of traction on the fracture table. A report of four cases. *J. Bone Joint Surg. [Am.]* **64**, 136–138.

Holme, J.B., Skajaa, K. and Holme, K. (1990) Incidence of lesions of the saphenous nerve after partial or complete stripping of the long saphenous vein. *Acta Chir. Scand.* **156**, 145–148.

Holtzman, R.N., Mark, M.H., Patel, M.R. and Wiener, L.M. (1984) Ulnar nerve entrapment neuropathy in the forearm. *J. Hand Surg. [Am.]* **9**, 576–578.

Hopf, H.C. (1974) Obturatorius-Lähmung unter der Geburt. [Obturator nerve paralysis during parturition.] *J. Neurol.* **207**, 165–166.

Hopkins, A. (1996) A novel cause of a pressure palsy: mobile telephone user's shoulder droop. *J. Neurol. Neurosurg. Psychiatry* **61**, 346.

Hopper, C.L. and Baker, J.B. (1968) Bilateral femoral neuropathy complicating vaginal hysterectomy. Analysis of contributing factors in 3 patients. *Obstet. Gynecol.* **32**, 543–547.

Horch, R.E., Allmann, K.H., Laubenberger, J., Langer, M. and Stark, G.B. (1997) Median nerve compression can be detected by magnetic resonance imaging of the carpal tunnel. *Neurosurgery* **41**, 76–82.

Hornig, C.R. and Dorndorf, W. (1983) Sensitive estimation of immunoglobulin M in cerebrospinal fluid by an immunoenzymatic technique. *Clin. Chim. Acta* **134**, 233–234.

Horowitz, S.H. (1984) Iatrogenic causalgia. Classification, clinical findings, and legal ramifications. *Arch. Neurol.* **41**, 821–824.

House, J.H. and Ahmed, K. (1977) Entrapment neuropathy of the infrapatellar branch of the saphenous nerve. *Am. J. Sports Med.* **5**, 217–224.

Howard, P.L. (1982) Gamba leg [letter]. *N. Engl. J. Med.* **306**, 1115.

Howe, F.A., Saunders, D.E., Filler, A.G., McLean, M.A., Heron, C., Brown, M.M. and Griffiths, J.R. (1994) Magnetic resonance neurography of the median nerve. *Br. J. Radiol.* **67**, 1169–1172.

Howell, A.E. and Leach, R.E. (1970) Bowler's thumb. Perineural fibrosis of the digital nerve. *J. Bone Joint Surg. [Am.]* **52**, 379–381.

Hsu, R.W. (1989) The study of Maquet dome high tibial osteotomy. Arthroscopic-assisted analysis. *Clin. Orthop.* 280–285.

Hudson, A.R., Hunter, G.A. and Waddell, J.P. (1979) Iatrogenic femoral nerve injuries. *Can. J. Surg.* **22**, 62–66.

Huffmann, G. (1973) Neuralgische Schulteramyotrophie – Klinik und Verlauf. [Neuralgic amyotrophy – clinical features and course.] *Z. Neurol.* **206**, 79–83.

Hughes, R.A.C., Cameron, J.S., Hall, S.M., Heaton, J., Payan, J. and Teoh, R. (1982) Multiple mononeuropathy as the initial presentation of systemic lupus erythematosus – nerve biopsy and response to plasma exchange. *J. Neurol.* **228**, 239–247.

Hunt, J.R. (1908) Occupation neuritis of the deep palmar branch of the ulnar nerve. A well defined clinical type of professional palsy of the hand. *J. Nerv. Ment. Dis.* **35**, 673–689.

Hustead, A.P., Mulder, D.W. and MacCarty, C.S. (1958) Non-traumatic progressive paralysis of the deep radial (posterior interosseous) nerve. *Arch. Neurol. Psych.* **79**, 269–274.

Iida, T. and Kobayashi, M. (1997) Tibial nerve entrapment at the tendinous arch of the soleus – a case report. *Clin. Orthop.* 265–269.

Ijichi, S., Niina, K., Tara, M., Nakamura, F., Ijichi, N., Izumo, S. and Osame, M. (1990) Mononeuropathy associated with hyperthyroidism [letter]. *J. Neurol. Neurosurg. Psychiatry* **53**, 1109–1110.

Irwin, L.R., Beckett, R. and Suman, R.K. (1996) Steroid injection for carpal tunnel syndrome. *J. Hand Surg. [Br.]* **21**, 355–357.

Ishikawa, H. and Hirohata, K. (1990) Posterior interosseous nerve syndrome associated with rheumatoid synovial cysts of the elbow joint. *Clin. Orthop.* 134–139.

Iyer, V.G. and Shields, C.B. (1989) Isolated injection injury to the posterior femoral cutaneous nerve. *Neurosurgery* **25**, 835–838.

Izzo, K.L., Aravabhumi, S., Jafri, A., Sobel, E. and Demopoulos, J.T. (1985) Medial and lateral antebrachial cutaneous nerves: standardization of technique, reliability and age effect on healthy subjects. *Arch. Phys. Med. Rehabil.* **66**, 592–597.

Jablecki, C.K., Andary, M.T., So, Y.T., Wilkins, D.E. and Williams, F.H. (1993) Literature review of the usefulness of nerve conduction studies and electromyography for the evaluation of patients with carpal tunnel syndrome. *Muscle Nerve* **16**, 1392–1414.

Jackson, D.A. and Clifford, J.C. (1989) Electrodiagnosis of mild carpal tunnel syndrome. *Arch.Phys.Med.Rehabil.* **70**, 199–204.

Jackson, D.L., Farrage, J., Hynninen, B.C. and Caborn, D.N. (1995) Suprascapular neuropathy in athletes: case reports. *Clin. J. Sport. Med.* **5**, 134–136.

Jackson, J.L., Gibbons, R., Meyer, G. and Inouye, L. (1997) The effect of treating herpes zoster with oral acyclovir in preventing postherpetic neuralgia – a meta-analysis. *Arch. Intern. Med.* **157**, 909–912.

Jackson, M. (1992) Post radiation monomelic amyotrophy [letter]. *J. Neurol. Neurosurg. Psychiatry* **55**, 629.

Jacobs, M.J., Gregoric, I.D. and Reul, G.J. (1992) Profunda femoral artery pseudoaneurysm after percutaneous transluminal procedures manifested by neuropathy. *J. Cardiovasc. Surg. Torino* **33**, 729–731.

Jacoulet, P. (1994) Double syndrome canalaire au membre superieur par tophi goutteux. A propos d'un cas. [Double tunnel syndrome of the upper limb in tophaceous gout. Apropos of a case.] *Ann. Chir. Main. Memb. Super.* **13**, 42–45.

Jamieson, P.W., Giuliani, M.J. and Martinez, A.J. (1991) Necrotizing angiopathy presenting with multifocal conduction blocks. *Neurology* **41**, 442–444.

Jamjoom, Z.A., al Bakry, A., al Momen, A., Malabary, T., Tahan, A.R. and Yacub, B. (1993) Bilateral femoral nerve compression by iliacus hematomas complicating anticoagulant therapy. *Surg. Today* **23**, 535–540.

Jelk, W. and Estape, R. (1995) Zyklische Ischialgie und extrauterine Endometriose. [Cyclic sciatica and extrauterine endometriosis.] *Schweiz. Rundsch. Med. Prax.* **84**, 1349–1355.

Jensen, M.C., Brant-Zawadzki, M.N., Obuchowski, N., Modic, M.T., Malkasian, D. and Ross, J.S. (1994) Magnetic resonance imaging of the lumbar spine in people without back pain. *N. Engl. J. Med.* **331**, 69–73.

Jerosch, J., Castro, W.H. and Colemont, J. (1989) A lesion of the musculocutaneous nerve. A rare complication of anterior shoulder dislocation. *Acta Orthop. Belg.* **55**, 230–232.

Jindal, R.M., Gordon, J., Schmitt, G., Carpinito, G. and Cho, S.I. (1993) Neuropathy of the lateral cutaneous nerve of the thigh: an avoidable complication of renal transplantation [letter]. *Postgrad. Med. J.* **69**, 328.

Job, C.K., Baskaran, B., Jayakumar, J. and Aschhoff, M. (1997) Pathologic changes in a tibial nerve with surviving *M. leprae* in a healed tuberculoid leprosy patient. *Int. J. Lepr. Other Mycobact. Dis.* **65**, 90–94.

Jog, M.S., Turley, J.E. and Berry, H. (1994) Femoral neuropathy in renal transplantation. *Can. J. Neurol. Sci.* **21**, 38–42.

Johnson, E.R., Kirby, K. and Lieberman, J.S. (1992) Lateral plantar nerve entrapment: foot pain in a power lifter. *Am. J. Sports Med.* **20**, 619–620.

Johnson, E.W. (1984) Axillary nerve injury [letter]. *Arch. Neurol.* **41**, 1022.

Johnson, E.W. (1993) Electrodiagnostic aspects of diabetic neuropathies: entrapments. *Muscle Nerve* **16**, 127–134.

Johnson, P.C., Rolak, L.A., Hamilton, R.H. and Laguna, J.F. (1979) Paraneoplastic vasculitis of nerve: a remote effect of cancer. *Ann. Neurol.* **5**, 437–444.

Johnson, R.K., Spinner, M. and Shrewsbury, M.M. (1979) Median nerve entrapment syndrome in the proximal forearm. *J. Hand Surg. [Am.]* **4**, 48–51.

Johr, M. (1987) Spate Komplikation der kontinuierlichen Blockade des N. femoralis. [A complication of continuous blockade of the femoral nerve.] *Reg. Anaesth.* **10**, 37–38.

Jones, H.R., Jr. (1988) Pizza cutter's palsy [letter]. *N. Engl. J. Med.* **319**, 450.

Jones, H.R., Jr. and Siekert, R.G. (1968) Embolic mononeuropathy and bacterial endocarditis. *Arch. Neurol.* **19**, 535–537.

Jones, H.R., Jr., Felice, K.J. and Gross, P.T. (1993) Pediatric peroneal mononeuropathy: a clinical and electromyographic study. *Muscle Nerve* **16**, 1167–1173.

Jones, H.R., Jr, Gianturco, L.E., Gross, P.T. and Buchhalter, J. (1988) Sciatic neuropathies in childhood: a report of ten cases and review of the literature. *J. Child Neurol.* **3**, 193–199.

Jones, J.R., Evans, D.M. and Kaushik, A. (1987) Synovial chondromatosis presenting with peripheral nerve compression-a report of two cases. *J. Hand Surg. [Br.]* **12**, 25–27.

Jones, N.A. (1978) Saphenous neuralgia: a complication of arterial surgery. *Br. J. Surg.* **65**, 465–466.

Jones, N.F. and Ming, N.L. (1988) Persistent median artery as a cause of pronator syndrome. *J. Hand Surg. [Am.]* **13**, 728–732.

Joplin, R.J. (1971) The proper digital nerve, vitallium stem arthroplasty, and some thoughts about foot surgery in general. *Clin. Orthop.* 199–212.

Joy, J.L. and Oh, S.J. (1989) Tomaculous neuropathy presenting as acute recurrent polyneuropathy. *Ann. Neurol.* **26**, 98–100.

Jugenheimer, M. and Junginger, T. (1992) Endoscopic subfascial sectioning of incompetent perforating veins in treatment of primary varicosis. *World J. Surg.* **16**, 971–975.

Kalisman, M., Laborde, K. and Wolff, T.W. (1982) Ulnar nerve compression secondary to ulnar artery false aneurysm at the Guyon's canal. *J. Hand Surg. [Am.]* **7**, 137–139.

Kang, H.J., Yoo, J.H. and Kang, E.S. (1996) Ulnar nerve compression syndrome due to an anomalous arch of the ulnar nerve piercing the flexor carpi ulnaris: A case report. *J. Hand Surg. [Am.]* **21**, 277–278.

Kao, J.T., Burton, D., Comstock, C., McClellan, R.T. and Carragee, E. (1993) Pudendal nerve palsy after femoral intramedullary nailing. *J. Orthop. Trauma* **7**, 58–63.

Kaplan, J.L. and Challenor, Y. (1993) Posttraumatic osseous tunnel formation causing sciatic nerve entrapment. *Arch. Phys. Med. Rehabil.* **74**, 552–554.

Karakousis, C.P., Hena, M.A., Emrich, L.J. and Driscoll, D.L. (1990) Axillary node dissection in malignant melanoma: results and complications. *Surgery* **108**, 10–17.

Karlsson, M.K., Lindau, T. and Hagberg, L. (1997) Ligament lengthening compared with simple division of the transverse carpal ligament in the open treatment of carpal tunnel syndrome. *Scand. J. Plast. Reconstr. Surg. Hand Surg.* **31**, 65–69.

Kars, H.Z., Topaktas, S. and Dogan, K. (1992) Aneurysmal peroneal nerve compression. *Neurosurgery* **30**, 930–931.

Kashani, S.R., Moon, A.H. and Gaunt, W.D. (1985) Tibial nerve entrapment by a Baker cyst: case report. *Arch. Phys. Med. Rehabil.* **66**, 49–51.

Katirji, B. and Hardy, R.W., Jr. (1995) Classic neurogenic thoracic outlet syndrome in a competitive swimmer: a true scalenus anticus syndrome. *Muscle Nerve* **18**, 229–233.

Katirji, M.B. and Wilbourn, A.J. (1988) Common peroneal mononeuropathy: a clinical and electrophysiologic study of 116 lesions. *Neurology* **38**, 1723–1728.

Katirji, B. and Wilbourn, A.J. (1994) High sciatic lesion mimicking peroneal neuropathy at the fibular head. *J. Neurol. Sci.* **121**, 172–175.

Katsuren, E., Ishikawa, S.E., Honda, K. and Saito, T. (1997) Galactorrhoea and amenorrhoea due to an intradural neurinoma originating from a thoracic intercostal nerve radicle. *Clin. Endocrinol. (Oxford)* **46**, 631–636.

Katz, M.R. and Lenobel, M.I. (1970) Intraneural ganglionic cyst of the peroneal nerve – case report. *J. Neurosurg.* **32**, 692–694.

Kauppila, L.I. and Vastamäki, M. (1996) Iatrogenic serratus anterior paralysis. Long-term outcome in 26 patients. *Chest* **109**, 31–34.

Kavoussi, L.R., Sosa, E., Chandhoke, P., *et al.* (1993) Complications of laparoscopic pelvic lymph node dissection. *J. Urol.* **149**, 322–325.

Kay, P.R., Abraham, J.S., Davies, D.R. and Bertfield, H. (1988) Ulnar artery aneurysms after injury mimicking acute infection in the hand. *Injury* **19**, 402–404.

Kchouk, M., Rabet, A.M., Ghedas, K., Nagi, S., Douik, M., Ben Romdhane, K., Touibi, S. and Sliman, N. (1993) Schwannome malin étendu du sciatique. Apport de l'imagerie. [Extensive malignant schwannoma of the sciatic nerve. Contribution of imaging techniques.] *J. Radiol.* **74**, 641–644.

Keegan, J.J. and Holyoke, E.A. (1962) Meralgia paraesthetica: anatomical and surgical study. *J. Neurosurg.* **19**, 341–345.

Keh, R.A., Ballew, K.K., Higgins, K.R., Odom, R. and Harkless, L.B. (1992) Long-term follow-up of Morton's neuroma. *J. Foot Surg.* **31**, 93–95.

Kempster, P., Gates, P., Byrne, E. and Wilson, A. (1991) Painful sciatic neuropathy following cardiac surgery. *Aust. N.Z. J. Med.* **21**, 732–735.

Kennedy, A.M., Grocott, M., Schwartz, M.S., Modarres, H., Scott, M. and Schon, F. (1997) Median nerve injury: an underrecognized complication of brachial artery catheterisation? *J. Neurol. Neurosurg. Psychiatry* **63**, 542–546.

Kernohan, J., Levack, B. and Wilson, J.N. (1985) Entrapment of the superficial peroneal nerve. Three case reports. *J. Bone Joint Surg. [Br.]* **67**, 60–61.

Kerr, R. and Frey, C. (1991) MR imaging in tarsal tunnel syndrome. *J. Comput. Assist. Tomogr.* **15**, 280–286.

Kerrigan, J.J., Bertoni, J.M., Jaeger, S.H. (1988) Ganglion cysts and carpal tunnel syndrome. *J. Hand Surg. [Am.]* **13**, 763–765.

Khella, L. (1979) Femoral nerve palsy: compression by lymph glands in the inguinal region. *Arch. Phys. Med. Rehabil.* **60**, 325–326.

Kikta, D.G., Breuer, A.C. and Wilbourn, A.J. (1982) Thoracic root pain in diabetes: the spectrum of clinical and electromyographic findings. *Ann. Neurol.* **11**, 80–85.

Kim, L.Y. (1987) Compression neuropathy of the radial nerve due to pentazocine-induced fibrous myopathy. *Arch. Phys. Med. Rehabil.* **68**, 49–50.

Kimura, J. (1979) The carpal tunnel syndrome: localization of conduction abnormalities within the distal segment of the median nerve. *Brain* **102**, 619–635.

Kincaid, J.C., Phillips, L.H. and Daube, J.R. (1986) The evaluation of suspected ulnar neuropathy at the elbow. *Arch. Neurol.* **43**, 44–47.

Kindstrand, E. (1995) Lyme borreliosis and cranial neuropathy. *J. Neurol.* **242**, 658–663.

King, R.B. (1993) Topical aspirin in chloroform and the relief of pain due to herpes zoster and postherpetic neuralgia. *Arch. Neurol.* **50**, 1046–1053.

King, R.B. and Bechtold, D.L. (1985) Warfarin-induced iliopsoas hemorrhage with subsequent femoral nerve palsy. *Ann. Emerg. Med.* **14**, 362–364.

Kirchof, J.K.J., Kumral, K. and Ertekin, C. (1962) Doppelseitige Radialis-lähmung imfolge

Lastentragens auf dem Rücken (Druckläsion). [Bilateral radial palsy due to carrying weights on the back.] *Nervenartzt* **33**, 536–538.

Kiss, G. and Kómár, J. (1990) Suprascapular nerve compression at the spinoglenoid notch. *Muscle Nerve* **13**, 556–557.

Kissel, J.T., Slivka, A.P., Warmolts, J.R. and Mendell, J.R. (1985) The clinical spectrum of necrotizing angiopathy of the peripheral nervous system. *Ann. Neurol.* **18**, 251–257.

Knezevic, W. and Mastaglia, F.L. (1984) Neuropathy associated with Brescia–Cimino arteriovenous fistulas. *Arch. Neurol.* **41**, 1184–1186.

Koehler, P.J., Jager, J., Verbiest, H. and Vecht, C.J. (1995) Anticoagulation for radiation injury [letter]. *Neurology* **45**, 1786.

Kómár, J. (1976) Eine wichtige Ursache des Schulterschmerzes: Incisura-scapulae-Syndrom. [An important cause of shoulder-pain: the 'incisura scapulae syndrome'.] *Fortschr. Neurol. Psychiatr. Grenzgeb.* **44**, 644–648.

Kompf, D., Neundorfer, B., Kayser-Gatchalian, C., Meyer-Wahl, L. and Ranft, K. (1976) Mononeuritis multiplex in Boeck's sarcoidosis. *Nervenartzt* **47**, 687–689.

Konishi, T., Saida, K., Ohnishi, A. and Nishitani, H. (1982) Perineuritis in mononeuritis multiplex with cryoglobulinemia. *Muscle Nerve* **5**, 173–177.

Konishiike, T., Hashizume, H., Nishida, K., Inoue, H. and Moriwaki, K. (1994) Cubital tunnel syndrome in a patient in long-term haemodialysis. *J. Hand Surg. Br.* **19**, 636–637.

Kopell, H.P. and Thompson, W.A.L. (1963) *Peripheral Entrapment Neuropathies.* Baltimore: Williams & Wilkins.

Kopell, H.P., Thompson, W.A.L. and Postel, A.H. (1962) Entrapment neuropathy of the ilioinguinal nerve. *N. Engl. J. Med.* **266**, 16–19.

Kori, S.H., Foley, K.M. and Posner, J.B. (1981) Brachial plexus lesions in patients with cancer: 100 cases. *Neurology* **31**, 45–50.

Kothari, M.J. and Preston, D.C. (1995) Comparison of flexed and extended elbow positions in localizing ulnar neuropathy at the elbow. *Muscle Nerve* **18**, 336–340.

Kothari, M.J., Preston, D.C. and Logigian, E.L. (1996) Lumbrical-interossei motor studies localize ulnar neuropathy at the wrist. *Muscle Nerve* **19**, 170–174.

Kraus, M.A. (1993) Nerve injury during laparoscopic inguinal hernia repair. *Surg. Laparosc. Endosc.* **3**, 342–345.

Krause, K.H. and Reuther, R. (1979) Electroneurographischer Nachweis des N. interosseus anterior–Syndroms. [Electroneurographic proof of the anterior interosseous nerve syndrome.] *EEG EMG Z. Elektroenzephalogr. Verwandte. Geb.* **10**, 140–142.

Krause, K.H., Flemming, M. and Scheglmann, K. (1987) Alopezie bei der Meralgia paraesthetica. [Alopecia in meralgia paraesthetica.] *Hautarzt.* **38**, 474–476.

Kremer, M., Gilliatt, R.W., Golding, J.S.R. and Wilson, T.G. (1953) Acroparaesthesia in the carpal tunnel syndrome. *Lancet* **ii**, 590–595.

Kreusser, K.L. and Volpe, J.J. (1984) Peroneal palsy produced by intravenous fluid infiltration in a newborn. *Dev. Med. Child Neurol.* **26**, 522–524.

Kruse, F. (1958) Paralysis of the dorsal interosseous nerve not due to direct trauma. A case showing spontaneous recovery. *Neurology* **8**, 307–308.

Kukowski, B. (1993) Suprascapular nerve lesion as an occupational neuropathy in a semiprofessional dancer. *Arch. Phys. Med. Rehabil.* **74**, 768–769.

Kumar, S., Anantham, J. and Wan, Z. (1992) Posttraumatic hematoma of iliacus muscle with paralysis of the femoral nerve. *J. Orthop. Trauma* **6**, 110–112.

Kurita, M., Niwa, Y., Hamada, E., *et al.* (1994) Churg–Strauss syndrome (allergic granulomatous angiitis) with multiple perforating ulcers of the small intestine, multiple ulcers of the colon, and mononeuritis multiplex. *J. Gastroenterol.* **29**, 208–213.

Kvist-Poulsen H. and Borel, J. (1982) Iatrogenic femoral neuropathy subsequent to abdominal hysterectomy: incidence and prevention. *Obstet. Gynecol.* **60**, 516–520.

Kwasny, O., Fuchs, M. and Schabus, R. (1994) Opening wedge osteotomy for malunion of the distal radius with neuropathy. 13 cases followed for 6 (1–11) years. *Acta Orthop. Scand.* **65**, 207–208.

Kyle, R.A. and Greipp, P.R. (1983) Amyloidosis (AL). Clinical and laboratory features in 229 cases. *Mayo Clin. Proc.* **58**, 665–683.

Laban, E. and Kon, M. (1990) Lesion of the long thoracic nerve during transaxillary breast augmentation: an unusual complication. *Ann. Plast. Surg.* **24**, 445–446.

Laban, M.M., Meerschaert, J.R. and Taylor, R.S. (1982) Electromyographic evidence of inferior gluteal nerve compromise: an early representation of recurrent colorectal carcinoma. *Arch. Phys. Med. Rehabil.* **63**, 33–35.

Lachance, D.H., O'Neill, B.P., Harper, C.M., Jr, Banks, P.M. and Cascino, T.L. (1991) Paraneoplastic brachial plexopathy in a patient with Hodgkin's disease. *Mayo Clin. Proc.* **66**, 97–101.

Lachiewicz, P.F. and Latimer, H.A. (1991) Rhabdomyolysis following total hip arthroplasty. *J. Bone Joint Surg. [Br.]* **73**, 576–579.

Lachmann, E.A., Rook, J.L., Tunkel, R. and Nagler, W. (1992) Complications associated with intermittent pneumatic compression. *Arch. Phys. Med. Rehabil.* **73**, 482–485.

Lagueny, A., Deliac, M.M., Deliac, P. and Durandeau, A. (1991) Diagnostic and prognostic value of electrophysiologic tests in meralgia paresthetica. *Muscle Nerve* **14**, 51–56.

Lalanandham, T. and Laurence, W.N. (1984) Entrapment of the ulnar nerve in the callus of a supracondylar fracture of the humerus. *Injury* **16**, 129–130.

Lamy, C., Mas, J.L., Varet, B., Ziegler, M. and de Recondo, J. (1991) Postradiation lower motor neuron syndrome presenting as monomelic amyotrophy. *J. Neurol. Neurosurg. Psychiatry* **54**, 648–649.

Lang, C., Druschky, K.F., Sturm, U., Neundorfer, B. and Fahlbusch, R. (1988) Lasionssyndrome des N. suprascapularis. [Suprascapular nerve entrapment syndrome.] *Dtsch. Med. Wochenschr.* **113**, 1349–1353.

Lang, W., Bockler, D., Meister, R. and Schweiger, H. (1995) Endoskopische Dissektion der Perforansvenen. [Endoscopic dissection of perforating veins.] *Chirurg.* **66**, 131–134.

Lange, D.J. (1994) Neuromuscular diseases associated with HIV-1 infection (AAEM Minimonograph No. 41). *Muscle Nerve* **17**, 16–30.

Lanzetta, M. and Foucher, G. (1993) Entrapment of the superficial branch of the radial nerve (Wartenberg's syndrome). A report of 52 cases. *Int. Orthop.* **17**, 342–345.

Large, D.F., Ludlam, C.A. and Macnicol, M.F. (1983) Common peroneal nerve entrapment in a hemophiliac. *Clin. Orthop.* 165–166.

Laroy, V., Spaans, F., Reulen, J. (1998) The sensory innervation pattern of the fingers. *J. Neurol.* **245**, 294–298.

Laulund, T., Fedders, O., Sogaard, I. and Kornum, M. (1984) Suprascapular nerve compression syndrome. *Surg. Neurol.* **22**, 308–312.

Laurent, L.E. (1975) Femoral nerve compression syndrome with paresis of the quadriceps muscle caused by radiotherapy of malignant tumours. A report of four cases. *Acta Orthop. Scand.* **46**, 804–808.

Lazaro, L.,III (1972) Carpal-tunnel syndrome from an insect sting. A case report. *J. Bone Joint Surg. [Am.]* **54**, 1095–1096.

Lazzarino, L.G., Nicolai, A. and Toppari, D. (1991) Neuropatia femorale, diabete mellito, ridotta tolleranza ai glicidi. Possibili correlazioni. [Femoral neuropathy, diabetes mellitus, reduced glucose tolerance. Possible correlations.] *Riv. Neurol.* **61**, 119–121.

Lazzarino, L.G., Nicolai, A. and Mesiano, T. (1994) Peripheral nervous system involvement as the only neurological manifestation of infective endocarditis. *Ital. J. Neurol. Sci.* **15**, 167–170.

Leach, R.E., Purnell, M.B. and Saito, A. (1989) Peroneal nerve entrapment in runners. *Am. J. Sports Med.* **17**, 287–291.

Lederman, R.J. (1989) Peripheral nerve disorders in instrumentalists. *Ann. Neurol.* **26**, 640–646.

Lederman, R.J. and Wilbourn, A.J. (1984) Brachial plexopathy: recurrent cancer or radiation? *Neurology* **34**, 1331–1335.

Lederman, R.J. and Wilbourn, A.J. (1996) Postpartum neuralgic amyotrophy. *Neurology* **47**, 1213–1219.

Lederman, R.J., Breuer, A.C., Hanson, M.R., Furlan, A.J., Loop, F.D., Cosgrove, D.M., Estafanous, F.G. and Greenstreet, R.L. (1982) Peripheral nervous system complications of coronary artery bypass graft surgery. *Ann. Neurol.* **12**, 297–301.

Leffert, R.D. (1982) Anterior submuscular transposition of the ulnar nerves by the Learmonth technique. *J. Hand Surg. [Am.]* **7**, 147–155.

Leibovic, S.J. and Hastings, H. (1992) Martin–Gruber revisited. *J. Hand Surg. [Am.]* **17**, 47–53.

Leinberry, C.F., Hammond, N.L. and Siegfried, J.W. (1997) The role of epineurotomy in the operative treatment of carpal tunnel syndrome. *J. Bone Joint Surg. [Am.]* **79A**, 555–557.

Lekos, A., Katirji, M.B., Cohen, M.L., Weisman, R., Jr and Harik, S.I. (1994) Mononeuritis multiplex. A harbinger of acute leukemia in relapse. *Arch. Neurol.* **51**, 618–622.

Lemont, H. and Cullen, R.W. (1984) Compression of the superficial peroneal nerve secondary to sleeping and sitting positions. *J. Am. Podiatr. Assoc.* **74**, 450–451.

Leon, J. and Marano, G. (1987) MRI of peroneal nerve entrapment due to a ganglion cyst. *Magn. Reson. Imaging* **5**, 307–309.

Le Roux, P.D., Ensign, T.D. and Burchiel, K.J. (1990) Surgical decompression without transposition for ulnar neuropathy: factors determining outcome. *Neurosurgery* **27**, 709–714.

Letourneau, L., Dessureault, M. and Carette, S. (1991) Rheumatoid iliopsoas bursitis presenting as unilateral femoral nerve palsy. *J. Rheumatol.* **18**, 462–463.

Levitt, L.P. and Prager, D. (1975) Mononeuropathy due to vincristine toxicity. *Neurology* **25**, 894–895.

Levy, L.A. (1977) Arteriosclerotic common iliac aneurysm causing sciatic pain [letter]. *Arch. Neurol.* **34**, 581.

Leys, D., Lafitte, J.J., Derollez, M., Niquet, G. and Petit, H. (1989) Paralysie diaphragmatique bilaterale: sequelle d'une nevralgie amyotrophique. [Bilateral diaphragmatic paralysis: sequelae of neuralgic amyotrophy.] *Rev. Neurol. (Paris)* **145**, 811–812.

Lidor, C., Lotem, M. and Hallel, T. (1992) Parosteal lipoma of the proximal radius: a report of five cases. *J. Hand Surg. [Am.]* **17**, 1095–1097.

Liguori, R. and Trojaborg, W. (1990) Are there motor fibers in the sural nerve? *Muscle Nerve* **13**, 12–15.

Lilly, C.J. and Magnell, T.D. (1985) Severance of the thenar branch of the median nerve as a complication of carpal tunnel release. *J. Hand Surg. [Am.]* **10**, 399–402.

Linden, D. and Berlit, P. (1994) The intrinsic foot muscles are purely innervated by the tibial nerve ('all tibial foot') – an unusual innervation anomaly [letter]. *Muscle Nerve* **17**, 5.

Lindenbaum, B.L. (1979) Ski boot compression syndrome. *Clin. Orthop.* 109–110.

Lindenbaum, S.D., Fleming, L.L. and Smith, D.W. (1982) Pudendal-nerve palsies associated with closed intramedullary femoral fixation. A report of two cases and a study of the mechanism of injury. *J. Bone Joint Surg. [Am.]* **64**, 934–938.

Lindscheid, R.L. (1965) Injuries to radial nerves at the wrist. *Arch. Surg.* **91**, 942–946.

Linker, C.S., Helms, C.A. and Fritz, R.C. (1993) Quadrilateral space syndrome: findings at MR imaging. *Radiology* **188**, 675–676.

Lister, G.D., Belsole, R.B., Kleinert, H.E. (1979) The radial tunnel syndrome. *J. Hand Surg. Am.* **4**, 52–59.

Liszka, T.G., Dellon, A.L. and Manson, P.N. (1994) Iliohypogastric nerve entrapment following abdominoplasty. *Plast. Reconstr. Surg.* **93**, 181–184.

Little, J.R. and Furlan, A.J. (1985) Resolving occlusive lesions of the basilar artery. *Neurosurgery* **17**, 811–814.

Liu, Z., Zhou, J. and Zhao, L. (1991) Anterior tarsal tunnel syndrome. *J. Bone Joint Surg. [Br.]* **73**, 470–473.

Liveson, J.A. (1984a) Nerve lesions associated with shoulder dislocation; an electrodiagnostic study of 11 cases. *J. Neurol. Neurosurg. Psychiatry* **47**, 742–744.

Liveson, J.A. (1984b) Thoracic radiculopathy related to collapsed thoracic vertebral bodies. *J. Neurol. Neurosurg. Psychiatry* **47**, 404–406.

Lockwood, A.H. (1989) Medical problems of musicians. *N. Engl. J. Med.* **320**, 221–227.

Lockwood, C.M. (1996) Small-vessel vasculitis. In: Weatherall, D.J., Ledingham, J.G.G. and Warrell, D.A. (eds), *Oxford Textbook of Medicine*, 3rd edn (CD version). Oxford: Oxford University Press.

Loening-Baucke, V., Read, N.W., Yamada, T. and Barker, A.T. (1994) Evaluation of the motor and sensory components of the pudendal nerve. *Electroencephalogr. Clin. Neurophysiol.* **93**, 35–41.

Logigian, E.L. and Steere, A.C. (1992) Clinical and electrophysiologic findings in chronic neuropathy of Lyme disease. *Neurology* **42**, 303–311.

Logigian, E.L., Berger, A.R. and Shahani, B.T. (1989) Injury to the tibial and peroneal nerves due to hemorrhage in the popliteal fossa. Two case reports. *J. Bone Joint Surg. [Am.]* **71**, 768–770.

Logigian, E.L., Shefner, J.M., Frosch, M.P., Kloman, A.S., Raynor, E.M., Adelman, L.S. and Hollander, D. (1993) Nonvasculitic, steroid-responsive mononeuritis multiplex. *Neurology* **43**, 879–883.

Loh, F.L., Herskovitz, S., Berger, A.R. and Swerdlow, M.L. (1992) Brachial plexopathy associated with interleukin-2 therapy. *Neurology* **42**, 462–463.

Longstreth, G.F. and Newcomer, A.D. (1977) Abdominal pain caused by diabetic radiculopathy. *Ann. Intern. Med.* **86**, 166–168.

Löser, R. and Schafer, E.R. (1972) Ein Ganglion der Ellenbeuge als Ursache einer dissozierten Radialisparese vom Unterarmtyp. Darstellung eines seltenen Falles. [A ganglion of the elbow as the cause of dissociated radial paresis of the forearm type. Description of a rare case.] *Neurochirurgia. Stuttg.* **15**, 182–186.

Lotem, M., Fried, A., Levy, M., Solzi, P., Najenson, T. and Nathan, H. (1971) Radial palsy following muscular effort. A nerve compression syndrome possibly related to a fibrous arch of the lateral head of the triceps. *J. Bone Joint Surg. [Br.]* **53**, 500–506.

Love, J.G. and Schorn, V.G. (1967) Thoracic disk protrusions. *Rheumatism.* **23**, 2–10.

Low, P.A., McLeod, J.G., Turtle, J.R., Donnelly, P. and Wright, R.G. (1974) Peripheral neuropathy in acromegaly. *Brain* **97**, 139–152.

Luboshitzky, R. and Barzilai, D. (1980) Bromocriptine for an acromegalic patient. Improvement in cardiac function and carpal tunnel syndrome. *JAMA* **244**, 1825–1827.

Lubowski, D.Z., Swash, M., Nicholls, R.J. and Henry, M.M. (1988) Increase in pudendal nerve terminal motor latency with defaecation straining. *Br. J. Surg.* **75**, 1095–1097.

Luchetti, R., Mingione, A., Monteleone, M. and Cristiani, G. (1988) Carpal tunnel syndrome in Madelung's deformity. *J. Hand Surg. [Br.]* **13**, 19–22.

Luerssen, T.G., Campbell, R.L., Defalque, R.J. and Worth, R.M. (1983) Spontaneous saphenous neuralgia. *Neurosurgery* **13**, 238–241.

Luethke, R. and Dellon, A.L. (1992) Accessory abductor digiti minimi muscle originating proximal to the wrist causing symptomatic ulnar nerve compression. *Ann. Plast. Surg.* **28**, 307–308.

Lumio, J., Jahkola, M., Vuento, R., Haikala, O. and Eskola, J. (1993) Diphtheria after visit to Russia [letter]. *Lancet* **342**, 53–54.

Lundborg, G. (1975) Structure and function of the intraneural microvessels as related to trauma, edema formation, and nerve function. *J. Bone Joint Surg. [Am.]* **57**, 938–948.

Lussiez, B., Courbier, R., Toussaint, B., Benichou, M., Gomis, R. and Allieu, Y. (1993) Paralysie radiale au bras apres effort musculaire. A propos de quatre cas. Etude clinique et physio-pathologique. [Radial paralysis of the arm after muscular effort. 4 case reports. Clinical and physiopathological study.] *Ann. Chir. Main. Memb. Super.* **12**, 130–135.

Luyendijk, W. (1960) Precordiale pijn. [Precordial pain.] *Ned. Tijdschr. Geneeskd.* **104**, 1569–1571.

Maas, J.J., Beersma, M.F.C., Haan, J., Jonkers, G.J.P.M. and Kroes, A.C.M. (1996) Bilateral brachial plexus neuritis following parvovirus B19 and cytomegalovirus infection. *Ann. Neurol.* **40**, 928–932.

Macaulay, R.A. (1978) Neurofibrosarcoma of the radial nerve in von Recklinghausen's disease

with metastatic angiosarcoma. *J. Neurol. Neurosurg. Psychiatry* **41**, 474–478.

MacDougal, B., Weeks, P.M. and Wray-RC, J. (1977) Median nerve compression and trigger finger in the mucopolysaccharidoses and related diseases. *Plast. Reconstr. Surg.* **59**, 260–263.

Macgregor, J. and Moncur, J.A. (1977) Meralgia paraesthetica – a sports lesion in girl gymnasts. *Br. J. Sports Med.* **11**, 16–19.

Mack, G.J. (1968) Watchpocket meralgia paresthetica. *Ind. Med. Surg.* **37**, 778–779.

MacKenzie, J.R., LaBan, M.M. and Sackeyfio, A.H. (1989) The prevalence of peripheral neuropathy in patients with anorexia nervosa. *Arch. Phys. Med. Rehabil.* **70**, 827–830.

MacKenzie, K. and DeLisa, J.A. (1981) Distal sensory latency measurement of the superficial radial nerve in normal subjects. *Arch. Phys. Med. Rehab.* **62**, 31–34.

Mackinnon, S.E., McCabe, S., Murray, J.F., Szalai, J.P., Kelly, L., Novak, C., Kin, B. and Burke, G.M. (1991) Internal neurolysis fails to improve the results of primary carpal tunnel decompression. *J. Hand Surg. [Am.]* **16**, 211–218.

Macnicol, M.F. and Thompson, W.J. (1990) Idiopathic meralgia paresthetica. *Clin. Orthop.* 270–274.

Macon, W.L.4th. and Futrell, J.W. (1973) Median-nerve neuropathy after percutaneous puncture of the brachial artery in patients receiving anticoagulants. *N. Engl. J. Med.* **288**, 1396.

Magistris, M.R. and Roth, G. (1985) Long-lasting conduction block in hereditary neuropathy with liability to pressure palsies. *Neurology* **35**, 1639–1641.

Mah, V., Vartavarian, L.M., Akers, M.A. and Vinters, H.V. (1988) Abnormalities of peripheral nerve in patients with human immunodeficiency virus infection. *Ann. Neurol.* **24**, 713–717.

Mahloudji, M., Teasdall, R.D., Adamkiewicz, J.J., Hartmann, W.H., Lambird, P.A. and McKusick, V.A. (1969) The genetic amyloidoses with particular reference to hereditary neuropathic amyloidosis, type II (Indiana or Rukavina type). *Med. Balt.* **48**, 1–37.

Maimaris, C. and Zadeh, H.G. (1990) Ulnar nerve compression in the cyclist's hand: two case reports and review of the literature. *Br. J. Sports Med.* **24**, 245–246.

Mainard, D., Saury, P. and Delagoutte, J.P. (1991) Compression du nerf cubital au coude par un kyste synovial d'origine rhumatoide. [Ulnar nerve compression at the elbow caused by synovial cyst of rheumatoid origin.] *Rev. Rhum. Mal. Osteoartic.* **58**, 611–614.

Makin, G.J. and Brown, W.F. (1985) Entrapment of the posterior cutaneous nerve of the arm [letter]. *Neurology* **35**, 1677–1678.

Makin, G.J., Brown, W.F. and Ebers, G.C. (1986) C7 radiculopathy: importance of scapular winging in clinical diagnosis. *J. Neurol. Neurosurg. Psychiatry* **49**, 640–644.

Malamut, R.I., Marques, W., England, J.D. and Sumner, A.J. (1994) Postsurgical idiopathic brachial neuritis. *Muscle Nerve* **17**, 320–324.

Malin, J.P. (1979) Familial meralgia paresthetica with an autosomal dominant trait. *J. Neurol.* **221**, 133–136.

Mallory, T.H. (1983) Sciatic nerve entrapment secondary to trochanteric wiring following total hip arthroplasty. A case report. *Clin. Orthop.* 198–200.

Malow, B.A. and Dawson, D.M. (1991) Neuralgic amyotrophy in association with radiation therapy for Hodgkin's disease. *Neurology* **41**, 440–441.

Mancardi, G.L., Mandich, P., Nassani, S., Schenone, A., James, R., Defferrari, R., Bellone, E., Giunchedi, M., Ajmar, F. and Abbruzzese, M. (1995) Progressive sensory-motor polyneuropathy with tomaculous changes is associated to 17p11.2 deletion. *J. Neurol. Sci.* **131**, 30–34.

Mandich, P., James, R., Nassani, S., *et al.* (1995) Molecular diagnosis of hereditary neuropathy with liability to pressure palsies (hnpp) by detection of 17p11.2 deletion in Italian patients. *J. Neurol.* **242**, 295–298.

Mann, R.A. (1974) Tarsal tunnel syndrome. *Orthop. Clin. North Am.* **5**, 109–115.

Manske, P.R., Johnston, R., Pruitt, D.L. and Strecker, W.B. (1992) Ulnar nerve decompression at the cubital tunnel. *Clin. Orthop.* 231–237.

Mansukhani, K.A. and D'Souza, C. (1991) Ulnar neuropathy at the elbow in diamond assorters. *Ind. J. Med. Res.* **94**, 433–436.

Marazzi, R., Pareyson, D., Boiardi, A., Corbo, M., Scaioli, V. and Sghirlanzoni, A. (1992) Peripheral nerve involvement in Churg–Strauss syndrome. *J. Neurol.* **239**, 317–321.

March, L.M., Francis, H. and Webb, J. (1988) Benign joint hypermobility with neuropathies: documentation and mechanism of median,

sciatic, and common peroneal nerve compression. *Clin. Rheumatol.* **7**, 35–40.

Marchiodi, L., Mignani, G. and Stilli, S. (1994) Mucous cysts of the external popliteal sciatic nerve during childhood: presentation of two cases and a review of the literature. *Chir. Organi. Mov.* **79**, 175–179.

Marchiori, P.E., Silva, H.C., Hirata, M.T., Lino, A.M. and Scaff, M. (1995) Acute multiple mononeuropathy after accidental exposure to oven microwaves. *Occup. Med. Oxf.* **45**, 276–277.

Margles, S.W. (1994) Palmar ganglion producing diminished sensation in the distribution of the radial digital nerve of the thumb: a case not previously reported. *Plast. Reconstr. Surg.* **93**, 1512–1513.

Marie, P. and Foix, Ch. (1913) Atrophie isolée de l'éminence thénar d'origine névritique: rôle du ligament annulaire antérieur du carpe dans la pathogénie de la lésion. [Isolated atrophy of the thenar eminence of neuritic origin: role of the anterior carpal ligament in the pathogenesis of the lesion.] *Rev. Neurol.* **26**, 647–649.

Mariette, X., Leche, J., Lecanuet, P., Fenelon, G. and Guillard, A. (1987) Paralysie de la branche posterieure du nerf radial due a un lipome. [Paralysis of the posterior branch of the radial nerve caused by a lipoma.] *Rev. Neurol. (Paris)* **143**, 690–692.

Marinacci, A.A. (1964) Diagnosis of 'all median hand'. *Bull. Los Angeles. Neurol. Soc.* **29**, 191–197.

Marinacci, A.A. (1968) Neurological syndromes of the tarsal tunnels. *Bull. Los Angeles. Neurol. Soc.* **33**, 90–100.

Marquez, S., Turley, J.J. and Peters, W.J. (1993) Neuropathy in burn patients. *Brain* **116**, 471–483.

Marra, T.R. (1987) The clinical and electrodiagnostic features of idiopathic lumbo-sacral and brachial plexus neuropathy: a review of 20 cases. *Electromyogr. Clin. Neurophysiol.* **27**, 305–315.

Martin, J.T. (1989) Postoperative isolated dysfunction of the long thoracic nerve: a rare entity of uncertain etiology. *Anesth. Analg.* **69**, 614–619.

Martin, K.W., Hyde, G.L., McCready, R.A. and Hull, D.A. (1986) Sciatic artery aneurysms: report of three cases and review of the literature. *J. Vasc. Surg.* **4**, 365–371.

Martinelli, P., Fabbri, R., Moretto, G., Gabellini, A.S., D'Alessandro, R. and Rizzuto, N. (1989)

Recurrent familial brachial plexus palsies as the only clinical expression of 'tomaculous' neuropathy. *Eur. Neurol.* **29**, 61–66.

Massey, E.W. and O'Brian, J.T. (1978) Cheiralgia paresthetica in diabetes mellitus. *Diabetes Care* **1**, 365–366.

Massey, E.W. and Tim, R.W. (1989) Femoral compression neuropathy from a mechanical pressure clamp. *Neurology* **39**, 1263.

Massey, E.W., Trofatter, L.P. and Hartwig, G.B. (1981) 'Hunkering'; and peroneal palsy [letter]. *Muscle Nerve* **4**, 445.

Mastaglia, F.L., Meythaler, J.M., Reddy, N.M. and Mitz, M. (1986) Musculocutaneous neuropathy after strenuous physical activity. *Med. J. Aust.* **67**, 770–772.

Mastroianni, P.P. and Roberts, M.P. (1983) Femoral neuropathy and retroperitoneal hemorrhage. *Neurosurgery* **13**, 44–47.

Matsuura, S., Kojima, T. and Kinoshita, Y. (1994) Cubital tunnel syndrome caused by abnormal insertion of triceps brachii muscle. *J. Hand Surg. [Br].* **19**, 38–39.

Matthews, W.B. (1993) Sarcoid neuropathy. In: Dyck, P.J., Thomas, P.K., Griffin, J.W., Low, P.A. and Poduslo, J.F. (eds), *Peripheral Neuropathy*, 3rd edn, pp. 1418–1423. Philadelphia: W.B. Saunders.

Mattio, T.G., Nishida, T. and Minieka, M.M. (1992) Lotus neuropathy: report of a case [letter]. *Neurology* **42**, 1636.

Maudsley, R.H. (1967) Fibular tunnel syndrome [abstract]. *J. Bone Joint Surg. [Br.]* **49**, 384.

Maynard, F.M. and Stolov, W.C. (1972) Experimental error in determination of nerve conduction velocity. *Arch. Phys. Med. Rehabil.* **53**, 362–372.

Mazeman, E., Wurtz, A., Gilliot, P. and Biserte, J. (1992) Extraperitoneal pelvioscopy in lymph node staging of bladder and prostatic cancer. *J. Urol.* **147**, 366–370.

McAlindon, T.E. and Ferguson, I.T. (1989) Mononeuritis multiplex and occipital infarction complicating giant cell arteritis. *Br. J. Rheumatol.* **28**, 257–258.

McAuliffe, T.B., Fiddian, N.J. and Browett, J.P. (1985) Entrapment neuropathy of the superficial peroneal nerve. A bilateral case. *J. Bone Joint Surg. [Br.]* **67**, 62–63.

McCombe, P.A., McLeod, J.G., Pollard, J.D., Guo, Y.P. and Ingall, T.J. (1987) Peripheral sensorimotor and autonomic neuropathy associated with systemic lupus erythematosus.

Clinical, pathological and immunological features. *Brain* **110**, 533–549.

McConnell, J.R. and Bush, D.C. (1990) Intraneural steroid injection as a complication in the management of carpal tunnel syndrome. A report of three cases. *Clin. Orthop.* 181–184.

McDonald, W.I. (1980) Physiological consequences of demyelination. In: Sumner, A.J. (ed) *The Physiology of Peripheral Nerve Disease*, pp. 265–286. Philadelphia: W.B. Saunders.

McDonnell, J.M., Makley, J.T. and Horwitz, S.J. (1987) Familial carpal-tunnel syndrome presenting in childhood. Report of two cases. *J. Bone Joint Surg. [Am.]* **69**, 928–930.

McKowen, H.C. and Voorhies, R.M. (1987) Axillary nerve entrapment in the quadrilateral space. Case report. *J. Neurosurg.* **66**, 932–934.

McManis, P.G. (1994) Sciatic nerve lesions during cardiac surgery. *Neurology* **44**, 684–687.

Meals, R.A. (1977) Peroneal-nerve palsy complicating ankle sprain. Report of two cases and review of the literature. *J. Bone Joint Surg. [Am.]* **59**, 966–968.

Meier, C. and Bischoff, A. (1977) Polyneuropathy in hypothyroidism. Clinical and nerve biopsy study of 4 cases. *J. Neurol.* **215**, 103–114.

Meier, C. and Moll, C. (1982) Hereditary neuropathy with liability to pressure palsies. Report of two families and review of the literature. *J. Neurol.* **228**, 73–95.

Meier, P.J. and Kenzora, J.E. (1985) The risks and benefits of distal first metatarsal osteotomies. *Foot Ankle* **6**, 7–17.

Meier, W. (1989) Erfahrungen mit dem 'epigastrischen Schmerzsyndrom' (EGS). [Experiences with the 'epigastric pain syndrome'.] *Helv. Chir. Acta* **55**, 731–736.

Melamed, N.B. and Satya Murti, S. (1983) Obturator neuropathy after total hip replacement [letter]. *Ann. Neurol.* **13**, 578–579.

Mendes, D.G., Nawalkar, R.R. and Eldar, S. (1991) Post-irradiation femoral neuropathy. A case report. *J. Bone Joint Surg. [Am.]* **73**, 137–140.

Merchut, M.P. and Gruener, G. (1996) Segmental zoster paresis of limbs. *Electromyogr. Clin. Neurophysiol.* **36**, 369–375.

Merlo, I.M., Poloni, T.E., Alfonsi, E., Messina, A.L. and Ceroni, M. (1997) Sciatic pain in a young sportsman. *Lancet* **349**, 846.

Merritt, G.N. and Subotnick, S.I. (1982) Medial plantar digital proper nerve syndrome (Joplin's neuroma) – typical presentation. *J. Foot Surg.* **21**, 166–169.

Meythaler, J.M., Reddy, N.M. and Mitz, M. (1986) Serratus anterior disruption: a complication of rheumatoid arthritis. *Arch. Phys. Med. Rehabil.* **67**, 770–772.

Michotte, A., Dierckx, R., Deleu, D., Herregodts, P., Schmedding, E., Bruyland, M. and Ebinger, G. (1988) Recurrent forms of sporadic brachial plexus neuropathy. A report of two cases. *Clin. Neurol. Neurosurg.* **90**, 71–74.

Middleton, W.D., Kneeland, J.B., Kellman, G.M., Cates, J.D., Sanger, J.R., Jesmanowicz, A., Froncisz, W. and Hyde, J.S. (1987) MR imaging of the carpal tunnel: normal anatomy and preliminary findings in the carpal tunnel syndrome. *Am. J. Roentgenol.* **148**, 307–316.

Millender, L.H., Nalebuff, E.A. and Holdsworth, D.E. (1973) Posterior interosseous-nerve syndrome secondary to rheumatoid synovitis. *J. Bone Joint Surg. [Am.]* **55**, 753–757.

Miller, R.G. (1979) The cubital tunnel syndrome: diagnosis and precise localization. *Ann. Neurol.* **6**, 56–59.

Miller, R.G. and Hummel, E.E. (1980) The cubital tunnel syndrome: treatment with simple decompression. *Ann. Neurol.* **7**, 567–569.

Millette, T.J., Subramony, S.H., Wee, A.S. and Harisdangkul, V. (1986) Systemic lupus erythematosus presenting with recurrent acute demyelinating polyneuropathy. *Eur. Neurol.* **25**, 397–402.

Mino, D.E. and Hughes, E.C., Jr (1984) Bony entrapment of the superficial peroneal nerve. *Clin. Orthop.* 203–206.

Mitra, A., Stern, J.D., Perrotta, V.J. and Moyer, R.A. (1995) Peroneal nerve entrapment in athletes. *Ann. Plast. Surg.* **35**, 366–368.

Mitsumoto, H., Wilbourn, A.J. and Goren, H. (1980) Perineurioma as the cause of localized hypertrophic neuropathy. *Muscle Nerve* **3**, 403–412.

Mitsunaga, M.M. and Nakano, K. (1988) High radial nerve palsy following strenuous muscular activity. A case report. *Clin. Orthop.* 39–42.

Miyazaki, F. and Shook, G. (1992) Ilioinguinal nerve entrapment during needle suspension for stress incontinence. *Obstet. Gynecol.* **80**, 246–248.

Mizuguchi, T. (1976) Division of the pyriformis muscle for the treatment of sciatica. Postlaminectomy syndrome and osteoarthritis of the spine. *Arch. Surg.* **111**, 719–722.

Mizuno, K., Fujita, K., Yamada, M., Saura, R. and Hirohata, K. (1992) Solitary paralysis of the triceps muscle due to trauma. *J. Orthop. Trauma.* **6**, 229–233.

Mochida, H. and Kikuchi, S. (1995) Injury to infrapatellar branch of saphenous nerve in arthroscopic knee surgery. *Clin. Orthop.* 88–94.

Mohan, S.R. and Grimley, R.P. (1987) Common iliac artery aneurysm presenting as acute sciatic nerve compression. *Postgrad. Med. J.* **63**, 903–904.

Monga, M. and Ghoniem, G.M. (1994) Ilioinguinal nerve entrapment following needle bladder suspension procedures. *Urology* **44**, 447–450.

Monnin, J.L., Pierrugues, R., Bories, P. and Michel, H. (1988) Le syndrome de Cyriax. Une cause d'erreur de diagnostic dans les douleurs abdominales. [Cyriax's syndrome. A cause of diagnostic error in abdominal pains.] *Presse Méd.* **17**, 25–29.

Montagna, P., Medori, R., Liguori, R. and Cortelli, P. (1985) Abdominal neuropathy after renal surgery [letter]. *Ital. J. Neurol. Sci.* **6**, 357–358.

Monteyne, P., Dupuis, M.J. and Sindic, C.J. (1994) Névrite du grand dentelé associée a une infection par Borrelia burgdorferi. [Neuritis of the serratus anterior muscle associated with Borrelia burgdorferi infection.] *Rev. Neurol. (Paris)* **150**, 75–77.

Montgomery, P.Q., Goddard, N.J. and Kemp, H.B. (1989) Solitary osteochondroma causing sural nerve entrapment neuropathy. *J. R. Soc. Med.* **82**, 761.

Moore, D.C. (1982) Anatomy of the intercostal nerve: its importance during thoracic surgery. *Am. J. Surg.* **144**, 371–373.

Moore, J.R. and Weiland, A.J. (1985) Gouty tenosynovitis in the hand. *J. Hand Surg. [Am.]* **10**, 291–295.

Moore, P.M. and Cupps, T.R. (1983) Neurological complications of vasculitis. *Ann. Neurol.* **14**, 155–167.

Moore, P.M. and Fauci, A.S. (1981) Neurologic manifestations of systemic vasculitis. A retrospective and prospective study of the clinicopathologic features and responses to therapy in 25 patients. *Am. J. Med.* **71**, 517–524.

Moore, P.M., Harley, J.B. and Fauci, A.S. (1985) Neurologic dysfunction in the idiopathic hypereosinophilic syndrome. *Ann. Intern. Med.* **102**, 109–114.

Moran, H., Chen, S.L., Muirden, K.D., Jiang, S.J., Gu, Y.Y., Hopper, J., Jiang, P.L., Lawler, G. and Chen, R.B. (1986) A comparison of rheumatoid arthritis in Australia and China. *Ann. Rheum. Dis.* **45**, 572–578.

Morris, A.H. (1974) Irreducible Monteggia lesion with radial-nerve entrapment. A case report. *J. Bone Joint Surg. [Am.]* **56**, 1744–1746.

Morris, H.H. and Peters, B.H. (1976) Pronator syndrome: clinical and electrophysiological features in seven cases. *J. Neurol. Neurosurg. Psychiatry* **39**, 461–464.

Moscona, A.R. and Hirshowitz, B. (1980) Meralgia paresthetica as a complication of the groin flap. *Ann. Plast. Surg.* **4**, 161–163.

Moscona, A.R. and Sekel, R. (1978) Post-traumatic meralgia paresthetica – an unusual presentation. *J. Trauma.* **18**, 288.

Muller-Vahl H. (1985) Isolated complete paralysis of the tensor fasciae latae muscle. *Eur. Neurol.* **24**, 289–291.

Mulvey, D.A., Aquilina, R.J., Elliott, M.W., Moxham, J. and Green, M. (1993) Diaphragmatic dysfunction in neuralgic amyotrophy: an electrophysiologic evaluation of 16 patients presenting with dyspnea. *Am. Rev. Respir. Dis.* **147**, 66–71.

Mumenthaler, A., Mumenthaler, M., Luciani, G. and Kramer, J. (1965) Das Ilioinguinalis-Syndrom – Beschreibung von sieben eigenen Beobachtungen. [The ilio-inguinal syndrome – description of seven personal observations.] *Dtsch. Med. Wochenschr.* **90**, 1073–1078.

Mumenthaler, M. (1961) *Die Ulnarisparesen*, Stuttgart: Thieme.

Mumenthaler, M. and Schliack, H. (1993) *Läsionen peripheren Nerven – Diagnostik und Therapie*, 6th edn. Stuttgart: Thieme.

Murai, H., Inaba, S., Kira, J., Yamamoto, A., Ohno, M. and Goto, I. (1995) Hepatitis C virus associated cryoglobulinemic neuropathy successfully treated with plasma exchange. *Artif. Organs* **19**, 334–338.

Murali, S.R., Ashcroft, P. and Scotland, T. (1995) Bilateral compression of the median nerve by supracondylar spurs. *J. Pediatr. Orthop. B* **4**, 118–120.

Murayama, K., Takeuchi, T. and Yuyama, T. (1991) Entrapment of the saphenous nerve by branches of the femoral vessels. A report of two cases. *J. Bone Joint Surg. [Am.]* **73**, 770–772.

Murphy, R.X., Jr, Chernofsky, M.A., Osborne, M.A. and Wolson, A.H. (1993) Magnetic resonance imaging in the evaluation of persistent carpal tunnel syndrome. *J. Hand Surg. Am.* **18**, 113–120.

Murphy, R.X., Jr, Jennings, J.F. and Wukich, D.K. (1994) Major neurovascular complications of endoscopic carpal tunnel release. *J. Hand Surg. [Am.]* **19**, 114–118.

Murphy, T.P. and Parkhill, W.S. (1990) Fracture-dislocation of the base of the fifth metacarpal with an ulnar motor nerve lesion: case report. *J. Trauma* **30**, 1585–1587.

Myers, K.G. and George, R.J.D. (1996) Painful neuropathy of the lateral cutaneous nerve of the thigh in patients with AIDS: successful treatment by injection with bupivacaine and triamcinolone. *AIDS* **10**, 1302–1303.

Naess, P.A. and Blom, H. (1991) Hemoragisk kompresjon av nervus medianus etter streptokinasebehandling. [Hemorrhagic compression of the median nerve after streptokinase treatment.] *Tidsskr. Nor. Laegeforen.* **111**, 1627–1628.

Nakamichi, K. and Tachibana, S. (1996) Carpal tunnel syndrome caused by a synovial nodule of the flexor digitorum profundus tendon of the index finger. *J. Hand Surg. [Am.]* **21**, 282–284.

Nakano, K.K. (1978) Entrapment neuropathy from Baker's cyst. *JAMA* **239**, 135.

Nakano, K.K., Lundergran, C. and Okihiro, M.M. (1977) Anterior interosseous nerve syndromes. Diagnostic methods and alternative treatments. *Arch. Neurol.* **34**, 477–480.

Nelson, G.A., Puhl, R.W. and Altman, M.I. (1985) Superficial dysesthesias secondary to epidermoid cyst of the foot. *J. Foot Surg.* **24**, 269–271.

Neundörfer, B. and Seiberth, R. (1975) The accessory deep peroneal nerve. *J. Neurol.* **209**, 125–129.

Neundörfer, B., Claus, D. and Waller, D. (1984) Brachial neuritis in salmonellosis. *J. Neurol.* **231**, 198–199.

Ng, K.K.P., Yeung, H.M., Loo, K.T., Chan, H.M., Wong, C.K. and Li, P.C.K. (1997) Acute fulminant neuropathy in a patient with Churg–Strauss syndrome. *Postgrad. Med. J.* **73**, 236–238.

Niakan, E., Carbone, J.E., Adams, M. and Schroeder, F.M. (1991) Anticoagulants, iliopsoas hematoma and femoral nerve compression. *Am. Fam. Physician.* **44**, 2100–2102.

Nigst, H. (1983) Ergebnisse der operativen Behandlung der Neuropathie des N. ulnaris im Ellenbogenbereich. [Results of the surgical treatment of ulnar nerve neuropathy in the elbow area.] *Handchir. Mikrochir. Plast. Chir.* **15**, 212–220.

Nishino, H., Rubino, F.A., De Remee, R.A., Swanson, J.W. and Parisi, J.E. (1993a) Neurological involvement in Wegener's granulomatosis: an analysis of 324 consecutive patients at the Mayo Clinic. *Ann. Neurol.* **33**, 4–9.

Nishino, H., Rubino, F.A. and Parisi, J.E. (1993b) The spectrum of neurologic involvement in Wegener's granulomatosis. *Neurology* **43**, 1334–1337.

Nitz, A.J., Dobner, J.J. and Kersey, D. (1985) Nerve injury and grades II and III ankle sprains. *Am. J. Sports Med.* **13**, 177–182.

Noordeen, S.K., Lopez Bravo, L. and Sundaresan, T.K. (1992) Estimated number of leprosy cases in the world. *Bull. WHO* **70**, 7–10.

Norman Taylor, F., Fixsen, J.A. and Sharrard, W.J. (1995) Hunter's syndrome as a cause of childhood carpal tunnel syndrome: a report of three cases. *J. Pediatr. Orthop. B* **4**, 106–109.

Noth, J., Dietz, V. and Mauritz, K.H. (1980) Cyclist's palsy: neurological and EMG study in 4 cases with distal ulnar lesions. *J. Neurol. Sci.* **47**, 111–116.

Nucci, F., Mastronardi, L., Artico, M., Ferrante, L. and Acqui, M. (1988) Tuberculoma of the ulnar nerve: case report. *Neurosurgery* **22**, 906–907.

Nucci, F., Artico, M., Santoro, A., Bardella, L., Delfini, R., Bosco, S. and Palma, L. (1990) Intraneural synovial cyst of the peroneal nerve: report of two cases and review of the literature. *Neurosurgery* **26**, 339–344.

Obach, J., Aragones, J.M. and Ruano, D. (1983) The infrapiriformis foramen syndrome resulting from intragluteal injection. *J. Neurol. Sci.* **58**, 135–142.

Oberpenning, F., Roth, S., Leusmann, D.B., van, A.H. and Hertle, L. (1994) The Alcock syndrome: temporary penile insensitivity due to compression of the pudendal nerve within the Alcock canal. *J. Urol.* **151**, 423–425.

O'Brien, D.F., Kaar, T.K. and McGuinness, A.J. (1995) Intraneural ganglion of the peroneal nerve: a case report. *Ir. Med. J.* **88**, 131.

Ochiai, N., Hayashi, T. and Ninomiya, S. (1992) High ulnar nerve palsy caused by the arcade of Struthers. *J. Hand Surg. Br.* **17**, 629–631.

Ochoa, J. and Hedley-White, T.E. (1995) MGH case records (case 38–1995). A 68-year-old man with paresthesias and severe pain in both hands. *N. Engl. J. Med.* **333**, 1625–1630.

Ochoa, J., Fowler, T.J. and Gilliatt, R.W. (1972) Anatomical changes in peripheral nerves compressed by a pneumatic tourniquet. *J. Anat.* **113**, 433–455.

Ochoa, J.L. and Yarnitsky, D. (1994) The triple cold syndrome. Cold hyperalgesia, cold hypoaesthesia and cold skin in peripheral nerve disease. *Brain* **117**, 185–197.

O'Duffy, J.D., Randall, R.V. and MacCarty, C.S. (1973) Median neuropathy (carpal-tunnel syndrome) in acromegaly. A sign of endocrine overactivity. *Ann. Intern. Med.* **78**, 379–383.

O'Duffy, J.D., Hunder, G.G. and Wahner, H.W. (1980) A follow-up study of polymyalgia rheumatica: evidence of chronic axial synovitis. *J. Rheumatol.* **7**, 685–693.

Ogino, T., Minami, A. and Kato, H. (1991) Diagnosis of radial nerve palsy caused by ganglion with use of different imaging techniques. *J. Hand Surg. [Am.]* **16**, 230–235.

Oh, S.J. and Lee, K.W. (1987) Medial plantar neuropathy. *Neurology* **37**, 1408–1410.

Oh, S.J., Kim, H.S. and Ahmad, B.K. (1984) Electrophysiological diagnosis of interdigital neuropathy of the foot. *Muscle Nerve* **7**, 218–225.

Oh, S.J., Kim, H.S. and Ahmad, B.K. (1985) The near-nerve sensory nerve conduction in tarsal tunnel syndrome. *J. Neurol. Neurosurg. Psychiatry* **48**, 999–1003.

Oh, S.J., Sarala, P.K., Kuba, T. and Elmore, R.S. (1979) Tarsal tunnel syndrome: electrophysiological study. *Ann. Neurol.* **5**, 327–330.

Ohnishi, A., Li, L.Y., Fukushima, Y., Mori, T., Mori, M., Endo, C., Yoshimura, T., Sonobe, M., Flandermeyer, R. and Lebo, R.V. (1995) Asian hereditary neuropathy patients with peripheral myelin protein-22 gene aneuploidy. *Am. J. Med. Genet.* **59**, 51–58.

Oleksak, M. and Edge, A.J. (1992) Compression of the sciatic nerve by methylmethacrylate cement after total hip replacement. *J. Bone Joint Surg. [Br.]* **74**, 729–730.

Olney, R.K. and Hanson, M. (1988) AAEE case report 15: ulnar neuropathy at or distal to the wrist. *Muscle Nerve* **11**, 8–32.

Olsen, N.K., Pfeiffer, P., Johannsen, L., Schroder, H. and Rose, C. (1993) Radiation-induced brachial plexopathy: neurological follow-up in 161 recurrence-free breast cancer patients. *Int. J. Radiat. Oncol. Biol. Phys.* **26**, 43–49.

Omdal, R., Mellgren, S.I. and Husby, G. (1988) Clinical neuropsychiatric and neuromuscular manifestations in systemic lupus erythematosus. *Scand. J. Rheumatol.* **17**, 113–117.

O'Neill, B.J., Flanders, A.E., Escandon, S.L. and Tahmoush,A.J. (1997) Treatable lumbosacral polyradiculitis masquerading as diabetic amyotrophy. *J. Neurol. Sci.* **151**, 223–225.

Opsomer, R.J., Caramia, M.D., Zarola, F., Pesce, F. and Rossini, P.M. (1989) Neurophysiological evaluation of central-peripheral sensory and motor pudendal fibres. *Electroencephalogr. Clin. Neurophysiol.* **74**, 260–270.

O'Rourke, P.J. and Quinlan, W. (1993) Fracture dislocation of the fifth metacarpal resulting in compression of the deep branch of the ulnar nerve. *J. Hand Surg. [Br.]* **18**, 190–191.

Oware, A., Herskovitz, S. and Berger, A.R. (1995) Long thoracic nerve palsy following cervical chiropractic manipulation [letter]. *Muscle Nerve* **18**, 1351.

Ozdogan, H. and Yazici, H. (1984) The efficacy of local steroid injections in idiopathic carpal tunnel syndrome: a double-blind study. *Br. J. Rheumatol.* **23**, 272–275.

Pace, N., Serafini, P., Lo Iacono, E., Castricini, R. and Zanoli, S. (1991) The tarsal and calcaneal tunnel syndromes. *Ital. J. Orthop. Traumatol.* **17**, 247–252.

Pachner, A.R. and Steere, A.C. (1985) The triad of neurologic manifestations of Lyme disease: meningitis, cranial neuritis, and radiculoneuritis. *Neurology* **35**, 47–53.

Packer, G.J., McLatchie, G.R. and Bowden, W. (1993) Scapula winging in a sports injury clinic. *Br. J. Sports Med.* **27**, 90–91.

Packer, J.W., Foster, R.R., Garcia, A. and Grantham, S.A. (1972) The humeral fracture with radial nerve palsy: is exploration warranted? *Clin. Orthop.* 34–38.

Padma, M.N. and Bhatia, V.N. (1983) 'Nose-blow' smears in multibacillary leprosy patients. *Lepr. India.* **55**, 640–647.

Padua, L., D'Aloya, E., LoMonaco, M., Padua, R., Gregori, B. and Tonali, P. (1997) Mononeuropathy of a distal branch of the femoral nerve in a body building champion. *J. Neurol. Neurosurg. Psychiatry* **63**, 669–671.

Pagliughi, G. (1980) Le metatarsalgie da compressione del nervo plantare interno. [Metatarsalgia caused by compression of the internal plantar nerve.] *Chir. Ital.* **32**, 90–93.

Pal, B., Keenan, J., Misra, H.N., Moussa, K. and Morris, J. (1996) Raynaud's phenomenon in idiopathic carpal tunnel syndrome. *Scand. J. Rheumatol.* **25**, 143–145.

Paladini, D., Dellantonio, R., Cinti, A. and Angeleri, F. (1996) Axillary neuropathy in volleyball players: report of two cases and literature review. *J. Neurol. Neurosurg. Psychiatry* **60**, 345–347.

Palande, D.D. and Azhaguraj, M. (1975) Surgical decompression of posterior tibial neurovascular complex in treatment of certain chronic plantar ulcers and posterior tibial neuritis in leprosy. *Int. J. Lepr. Other Mycobact. Dis.* **43**, 36–40.

Pallis, C.A. and Scott, J.T. (1965) Peripheral neuropathy in rheumatoid arthritis. *Br. Med. J.* **i**, 1141–1147.

Palliyath, S. and Buday, J. (1989) Sciatic nerve compression: diagnostic value of electromyography and computerized tomography. *Electromyogr. Clin. Neurophysiol.* **29**, 9–11.

Palmer, R.A. and Collin, J. (1994) Preventing the hand-arm vibration syndrome [letter]. *Br. Med. J.* **308**, 655.

Papadopoulos, S.M., McGillicuddy, J.E. and Messina, L.M. (1989) Pseudoaneurysm of the inferior gluteal artery presenting as sciatic nerve compression. *Neurosurgery* **24**, 926–928.

Papilion, J.D., Neff, R.S. and Shall, L.M. (1988) Compression neuropathy of the radial nerve as a complication of elbow arthroscopy: a case report and review of the literature. *Arthroscopy* **4**, 284–286.

Parry, G.J. and Floberg, J. (1989) Diabetic truncal neuropathy presenting as abdominal hernia. *Neurology* **39**, 1488–1490.

Parsonage, M.J. and Turner, J.W.A. (1948) Neuralgic amyotrophy: the shoulder-girdle syndrome. *Lancet* **i**, 973–978.

Pasternack, W.A. and Lipp, R.M. (1992) Idiopathic sural neuroma. A case report. *J. Am. Podiatr. Med. Assoc.* **82**, 424–427.

Patel, M.E., Silver, J.W., Lipton, D.E. and Pearlman, H.S. (1979) Lipofibroma of the median nerve in the palm and digits of the hand. *J. Bone Joint Surg. [Am.]* **61**, 393–397.

Patel, M.R., Mody, K. and Moradia, V.J. (1996) Multiple schwannomas of the ulnar nerve: a case report. *J. Hand Surg. [Am.]* **21**, 875–876.

Pattrick, M.G., Watt, I., Dieppe, P.A. and Doherty, M. (1988) Peripheral nerve entrapment at the wrist in pyrophosphate arthropathy. *J. Rheumatol.* **15**, 1254–1257.

Paul, E. and Thiel, T. (1996) Zur Epidemiologie des Varizella-Zoster Infektion. Ergebnisse in der prospectiven Erhebung im Landkreis Ansbach. [Epidemiology of varicella zoster infection.

Results of a prospective study in the Ansbach area]. *Hautarzt* **47**, 604–609.

Pecina, M. (1979) Contribution to the etiological explanation of the piriformis syndrome. *Acta Anat. (Basel)* **105**, 181–187.

Pecina, M. and Bojanic, I. (1993) Musculocutaneous nerve entrapment in the upper arm. *Int. Orthop.* **17**, 232–234.

Pedersen, E., Harving, H., Klemar, B. and Torring, J. (1978) Human anal reflexes. *J. Neurol. Neurosurg. Psychiatry* **41**, 813–818.

Pedersen, E., Klemar, B., Schroder, H.D. and Torring, J. (1982) Anal sphincter responses after perianal electrical stimulation. *J. Neurol. Neurosurg. Psychiatry* **45**, 770–773.

Pellas, F., Olivares, J.P., Zandotti, C. and Delarque, A. (1993) Neuralgic amyotrophy after parvovirus B19 infection [letter]. *Lancet* **342**, 503–504.

Pellegrino, J.E., Rebbeck, T.R., Brown, M.J., Bird, T.D. and Chance, P.F. (1996) Mapping of hereditary neuralgic amyotrophy (familial brachial plexus neuropathy) to distal chromosome 17q. *Neurology* **46**, 1128–1132.

Pellegrino, M.J. and Johnson, E.W. (1988) Bilateral obturator nerve injuries during urologic surgery. *Arch. Phys. Med. Rehabil.* **69**, 46–47.

Penkert, G. and Schwandt, D. (1979) Beidseitige, nicht traumatische Radialis-profundus-Läsion. [Bilateral, non-traumatic palsy of the posterior interosseus nerve [author's transl.].] *Nervenarzt* **50**, 783–787.

Peppard, R.F., Byrne, E., Anderson, R.M. and Clarke, B.G. (1986) Cryoglobulinaemic neuropathy – a clinical spectrum. *Clin. Exp. Neurol.* **22**, 113–121.

Perlman, M.D. (1990) Os peroneum fracture with sural nerve entrapment neuritis. *J. Foot Surg.* **29**, 119–121.

Persing, J.A., Nachbar, J. and Vollmer, D.G. (1988) Tarsal tunnel syndrome caused by sciatic nerve schwannoma. *Ann. Plast. Surg.* **20**, 252–255.

Petrera, J.E. and Trojaborg, W. (1984) Conduction studies of the long thoracic nerve in serratus anterior palsy of different etiology. *Neurology* **34**, 1033–1037.

Petrucci, F.S., Morelli, A. and Raimondi, P.L. (1982) Axillary nerve injuries – 21 cases treated by nerve graft and neurolysis. *J. Hand Surg.* **7**, 271–278.

Peyronnard, J.M., Charron, L., Beaudet, F. and Couture, F. (1982) Vasculitic neuropathy in rheumatoid disease and Sjögren syndrome. *Neurology* **32**, 839–845.

Phalen, G.S. (1966) The carpal-tunnel syndrome. Seventeen years' experience in diagnosis and treatment of six hundred fifty-four hands. *J. Bone Joint Surg. Am.* **48**, 211–228.

Phalen, G.S. (1970) Reflections on 21 years' experience with the carpal-tunnel syndrome. *JAMA* **212**, 1365–1367.

Phillips, L.H.,II (1986) Familial long thoracic nerve palsy: a manifestation of brachial plexus neuropathy. *Neurology* **36**, 1251–1253.

Phillips, L.H.,II, Persing, J.A. and Vandenberg, S.R. (1991) Electrophysiological findings in localized hypertrophic mononeuropathy. *Muscle Nerve* **14**, 335–341.

Pickett, J.B. (1984) Localizing peroneal nerve lesions to the knee by motor conduction studies. *Arch. Neurol.* **41**, 192–195.

Pickett, J.B., Layzer, R.B., Levin, S.R., Scheider, V., Campbell, M.J. and Sumner, A.J. (1975) Neuromuscular complications of acromegaly. *Neurology* **25**, 638–645.

Pierallini, A., Bastianello, S., Antonini, G., Giuliani, S., Artico, M., Nucci, F., Millefiorini, M., Fantozzi, L.M. and Bozzao, L. (1993) CT findings in peripheral mononeuropathies. *Zentralbl. Neurochir.* **54**, 66–71.

Pierre, P.A., Laterre, C.E. and Van den Bergh, P.Y. (1990) Neuralgic amyotrophy with involvement of cranial nerves IX, X, XI and XII. *Muscle Nerve* **13**, 704–707.

Pierre-Jerome, C., Bekkelund, S.I., Mellgren, S.I. and Nordstrom, R. (1997) Bilateral fast magnetic resonance imaging of the operated carpal tunnel. *Scand. J. Plast. Reconstr. Surg. Hand Surg.* **31**, 171–177.

Pillay, P.K., Hardy, R.W., Jr., Wilbourn, A.J., Tubbs, R.R. and Lederman, R.J. (1988) Solitary primary lymphoma of the sciatic nerve: case report. *Neurosurgery* **23**, 370–371.

Pisani, R., Stubinski, R. and Datti, R. (1997) Entrapment neuropathy of the internal pudendal nerve – report of two cases. *Scand. J. Urol. Nephrol.* **31**, 407–410.

Pleet, A.B. and Massey, E.W. (1978) Notalgia paresthetica. *Neurology* **28**, 1310–1312.

Po, H.L. and Mei, S.N. (1992) Meralgia paresthetica: the diagnostic value of somatosensory evoked potentials. *Arch. Phys. Med. Rehabil.* **73**, 70–72.

Poilvache, P., Carlier, A., Rombouts, J.J., Partoune, E. and Lejeune, G. (1989) Carpal tunnel syndrome in childhood: report of five new cases. *J. Pediatr. Orthop.* **9**, 687–690.

Poisel, S. (1974) Ursprung und Verlauf des Ramus muscularis des Nervus digitalis palmaris communis I (N. medianus). [Origin and cause of the muscular branch of the common palmar digital nerve I.] *Chir. Praxis* **18**, 471–474.

Pollard, J.D., McLeod, J.G., Honnibal, T.G. and Verheijden, M.A. (1982) Hypothyroid polyneuropathy. Clinical, electrophysiological and nerve biopsy findings in two cases. *J. Neurol. Sci.* **53**, 461–471.

Ponsford, S.N. (1988) Sensory conduction in medial and lateral plantar nerves. *J. Neurol. Neurosurg. Psychiatry* **51**, 188–191.

Pontin, A.R., Donaldson, R.A. and Jacobson, J.E. (1978) Femoral neuropathy after renal transplantation. *S. Afr. Med. J.* **53**, 376–378.

Poppi, M., Giuliani, G., Pozzati, E., Acciarri, N. and Forti, A. (1989) Tarsal tunnel syndrome secondary to intraneural ganglion [letter]. *J. Neurol. Neurosurg. Psychiatry* **52**, 1014–1015.

Post, M. and Mayer, J. (1987) Suprascapular nerve entrapment. Diagnosis and treatment. *Clin. Orthop.* 126–136.

Prabhakar, Y., Bahadur, R.A., Mohanty, P.R. and Sharma, S. (1989) Meralgia paraesthetica. *J. Ind. Med. Assoc.* **87**, 140–141.

Pradhan, S. and Taly, A. (1989) Intercostal nerve conduction study in man. *J. Neurol. Neurosurg. Psychiatry* **52**, 763–766.

Preston, D. and Logigian, E. (1988) Iatrogenic needle-induced peroneal neuropathy in the foot. *Ann. Intern. Med.* **109**, 921–922.

Preston, D.C. and Logigian, E.L. (1992) Lumbrical and interossei recording in carpal tunnel syndrome. *Muscle Nerve* **15**, 1253–1257.

Preston, D.C. and Shapiro, B.E. (1997) Meeting badge neuropathy. *Neurology* **48**, 289–290.

Preston, D.N. and Grimes, J.D. (1985) Radial compression neuropathy in advanced Parkinson's disease. *Arch. Neurol.* **42**, 695–696.

Prince, H., Ispahani, P., and Baker, M. (1988) A *Mycobacterium malmoense* infection of the hand presenting as carpal tunnel syndrome. *J. Hand Surg. [Br.]* **13**, 328–330.

Pringle, R.M., Protheroe, K. and Mukherjee, S.K. (1974) Entrapment neuropathy of the sural nerve. *J. Bone Joint Surg. [Br.]* **56**, 465–468.

Privat, J.M., Allieu, Y., Bonnel, F., Frerebeau, P., Bonis, J.L., Benezech, J. and Gros, C. (1978) Chirurgie directe des lésions traumatiques du nerf radial. Indications, technique et résultats. [Direct surgery of traumatic injuries of the radial nerve.] *Neurochirurgie.* **24**, 375–379.

Probst, A., Harder, F., Hofer, H. and Thiel, G. (1982) Femoral nerve lesion subsequent to renal transplantation. *Eur. Urol.* **8**, 314–316.

Proschek, R., Fowles, J.V. and Bruneau, L. (1983) A case of post-traumatic false aneurysm of the superior gluteal artery with compression of the sciatic nerve. *Can. J. Surg.* **26**, 554–555.

Prosser, A.J. and Hooper, G. (1986) Entrapment of the ulnar nerve in a greenstick fracture of the ulna. *J. Hand Surg. [Br.]* **11**, 211–212.

Pryse-Phillips, W.E. (1984) Validation of a diagnostic sign in carpal tunnel syndrome. *J. Neurol. Neurosurg. Psychiatry* **47**, 870–872.

Psathakis, D. and Psathakis, N. (1991) Popliteales Kompressionssyndrom: Eine uberproportionale Haufung. [Popliteal compression syndrome: an overproportional incidence.] *Vasa.* **20**, 256–260.

Puduvalli, V.K., Sella, A., Austin, S.G. and Forman, A.D. (1996) Carpal tunnel syndrome associated with interleukin-2 therapy. *Cancer* **77**, 1189–1192.

Puechal, X., Said, G., Hilliquin, P., Coste, J., Job Deslandre, C., Lacroix, C. and Menkes, C.J. (1995) Peripheral neuropathy with necrotizing vasculitis in rheumatoid arthritis. A clinicopathologic and prognostic study of thirty-two patients. *Arthritis Rheum.* **38**, 1618–1629.

Pugliese, G.N., Green, R.F. and Antonacci, A. (1987) Radiation-induced long thoracic nerve palsy. *Cancer* **60**, 1247–1248.

Purves, J.K. and Miller, J.D. (1986) Inguinal neuralgia: a review of 50 patients. *Can. J. Surg.* **29**, 43–45.

Puschmann, E., Neundorfer, B. and Bauer, J. (1991) Nervus femoralis-Lasion unter Heparintherapie. [Femoral nerve lesion in heparin therapy.] *Fortschr. Neurol. Psychiatr.* **59**, 286–292.

Radford, P.J. and Matthewson, M.H. (1987) Hypoplastic scaphoid – an unusual cause of carpal tunnel syndrome. *J. Hand Surg. [Br.]* **12**, 236–238.

Raff, M.C. and Asbury, A.K. (1968) Ischemic mononeuropathy and mononeuropathy multiplex in diabetes mellitus. *N. Engl. J. Med.* **279**, 17–21.

Rahimizadeh, A. (1992) Unusual delayed radial nerve palsy caused by a traumatic aneurysm of a collateral radial artery: report of two cases. *Neurosurgery* **30**, 628–630.

Ramesh, M., O'Byrne, J.M., McCarthy, N., Jarvis, A., Mahalingham, K. and Cashman, W.F. (1996)

Damage to the superior gluteal nerve after the Hardinge approach to the hip. *J. Bone Joint Surg. [Br.]* **78**, 903–906.

Randall, G., Smith, P.W., Korbitz, B. and Owen, D.R. (1982) Carpal tunnel syndrome caused by Mycobacterium fortuitum and Histoplasma capsulatum. Report of two cases. *J. Neurosurg.* **56**, 299–301.

Rappaport, W.D., Valente, J., Hunter, G.C., Rance, N.E., Lick, S., Lewis, T. and Neal, D. (1993) Clinical utilization and complications of sural nerve biopsy. *Am. J. Surg.* **166**, 252–256.

Rask, M.R. (1978) Medial plantar neurapraxia (jogger's foot): report of 3 cases. *Clin. Orthop.* 193–195.

Rask, M.R. (1980) Superior gluteal nerve entrapment syndrome. *Muscle Nerve* **3**, 304–307.

Rawlings, C.E.3rd., Bullard, D.E. and Caldwell, D.S. (1986) Peripheral nerve entrapment due to steroid-induced lipomatosis of the popliteal fossa. Case report. *J. Neurosurg.* **64**, 666–668.

Rayan, G.M. and O'Donoghue, D.H. (1983) Ulnar digital compression neuropathy of the thumb caused by splinting. *Clin. Orthop.* 170–172.

Raynor, E.M., Shefner, J.M., Preston, D.C. and Logigian E.L. (1994) Sensory and mixed nerve conduction studies in the evaluation of ulnar neuropathy at the elbow. *Muscle Nerve* **17**, 785–792.

Read, N.W. and Sun, W.M. (1992) Anorectal manometry. In: Henry, M.M. and Swash, M., (eds), *Coloproctology and the Pelvic Floor,* pp. 119–145. Oxford: Butterworth Heinemann.

Redler, M.R., Ruland, L.J.,III and McCue, F.C.,III (1986) Quadrilateral space syndrome in a throwing athlete. *Am. J. Sports Med.* **14**, 511–513.

Redmond, J.M.T., Cros, D., Martin, J.B. and Shahani, B.T. (1989) Relapsing bilateral brachial plexopathy during pregnancy. Report of a case. *Arch. Neurol.* **46**, 462–464.

Redwine, D.B. and Sharpe, D.R. (1990) Endometriosis of the obturator nerve. A case report. *J. Reprod. Med.* **35**, 434–435.

Reed, S.C. and Wright, C.S. (1995) Compression of the deep branch of the peroneal nerve by the extensor hallucis brevis muscle: a variation of the anterior tarsal tunnel syndrome. *Can. J. Surg.* **38**, 545–546.

Refisch, A. and van Laack, W. (1989) Neuralgic amyotrophy of the lumbar area. Case report. *Arch. Orthop. Trauma. Surg.* **108**, 329–332.

Regan, P.J., Roberts, J.O. and Bailey, B.N. (1988) Ulnar nerve compression caused by a reversed palmaris longus muscle. *J. Hand Surg. [Br.]* **13**, 406–407.

Regan, P.J., Feldberg, L. and Bailey, B.N. (1991) Accessory palmaris longus muscle causing ulnar nerve compression at the wrist. *J. Hand Surg. [Am.]* **16**, 736–738.

Reik, L., Jr., Burgdorfer, W. and Donaldson, J.O. (1986) Neurologic abnormalities in Lyme disease without erythema chronicum migrans. *Am. J. Med.* **81**, 73–78.

Reinstein, L. and Eckholdt, J.W. (1983) Sciatic nerve compression by preexisting heterotopic ossification during general anesthesia in the dorsal lithotomy position. *Arch. Phys. Med. Rehabil.* **64**, 65–68.

Reisecker, F., Brugger, G., Leblhuber, F., Olschowski, A. and Deisenhammer, E. (1987) Zur Pathogenese und Therapie nicht-traumatischer kompressiver Radialislahmungen – Bericht uber einen ungewohnlichen Fall. [Pathogenesis and therapy of nontraumatic compressive radial nerve paralyses – report of an unusual case.] *Neurochirurgia. Stuttg.* **30**, 127–128.

Reisecker, F., Leblhuber, F., Lexner, R., Radner, G., Rosenkranz, W. and Wagner, K. (1994) A sporadic form of hereditary neuropathy with liability to pressure palsies: clinical, electrodiagnostic, and molecular genetic findings. *Neurology* **44**, 753–755.

Reisin, R., Pardal, A., Ruggieri, V. and Gold, L. (1994) Sural neuropathy due to external pressure: report of three cases. *Neurology* **44**, 2408–2409.

Reneman, R.S. (1975) The anterior and the lateral compartmental syndrome of the leg due to intensive use of muscles. *Clin. Orthop.* 69–80.

Rengachary, S.S., Burr, D., Lucas, S. and Brackett, C.E. (1979) Suprascapular entrapment neuropathy: a clinical, anatomical, and comparative study. Part 3: comparative study. *Neurosurgery* **5**, 452–455.

Rennels, G.D. and Ochoa, J.L. (1980) Neuralgic amyotrophy manifesting as anterior interosseous nerve palsy. *Muscle Nerve* **3**, 160–164.

Rettig, A.C. and Ebben, J.R. (1993) Anterior subcutaneous transfer of the ulnar nerve in the athlete. *Am. J. Sports Med.* **21**, 836–839.

Rhodes, Ph. (1957) Meralgia paraesthetica in pregnancy. *Lancet* **ii**, 831.

Richards, A.J. (1980) Carpal tunnel syndrome in polymyalgia rheumatica. *Rheumatol. Rehabil.* **19**, 100–102.

Richards, B.J., Gillett, W.R. and Pollock, M. (1991) Reversal of foot drop in sciatic nerve endometriosis [letter]. *J. Neurol. Neurosurg. Psychiatry* **54**, 935–936.

Richardus, J.H., Finlay, K.M., Croft, R.P. and Smith, W.C. (1996) Nerve function impairment in leprosy at diagnosis and at completion of MDT: a retrospective cohort study of 786 patients in Bangladesh. *Lepr. Rev.* **67**, 297–305.

Richman, J.A., Gelberman, R.H., Rydevik, B.L., Gylys Morin, V.M., Hajek, P.C. and Sartoris, D.J. (1987) Carpal tunnel volume determination by magnetic resonance imaging three-dimensional reconstruction. *J. Hand Surg. Am.* **12**, 712–717.

Richmond, D.A. (1963) Carpal ganglion with ulnar nerve compression. *J. Bone Joint Surg. [Br.]* **45**, 513–515.

Rietz, K.A. and Onne, L. (1967) Analysis of sixty-five operated cases of carpal tunnel syndrome. *Acta Chir. Scand.* **133**, 443–447.

Riley, D.E. and Shields, R.W. (1984) Diabetic amyotrophy with upper extremity involvement [abstract]. *Neurology* **34**, 216.

Rinaldi, E. (1983) Peroneal paralysis due to exostosis of the fibula. Report of 2 cases. *Ital. J. Orthop. Traumatol.* **9**, 259–262.

Ringel, S.P. and Treihaft, M.C. (1988) A pitcher's peril: suprascapular nerve injury [abstract]. *Neurology* **38**(Suppl. 1), 223.

Rinkel, G.J.E. and Wokke, J.H.J. (1990) Meralgia paraesthetica as the first symptom of a metastatic tumor in the lumbar spine. *Clin. Neurol. Neurosurg.* **92**, 365–367.

Ritts, G.D., Wood, M.B. and Linscheid, R.L. (1987) Radial tunnel syndrome. A ten-year surgical experience. *Clin. Orthop.* 201–205.

Roberts, A.P. and Allan, D.B. (1988) Digital nerve injuries in orthopaedic surgeons. *Injury* **19**, 233–234.

Robinson, D., Aghasi, M.K. and Halperin, N. (1989) Ulnar tunnel syndrome caused by an accessory palmaris muscle. *Orthop. Rev.* **18**, 345–347.

Robinson, D.R. (1947) Piriformis syndrome in relation to sciatic pain. *Am. J. Surg.* **73**, 355–358.

Roder, O.C., Kamper, A. and Jorgensen, S.J. (1984) Incidence of saphenous neuralgia in arterial surgery. *Acta Chir. Scand.* **150**, 23–24.

Rogers, L.R., Wilbourn, A.J., Lesser, M.L. and Sweeney, P.J. (1983) Spontaneous severe sciatic and gluteal mononeuropathies (gluteal compartment syndrome): a peripheral nerve complication of anticoagulation [abstract]. *Ann. Neurol.* **14**, 142.

Rogers, M.R., Bergfield, T.G. and Aulicino, P.L. (1991) The failed ulnar nerve transposition. Etiology and treatment. *Clin. Orthop.* 193–200.

Roig, J.V., Villoslada, C., Lledo, S., Solana, A., Buch, E., Alos, R. and Hinojosa, J. (1995) Prevalence of pudendal neuropathy in fecal incontinence. Results of a prospective study. *Dis. Colon Rectum* **38**, 952–958.

Roig, M., Santamaria, J., Fernandez, E. and Colomer, J. (1985) Peripheral neuropathy in meningococcal septicemia. *Eur. Neurol.* **24**, 310–313.

Roles, N.C. and Maudsley, R.H. (1972) Radial tunnel syndrome: resistant tennis elbow as a nerve entrapment. *J. Bone Joint Surg. [Br.]* **54**, 499–508.

Roncaroli, F., Poppi, M., Riccioni, L. and Frank, F. (1997) Primary non-Hodgkin's lymphoma of the sciatic nerve followed by localization in the central nervous system: Case report and review of the literature. *Neurosurgery* **40**, 618–621.

Ropert, A. and Metral, S. (1990) Conduction block in neuropathies with necrotizing vasculitis. *Muscle Nerve* **13**, 102–105.

Rorabeck, C.H. (1984) The treatment of compartment syndromes of the leg. *J. Bone Joint Surg. [Br.]* **66**, 93–97.

Rosenbaum, R.B. and Ochoa, J.L. (1993) *Carpal Tunnel Syndrome and Other Disorders of the Median Nerve.* Boston: Butterworth-Heinemann.

Rosenberg, J.N. (1990) Anterior interosseous/median nerve latency ratio. *Arch. Phys. Med. Rehabil.* **71**, 228-230.

Ross, D., Jones, R., Jr, Fisher, J. and Konkol, R.J. (1983) Isolated radial nerve lesion in the newborn. *Neurology* **33**, 1354–1356.

Rosset, P., Mir, A. and Wassmer, F.A. (1991) Anticoagulants et hematome du psoas. [Anticoagulants and psoas hematoma.] *Helv. Chir. Acta* **58**, 167–168.

Roth, V.K. (1895) *Meralgia Paraesthetica.* Berlin: Karger

Roullet, E., Assuerus, V., Gozlan, J., Ropert, A., Said, G., Baudrimont, M., el Amrani, M., Jacomet, C., Duvivier, C. and Gonzales-Canali, G. (1994) Cytomegalovirus multifocal neuropathy in AIDS: analysis of 15 consecutive cases. *Neurology* **44**, 2174–2182.

Rousou, J.A., Parker, T., Engelman, R.M. and Breyer, R.H. (1985) Phrenic nerve paresis associated with the use of iced slush and the cooling jacket for topical hypothermia. *J. Thorac. Cardiovasc. Surg.* **89**, 921–925.

Rousseau, J.J., Reznik, M., LeJeune, G.N. and Franck, G. (1979) Sciatic nerve entrapment by pentazocine-induced muscle fibrosis: a case report. *Arch. Neurol.* **36**, 723–724.

Roux, S., Grossin, M., De Bandt, M., Palazzo, E., Vachon, F. and Kahn, M.F. (1995) Angiotropic large cell lymphoma with mononeuritis multiplex mimicking systemic vasculitis. *J. Neurol. Neurosurg. Psychiatry* **58**, 363–366.

Rowbotham, M.C., Davies, P.S. and Fields, H.L. (1995) Topical lidocaine gel relieves postherpetic neuralgia. *Ann. Neurol.* **37**, 246–253.

Rowntree, T. (1949) Anomalous innervation of the hand muscles. *J. Bone Joint Surg. [Br.]* **31**, 505–510.

Rubin, M., Menche, D. and Pitman, M. (1991) Entrapment of an accessory superficial peroneal sensory nerve. *Can. J. Neurol. Sci.* **18**, 342–343.

Ruderman, M.I., Palmer, R.H., Olarte, M.R., Lovelace, R.E., Haas, R. and Rowland, L.P. (1983) Tarsal tunnel syndrome caused by hyperlipidemia. Reversal after plasmapheresis. *Arch. Neurol.* **40**, 124–125.

Sabin, T.D., Swift, T.R. and Jacobson, R.R. (1993) Leprosy. In: Dyck, P.J., Thomas, P.K., Griffin, J.W., Low, P.A. and Poduslo, J.F. (eds), *Peripheral Neuropathy*, 3rd edn, pp. 1354–1379. Philadelphia: W.B. Saunders.

Saeed, W.R. and Davies, D.M. (1995) Sensory innervation of the little finger by an anomalous branch of the median nerve associated with recurrent, atypical carpal tunnel syndrome. *J. Hand Surg. [Br.]* **20**, 42–43.

Said, G., Lacroix Ciaudo, C., Fujimura, H., Blas, C. and Faux, N. (1988) The peripheral neuropathy of necrotizing arteritis: a clinicopathological study. *Ann. Neurol.* **23**, 461–465.

Said, G., Goulon-Goeau, C., Lacroix, C. and Moulonguet, A. (1994) Nerve biopsy findings in different patterns of proximal diabetic neuropathy. *Ann. Neurol.* **35**, 559–569.

Salazar Grueso, E. and Roos, R. (1986) Sciatic endometriosis: a treatable sensorimotor mononeuropathy. *Neurology* **36**, 1360–1363.

Salisbury, R.E. and Dingeldein, G.P. (1982) Peripheral nerve complications following burn injury. *Clin. Orthop.* 92–97.

Salner, A.L., Botnick, L.E., Herzog, A.G., Goldstein, M.A., Harris, J.R., Levene, M.B. and Hellman, S. (1981) Reversible brachial plexopathy following primary radiation therapy for breast cancer. *Cancer Treat. Rep.* **65**, 797–802.

Samii, K., Cassinotti, P., De Freudenreich, J., Gallopin, Y., Le Fort, D. and Stalder, H. (1996) Acute bilateral carpal tunnel syndrome associated with human parvovirus B19 infection. *Clin. Infect. Dis.* **22**, 162–164.

San Augustin, M., Nitowski, H.M. and Borden, J.M. (1962) Neonatal sciatic palsy after umbilical vessel injection. *J. Pediatr.* **60**, 408–413.

Sander, H.W., Quinto, C.M., Elinzano, H., Chokroverty, S. (1997) Carpet carrier's palsy: musculocutaneous neuropathy. *Neurology* **48**, 1731–1732.

Sander, J.E. and Sharp, F.R. (1981) Lumbosacral plexus neuritis. *Neurology* **31**, 470–473.

Sanders, E.A.C.M., van den Neste, V.M.H. and Hoogenraad, T.U. (1988) Brachial plexus neuritis and recurrent laryngeal nerve palsy [letter]. *J.Neurol.* **235**, 323.

Sandhu, H.S. and Sandhey, B.S. (1976) Occupational compression of the common peroneal nerve at the neck of the fibula. *Aust. N.Z. J. Surg.* **46**, 160–163.

Sanger, J.R., Matloub, H.S., Yousif, N.J. and Komorowski, R. (1992) Silicone gel infiltration of a peripheral nerve and constrictive neuropathy following rupture of a breast prosthesis. *Plast. Reconstr. Surg.* **89**, 949–952.

Saragaglia, D., Farizon, F., Drevet, J.G. and Butel, J. (1986) Le syndrome du nerf musculo-cutane au dos du pied. Guerison par neurolyse. A propos d'un cas bilateral. [Peroneal nerve entrapment syndrome of the front of the foot. Treatment by neurolysis. Apropos of a bilateral case.] *Rev. Chir. Orthop.* **72**, 579–581.

Sarala, P.K., Nishihara, T. and Oh, S.J. (1979) Meralgia paresthetica: electrophysiologic study. *Arch. Phys. Med. Rehabil.* **60**, 30–31.

Sarin, S., Scurr, J.H. and Coleridge Smith, P.D. (1992) Assessment of stripping the long saphenous vein in the treatment of primary varicose veins. *Br. J. Surg.* **79**, 889–893.

Sasse, A., Malfait, P., Padron, T., Erikashvili, M., Freixa, E. and Moren, A. (1994) Outbreak of diphtheria in Republic of Georgia [letter]. *Lancet* **343**, 1358–1359.

Savitsky, U. and Gerson, M.J. (1942) Peripheral nerve injury following electrical trauma: axillary and radial nerve involvement. *J. Nerv. Ment. Dis.* **96**, 635–640.

Sawin, P.D. and Loftus, C.M. (1995) Posterior interosseous nerve palsy after brachiocephalic arteriovenous fistula construction: report of two cases. *Neurosurgery* **37**, 537–539.

Sayson, S.C., Ducey, J.P., Maybrey, J.B., Wesley, R.L. and Vermilion, D. (1994) Sciatic entrapment neuropathy associated with an anomalous piriformis muscle. *Pain* **59**, 149–152.

Schantz, K. and Riegels Nielsen, P. (1992) The anterior interosseous nerve syndrome. *J. Hand Surg. Br.* **17**, 510–512.

Schärli, A.F. and Ayer, G. (1984) Meralgia paraesthetica im Kindesalter: Jeans-Krankheit. [Meralgia paraesthetica in childhood: Jeans disease] *Kinderartzt* **15**, 9–12.

Scheid, W. (1952) Diphtherial paralysis. An analysis of 2292 cases of diphtheria in adults which included 174 cases of polyneuritis. *J. Nerv. Ment. Dis.* **116**, 1095–1101.

Schiller, F. (1985) Sigmund Freud's meralgia paresthetica. *Neurology* **35**, 557–558.

Schmalzried, T.P., Amstutz, H.C. and Dorey, F.J. (1991) Nerve palsy associated with total hip replacement. Risk factors and prognosis. *J. Bone Joint Surg. [Am.]* **73**A, 1074–1080.

Schmalzried, T.P., Neal, W.C. and Eckardt, J.J. (1992) Gluteal compartment and crush syndromes. Report of three cases and review of the literature. *Clin. Orthop.* 161–165.

Schmitz, U., Honisch, C. and Zierz, S. (1991) Pseudotumour cerebri and carpal tunnel syndrome associated with danazol therapy [letter]. *J. Neurol.* **238**, 355.

Schmutzhard, E., Poewe, W. and Gerstenbrand, F. (1984) Neurologische Symptomatik bei 79 Lepra Patienten in Tanzania. [Neurologic symptoms in 79 leprosy patients in Tanzania.] *Nervenarzt.* **55**, 637–639.

Schneider, H.A., Yonker, R.A., Katz, P., Longley, S. and Panush, R.S. (1985) Rheumatoid vasculitis: experience with 13 patients and review of the literature. *Semin. Arthritis Rheum.* **14**, 280–286.

Schon, L.C. and Baxter, D.E. (1990) Neuropathies of the foot and ankle in athletes. *Clin. Sports Med.* **9**, 489–509.

Schon, L.C., Glennon, T.P. and Baxter, D.E. (1993) Heel pain syndrome: electrodiagnostic support for nerve entrapment. *Foot Ankle* **14**, 129–135.

Schott, G.D. (1995) An unsympathetic view of pain. *Lancet* **345**, 634–636.

Schottland, J.R. (1996) Femoral neuropathy from inadvertent suturing of the femoral nerve. *Neurology* **47**, 844–845.

Schroter, C., Braune, H.J. and Huffmann, G. (1990) Die sogenannte Rubenzieherlahmung – eine heute seltene Differentialdiagnose. [The so-called turnip-harvester palsy – a rare differential diagnosis today.] *Fortschr. Neurol. Psychiatr.* **58**, 351–353.

Schuchmann, J.A. (1977) Sural nerve conduction: a standardized technique. *Arch. Phys. Med. Rehabil.* **58**, 166–168.

Schuhl, J.F. (1991) Compression du median au carpe par un petit palmaire intra-canalaire. [Compression of the median nerve in the carpal tunnel due to an intra-canal palmar muscle.] *Ann. Chir. Main. Memb. Super.* **10**, 171–173.

Schulak, D.J., Bear, T.F. and Summers, J.L. (1980) Transient impotence from positioning on the fracture table. *J. Trauma* **20**, 420–421.

Schultz, J.S. and Leonard, J.A., Jr (1992) Long thoracic neuropathy from athletic activity. *Arch. Phys. Med. Rehabil.* **73**, 87–90.

Schwartz, M.S., Mackworth, Y.C. and McKeran, R.O. (1983) The tarsal tunnel syndrome in hypothyroidism. *J. Neurol. Neurosurg. Psychiatry* **46**, 440–442.

Schweitzer, G. and Lewis, J.S. (1981) Puff adder bite – an unusual cause of bilateral carpal tunnel syndrome. A case report. *S Afr. Med. J.* **60**, 714–715.

Schwind, F. and Solcher, H. (1958) Durch Influenza-Virus hervorgerufene peripher-nervöse Krankheitsbilder. [Peripheral neuropathies caused by influenza virus.] *Nervenartzt* **29**, 414–416.

Scott, T.F., Yager, J.G. and Gross, J.A. (1989) Handcuff neuropathy revisited. *Muscle Nerve* **12**, 219–220.

Scott, T.S., Brillman, J. and Gross, J.A. (1993) Sarcoidosis of the peripheral nervous system. *Neurol. Res.* **15**, 389–390.

Segal, R., Machiraju, U. and Larkins, M. (1992) Tortuous peripheral arteries: a cause of focal neuropathy. Case report. *J. Neurosurg.* **76**, 701–704.

Seid, A.S. and Amos, E. (1994) Entrapment neuropathy in laparoscopic herniorrhaphy. *Surg. Endosc.* **8**, 1050–1053.

Seifert, V., Zumkeller, M., Stolke, D. and Dietz, H. (1987) Carpaltunnelsyndrom nach arterio-venosem Unterarmshunt bei chronischen Dialysepatienten – Eine Ubersicht uber 24 operierte Falle. [Carpal tunnel syndrome following arteriovenous forearm shunt in chronic dialysis patients – a review of 24 surgically treated patients.] *Z. Orthop.* **125**, 85–90.

Selby, R.C. (1974) Neurosurgical aspects of leprosy. *Surg. Neurol.* **2**, 165–177.

Semer, N., Crimmins, C. and Jones, N.F. (1996) Compression neuropathy of the palmar cutaneous branch of the median nerve by the antebrachial fascia. *J. Hand Surg. [Br.]* **21**, 666–667.

Senegor, M. (1991) Iatrogenic saphenous neuralgia: successful therapy with neuroma resection. *Neurosurgery* **28**, 295–298.

Senveli, M.E., Turker, A., Arda, M.N. and Altinors, M.N. (1987) Bilateral carpal tunnel syndrome in a young carpet weaver. *Clin. Neurol. Neurosurg.* **89**, 281–282.

Seppalainen, A.M., Aho, K. and Uusitupa, M. (1977) Strawberry pickers' foot drop [letter]. *Br. Med. J.* **2**, 767.

Seradge, H. and Seradge, E. (1990) Median innervated hypothenar muscle: anomalous branch of median nerve in the carpal tunnel. *J. Hand Surg. Am.* **15**, 356–359.

Serdaroglu, P., Yazici, H., Ozdemir, C., Yurdakul, S., Bahar, S. and Aktin, E. (1989) Neurologic involvement in Behcet's syndrome: a prospective study. *Arch. Neurol.* **46**, 265–269.

Serratrice, G., Baudoin, D., Pouget, J., Blin, O. and Guieu, R. (1992) Formes typiques et atypiques de nevralgie amyotrophiante de l'epaule: 86 cas. [Typical and atypical forms of neuralgic amyotrophy of the shoulder: 86 cases.] *Rev. Neurol. (Paris)* **148**, 47–50.

Shaffer, J.W. (1994) Suprascapular nerve injury during spine surgery. A case report. *Spine* **19**, 70–71.

Shaffrey, M.E., Jane, J.A., Persing, J.A., Shaffrey, C.I. and Phillips, L.H. (1992) Surgeon's foot: a report of sural nerve palsy. *Neurosurgery* **30**, 927–930.

Shapiro, P.P. and Shapiro, S.L. (1995) Sonographic evaluation of interdigital neuromas. *Foot Ankle Int.* **16**, 604–606.

Sharara, K.H. and Nairn, D.S. (1983) Metastatic calcification as a cause of ulnar nerve compression at the wrist. *Hand* **15**, 300–304.

Shea, J.D. and McClain, E.J. (1969) Ulnar-nerve compression syndromes at and below the wrist. *J. Bone Joint Surg. [Am.]* **51**, 1095–1103.

Sheean, G. and Morris, J.G. (1993) Handcuff neuropathy involving the dorsal ulnar cutaneous nerve [letter]. *Muscle Nerve* **16**, 325.

Sheldon, P. (1994) Cryptic Wegener's granulomatosis revealed after 18 years. *Br. J. Rheumatol.* **33**, 296–298.

Shepard, C.C. (1982) Leprosy today. *N. Engl. J. Med.* **307**, 1640–1641.

Shields, R.W., Jr. and Jacobs, I.B. (1986) Median palmar digital neuropathy in a cheerleader. *Arch. Phys. Med. Rehabil.* **67**, 824–826.

Shimizu, J., Nishiyama, K., Takeda, K., Ichiba, T. and Sakuta, M. (1990) A case of long thoracic nerve palsy, with winged scapula, as a result of prolonged exertion on practicing archery. *Rinsho. Shinkeigaku.* **30**, 873–876.

Shintani, S., Tsuruoka, S. and Yamada, M. (1995) Churg–Strauss syndrome associated with third nerve palsy and mononeuritis multiplex of the legs. *Clin. Neurol. Neurosurg.* **97**, 172–174.

Shiozawa, S., Ogawa, R., Morimoto, I., Tanaka, Y., Kanda, N., Tatsumi, E., Yamaguchi, N. and Fujita, T. (1991) Polyarthritis, mononeuritis multiplex and eczematous ulcerative skin rash in a patient with myelodysplastic syndrome and peripheral large granular lymphocytosis. *Clin. Exp. Rheumatol.* **9**, 629–633.

Shyu, W.C., Lin, J.C., Chang, M.K. and Tsao, W.L. (1993) Compressive radial nerve palsy induced by military shooting training: clinical and electrophysiological study. *J. Neurol. Neurosurg. Psychiatry* **56**, 890–893.

Siegler, M. and Refetoff, S. (1976) Pretibial myxedema – a reversible cause of foot drop due to entrapment of the peroneal nerve. *N. Engl. J. Med.* **294**, 1383–1384.

Siliski, J.M. and Scott, R.D. (1985) Obturator-nerve palsy resulting from intrapelvic extrusion of cement during total hip replacement. Report of four cases. *J. Bone Joint Surg. [Am.]* **67**, 1225–1228.

Silva, M., Mallinson, C. and Reynolds, F. (1996) Sciatic nerve palsy following childbirth. *Anaesthesia* **51**, 1144–1148.

Silverstein, A. (1964) Neuropathy in haemophilia. *JAMA* **190**, 554–555.

Silverstein, B.A., Fine, L.J. and Armstrong, T.J. (1987) Occupational factors and carpal tunnel syndrome. *Am. J. Ind. Med.* **11**, 343–358.

Simon, M.A. and Rosenberg, A.E. (1992) MGH case records (case 32–1992). A 72-year-old man with a mass in the posterior thigh. *N. Engl. J. Med.* **327**, 412–418.

Simpson, D.M. and Olney, R.K. (1992) Peripheral neuropathies associated with human immunodeficiency virus infection. *Neurol. Clin.* **10**, 685–711.

Sinson, G., Zager, E.L. and Kline, D.G. (1994) Windmill pitcher's radial neuropathy. *Neurosurgery* **34**, 1087–1089.

Sippo, W.C., Burghardt, A. and Gomez, A.C. (1987) Nerve entrapment after Pfannenstiel incision. *Am. J. Obstet. Gynecol.* **157**, 420–421.

Sisto, D., Chiu, W.S., Geelhoed, G.W. and Lewis, R. (1980) Femoral neuropathy after renal transplantation. *South. Med. J.* **73**, 1464–1466.

Skie, M., Zeiss, J., Ebraheim, N.A. and Jackson, W.T. (1990) Carpal tunnel changes and median nerve compression during wrist flexion and extension seen by magnetic resonance imaging. *J. Hand Surg. [Am.]* **15**, 934–939.

Smith, B.E. and Litchy, W.J. (1989) Sural mononeuropathy: a clinical and electrophysiological study [abstract]. *Neurology* **39**(Suppl. 1), 296.

Smith, B.H. and Herbst, B.A. (1974) Anterior interosseous nerve palsy. *Arch. Neurol.* **30**, 330–331.

Smith, G.P., Rudge, P.J. and Peters, T.J. (1984) Biochemical studies of pyridoxal and pyridoxal phosphate status and therapeutic trial of pyridoxine in patients with carpal tunnel syndrome. *Ann. Neurol.* **15**, 104–107.

Smith, S.E., DeLee, J.C. and Ramamurthy, S. (1984) Ilioinguinal neuralgia following iliac bone-grafting. Report of two cases and review of the literature. *J. Bone Joint Surg. [Am.]* **66**, 1306–1308.

Snooks, S.J., Barnes, P.R. and Swash, M. (1984) Damage to the innervation of the voluntary anal and periurethral sphincter musculature in incontinence: an electrophysiological study. *J. Neurol. Neurosurg. Psychiatry* **47**, 1269–1273.

Snooks, S.J., Henry, M.M. and Swash, M. (1985) Faecal incontinence due to external anal sphincter division in childbirth is associated with damage to the innervation of the pelvic floor musculature: a double pathology. *Br. J. Obstet. Gynaecol.* **92**, 824–828.

Snooks, S.J., Swash, M., Henry, M.M. and Setchell, M. (1986) Risk factors in childbirth causing damage to the pelvic floor innervation. *Int. J. Colorectal. Dis.* **1**, 20–24.

Somell, A., Ljungdahl, I. and Spangen, L. (1976) Thigh neuralgia as a symptom of obturator hernia. *Acta Chir. Scand.* **142**, 457–459.

Sommer, C. and Ferbert, A. (1992) Schädigung des N. cutaneus femoris lateralis nach transfemoraler Angiographie. [Damage to the lateral cutaneous femoral nerve after transfemoral angiography.] *Nervenarzt* **63**, 633–635.

Sorell, D.A., Hinterbuchner, C., Green, R.F. and Kalisky, Z. (1976) Traumatic common peroneal nerve palsy: a retrospective study. *Arch. Phys. Med. Rehabil.* **57**, 361–365.

Sotaniemi, K.A. (1983) Neurologic complications associated with Yersiniosis. *Neurology* **33**, 95–97.

Sourkes, M. and Stewart, J.D. (1991) Common peroneal neuropathy: a study of selective motor and sensory involvement. *Neurology* **41**, 1029–1033.

Spaans, F. (1984) Lesions of the brachial plexus and upper limb nerves. In: Notermans, S.L.H. (ed.), *Current Practice of Clinical Electromyography*, pp. 213–253. Amsterdam: Elsevier.

Spaans, F. (1987) Compression and entrapment neuropathies. In: Vinken, P.J., Bruyn, G.W. and Klawans, H.L. (eds), *Handbook of Clinical Neurology*, pp. 100–101. Amsterdam: Elsevier.

Spevak, M.K. and Prevec, T.S. (1995) A noninvasive method of neurography in meralgia paraesthetica. *Muscle Nerve* **18**, 601–605.

Spindler, H.A. and Dellon, A.L. (1990) Nerve conduction studies in the superficial radial nerve entrapment syndrome. *Muscle Nerve* **13**, 1–5.

Spindler, H.A. and Felsenthal, G. (1978) Sensory conduction in the musculocutaneous nerve. *Arch. Phys. Med. Rehabil.* **59**, 20–23.

Spinner, R.J. and Spinner, M. (1996a) Superficial radial nerve compression at the elbow due to an accessory brachioradialis muscle: a case report. *J. Hand Surg. [Am.]* **21**, 369–372.

Spinner, R.J. and Spinner, M. (1996b) Superficial radial nerve compression following flexor digitorum superficialis opposition transfer: a case report. *J. Hand Surg. [Am.]* **21**, 1091–1093.

Spinner, R.J., Carmichael, S.W. and Spinner, M. (1991) Infraclavicular ulnar nerve entrapment due to a chondroepitrochlearis muscle. *J. Hand Surg. [Br.]* **16**, 315–317.

Spinner, R.J., Lins, R.E. and Spinner, M. (1996) Compression of the medial half of the deep branch of the ulnar nerve by an anomalous origin of the flexor digiti minimi – a case report. *J. Bone Joint Surg. [Am.]* **78**, 427–430.

Sprofkin, B.E. (1958) Peroneal paralysis: a hazard of weight reduction. *Arch. Intern. Med.* **102**, 82–87.

Sreeram, S., Lumsden, A.B., Miller, J.S., Salam, A.A., Dodson, T.F. and Smith, R.B. (1993) Retroperitoneal hematoma following femoral arterial catheterization: a serious and often fatal complication. *Am. Surg.* **59**, 94–98.

Sridhara, C.R. and Izzo, K.L. (1985) Terminal sensory branches of the superficial peroneal nerve: an entrapment syndrome. *Arch. Phys. Med. Rehabil.* **66**, 789–791.

Srinivasan, R. and Rhodes, J. (1981) The median–ulnar anastomosis (Martin–Gruber) in normal and congenitally abnormal fetuses. *Arch. Neurol.* **38**, 418–419.

Staal, A. and van Voorthuisen, A.E. (1969) Neurologic complications of percutaneous axillary catheterisation. *Cardiol. Digest* **4**, 33–37.

Staal, A., de Weerdt, C.J. and Went, L.N. (1965) Hereditary compression syndromes of peripheral nerves. *Neurology* **15**, 1008–1017.

Staal, A., van Voorthuisen, A.E. and van Dijk, L.M. (1966) Neurological complications following arterial catheterisation by the axillary approach. *Br. J. Radiol.* **39**, 115–116.

Stadelmann, A., Waldis, M., von Hochstetter, A. and Schreiber, A. (1992) Nervenkompressionssyndrom durch Synovialzyste am Huftgelenk. [Nerve compression syndrome caused by synovial cyst of the hip joint.] *Z. Orthop. Ihre. Grenzgeb.* **130**, 125–128.

Stafford, C.R., Bogdanoff, B.M., Green, L. and Spector, H.B. (1975) Mononeuropathy multiplex as a complication of amphetamine angiitis. *Neurology* **25**, 570–572.

Stahl, S. and Kaufman, T. (1997) Ulnar nerve injury at the elbow after steroid injection for medial epicondylitis. *J. Hand Surg. [Br.]* **22**, 69–70.

Stahl, S., Blumenfeld, Z. and Yarnitsky, D. (1996) Carpal tunnel syndrome in pregnancy: Indications for early surgery. *J. Neurol. Sci.* **136**, 182–184.

Stallings, S.P., Kasdan, M.L., Soergel, T.M. and Corwin, H.M. (1997) A case-control study of obesity as a risk factor for carpal tunnel syndrome in a population of 600 patients presenting for independent medical examination. *J. Hand Surg. [Am.]* **22**, 211–215.

Starling, J.R. and Harms, B.A. (1989) Diagnosis and treatment of genitofemoral and ilioinguinal neuralgia. *World J. Surg.* **13**, 586–591.

Starling, J.R., Harms, B.A., Schroeder, M.E. and Eichman, P.L. (1987) Diagnosis and treatment of genitofemoral and ilioinguinal entrapment neuralgia. *Surgery* **102**, 581–586.

Stauffer, R.N. (1976) Editorial comment (Division of pyriformis muscle for sciatica). *Arch. Surg.* **111**, 722.

Steere, A.C. (1989) Lyme disease. *N. Engl. J. Med.* **321**, 586–596.

Stefenelli, T., Wimberger, D., Harmuth, P., Engel, A., Lack, W., Samec, P. and Silberbauer, K. (1990) Angiologische, neurologische und orthopadische Befunde bei vibrationsexponierten Kettensagenarbeitern. [Angiologic, neurologic and orthopedic findings in vibration exposed chain saw operators.] *Wien Klin. Wochenschr.* **102**, 24–27.

Steffens, K. and Koob, E. (1988) Kompression des Nervus medianus durch ein Chondrosarkom der Hand. [Compression of the median nerve by chondrosarcoma of the hand.] *Handchir. Mikrochir. Plast. Chir.* **20**, 220–222.

Stellbrink, G. (1972) Kompression des R. palmaris ni. mediani M. palmaris longus. [Compression of the palmar branch of the median nerve by the atypical palmaris longus muscle.] *Handchirurgie.* **4**, 155–157.

Stern, B.J., Krumholz, A., Johns, C., Scott, P. and Nissim, J. (1985) Sarcoidosis and its neurological manifestations. *Arch. Neurol.* **42**, 909–917.

Stevens, J.C., Sun, S., Beard, C.M., O'Fallon, W.M. and Kurland, L.T. (1988) Carpal tunnel syndrome in Rochester, Minnesota, 1961 to 1980. *Neurology* **38**, 134–138.

Stewart, J.D. (1981) Medial plantar neuropathy [abstract]. *Neurology* **31**(Suppl. 2), 149–150.

Stewart, J.D. (1987) The variable clinical manifestations of ulnar neuropathies at the elbow. *J. Neurol. Neurosurg. Psychiatry* **50**, 252–258.

Stewart, J.D. (1989) Diabetic truncal neuropathy: topography of the sensory deficit. *Ann. Neurol.* **25**, 233–238.

Stewart, J.D. (1993) *Focal Peripheral Neuropathies*, 2nd edn. New York: Raven.

Stewart, J.D. and Aguao, X.X. (1984) Compression neuropathies. In: Dyck, P.J., Thomas, P.K. and Lambert, E.H. (eds), *Peripheral Neuropathy*, pp. 1435–1457. Philadelphia: W.B. Saunders.

Stewart, J.D., Schmidt, B. and Wee, R. (1983) Computed tomography in the evaluation of plexopathies and proximal neuropathies. *Can. J. Neurol. Sci.* **10**, 244–247.

Stiehl, J.B. and Hanel, D.P. (1993) Knee arthrodesis using combined intramedullary rod and plate fixation. *Clin. Orthop.* 238–241.

Stoelting, R.K. (1993) Postoperative ulnar nerve palsy – is it a preventable complication? *Anesth. Analg.* **76**, 7–9.

Stoff, M.D. and Greene, A.F. (1982) Common peroneal nerve palsy following inversion ankle injury: a report of two cases. *Phys. Ther.* **62**, 1463–1464.

Stögbauer, F., Young, P., Timmerman, V., Spoelders, P., Ringelstein, E.B., Van Broeckhoven, C. and Kurlemann, G. (1997) Refinement of the hereditary neuralgic amyotrophy (HNA) locus to chromosome 17q24-q25. *Hum. Genet.* **99**, 685–687.

Stöhr, M. (1976) Lagerungsbedingte Ischiadicus-und Glutaeus-Paresen. [Sciatic and gluteal nerve lesions during coma and anesthesia.] *Fortschr. Neurol. Psychiatr. Grenzgeb.* **44**, 706–708.

Stöhr, M. and Reill, P. (1980) Chronic compression syndrome of the radial nerve above the elbow [letter]. *Muscle Nerve* **3**, 446–447.

Stöhr, M., Schumm, F. and Ballier, R. (1978) Normal sensory conduction in the saphenous nerve in man. *Electroencephalogr. Clin. Neurophysiol.* **44**, 172–178.

Stone, D.A. and Laureno, R. (1991) Handcuff neuropathies. *Neurology* **41**, 145–147.

Stratton, C.W., Lichtenstein, K.A., Lowenstein, S.R., Phelps, D.B. and Reller, L.B. (1981) Granulomatous tenosynovitis and carpal tunnel syndrome caused by *Sporothrix schenckii*. *Am. J. Med.* **71**, 161–164.

Straus, S.E. (1994) Overview: the biology of varicella-zoster virus infection. *Ann. Neurol.* **35**(Suppl.), S4–S8.

Streib, E. (1992) Upper arm radial nerve palsy after muscular effort: report of three cases. *Neurology* **42**, 1632–1634.

Streib, E.W. and Sun, S.F. (1984) Distal ulnar neuropathy in meat packers. An occupational disease? *J. Occup. Med.* **26**, 842–843.

Stricker, R.B., Sanders, K.A., Owen, W.F., Kiprov, D.D. and Miller, R.G. (1992) Mononeuritis multiplex associated with cryoglobulinemia in HIV infection. *Neurology* **42**, 2103–2105.

Strickland, J.W. and Steichen, J.B. (1977) Nerve tumors of the hand and forearm. *J. Hand Surg. [Am.]* **2**, 285–291.

Stulz, P. and Pfeiffer, K.M. (1982) Peripheral nerve injuries resulting from common surgical procedures in the lower portion of the abdomen. *Arch. Surg.* **117**, 324–327.

Sturzenegger, M. and Rutz, M. (1990) Die beidseitige Radialisparese. Diagnostische und differentialdiagnostische Aspekte. [Bilateral radial nerve paralysis. Diagnostic and differential diagnostic aspects.] *Schweiz. Med. Wochenschr.* **120**, 1325–1334.

Sturzenegger, M. and Rutz, M. (1991) Die Radialisparesen – Ursachen, Lokalisation und Diagnostik. Analyse von 103 Fällen. [Radial nerve paralysis – causes, site and diagnosis. analysis of 103 cases.] *Nervenarzt.* **62**, 722–729.

Styf, J. (1989) Entrapment of the superficial peroneal nerve. Diagnosis and results of decompression. *J. Bone Joint Surg. [Br.]* **71**, 131–135.

Styf, J.R. and Korner, L.M. (1986) Chronic anterior-compartment syndrome of the leg. Results of treatment by fasciotomy. *J. Bone Joint Surg. [Am.]* **68**, 1338–1347.

Suarez, G.A., Giannini, C., Bosch, E.P., Barohn, R.J., Wodak, J., Ebeling, P., Anderson, R., McKeever, P.E., Bromberg, M.B. and Dyck, P.J. (1996) Immune brachial plexus neuropathy: suggestive evidence for an inflammatory-immune pathogenesis. *Neurology* **46**, 559–561.

Suber, D.A. and Massey, E.W. (1979) Pelvic mass presenting as meralgia paresthetica. *Obstet. Gynecol.* **53**, 257–258.

Subin, G.D., Mallon, W.J. and Urbaniak, J.R. (1989) Diagnosis of ganglion in Guyon's canal by magnetic resonance imaging. *J. Hand Surg.[Am.]* **14**, 640–643.

Suh, J.S., Abenoza, P., Galloway, H.R., Everson, L.I. and Griffiths, H.J. (1992) Peripheral (extracranial) nerve tumours: correlation of MR imaging and histologic findings. *Radiology* **183**, 341–346.

Sultan, A.H., Kamm, M.A. and Hudson, C.N. (1994) Pudendal nerve damage during labour: prospective study before and after childbirth. *Br. J. Obstet. Gynaecol.* **101**, 22–28.

Sunderland, S. (1978) *Nerves and Nerve Injuries*, 2nd edn. Edinburgh: Churchill Livingstone.

Swash, M. (1992) Electromyography in pelvic disorders. In: Henry, M.M. and Swash, M. (eds), *Coloproctology and the Pelvic Floor*. pp. 184–195. Oxford: Butterworth Heinemann.

Swash, M. and Leigh, N. (1992) Criteria for diagnosis of familial amyotrophic lateral sclerosis. European FALS collaborative group. *Neuromusc. Disord.* **2**, 7–9.

Szewczyk, J., Hoffmann, M. and Kabelis, J. (1994) Meralgia paraesthetica beim Bodybuilder. [Meralgia paraesthetica in a body-builder.] *Sportverletz. Sportschaden.* **8**, 43–45.

Tada, K., Yonenobu, K. and Swanson, A.B. (1984) Congenital constriction band syndrome. *J. Pediatr. Orthop.* **4**, 726–730.

Takebe, K. and Hirohata, K. (1981) Peroneal nerve palsy due to fabella. *Arch. Orthop. Trauma. Surg.* **99**, 91–95.

Takeuchi, A., Kodama, M., Takatsu, M., Hashimoto, T. and Miyashita, H. (1989) Mononeuritis multiplex in incomplete Behcet's disease: a case report and the review of the literature. *Clin. Rheumatol.* **8**, 375–380.

Taras, J. and Melone, C.P. (1995) Hypertrophic neuropathy presenting with ulnar nerve compression: a case report. *J. Hand Surg. [Am.]* **20**, 233–234.

Tassin, S., Ferriere, G. and Laterre, E.C. (1980) Mononévrite multiple dans un cas de macroglobulinemie de Waldenstrom. [Mononeuritis multiplex in a case of primary macroglobulinemia [author's transl].] *Acta Neurol. Belg.* **80**, 287–297.

Tavares, S.P. and Giddins, G.E.B. (1996) Nerve injury following steroid injection for carpal tunnel syndrome – a report of two cases. *J. Hand Surg. [Br.]* **21**, 208–209.

Teitze, K., Glatzel, W., Krauss, J. and Schober, K.L. (1979) Läsionen von Interkostalnerven durch abdominelle Eingriffe. [Intercostal nerve lesions caused by abdominal interventions.] *Z. Arztl. Fortbild. Jena.* **73**, 1113–1115.

Tesio, L., Bassi, L. and Galardi, G. (1990) Transient palsy of hip abductors after a fall on the buttocks. *Arch. Orthop. Trauma. Surg.* **109**, 164–165.

Thanikachalam, M., Petros, J.G. and O'Donnell, S. (1995) Avulsion fracture of the anterior superior iliac spine presenting as acute-onset meralgia paresthetica. *Ann. Emerg. Med.* **26**, 515–517.

Thiebot, J., Laissy, J.P., Delangre, T., Biga, N. and Liotard, A. (1991) Benign solitary neurinomas of the sciatic popliteal nerves CT study. *Neuroradiology.* **33**, 186–188.

Thomas, F.P., Lovelace, R.E., Ding, X.S., Sadiq, S.A., Petty, G.W., Sherman, W.H., Latov, N. and Hays, A.P. (1992) Vasculitic neuropathy in a patient with cryoglobulinemia and anti-MAG IGM monoclonal gammopathy. *Muscle Nerve* **15**, 891–898.

Thomas, J.E. and Howard, F.M., Jr (1972) Segmental zoster paresis – a disease profile. *Neurology* **22**, 459–466.

Thomas, J.E., Cascino, T.L. and Earle, J.D. (1985) Differential diagnosis between radiation and tumour plexopathy of the pelvis. *Neurology* **35**, 1–7.

Thomas, P.K. and Tomlinson, D.R. (1993) Diabetic and hypoglycemic neuropathy. In: Dyck, P.J., Thomas, P.K., Griffin, J.W., Low, P.A. and Poduslo, J.F. (eds), *Peripheral Neuropathies*, 3rd edn, pp. 1219–1250. Philadelphia: W.B. Saunders.

Thorleifsson, R., Karlsson, J. and Thorsteinsson, T. (1988) Median nerve entrapment in bone after supracondylar fracture of the humerus. Case report. *Arch. Orthop. Trauma. Surg.* **107**, 183–185.

Thul, J.R. and Hoffman, S.J. (1985) Neuromas associated with tailor's bunion. *J. Foot Surg.* **24**, 342–344.

Thurman, R.T., Jindal, P. and Wolff, T.W. (1991) Ulnar nerve compression in Guyon's canal caused by calcinosis in scleroderma. *J. Hand Surg. [Am.]* **16**, 739–741.

Thyagarajan, D., Cascino, T. and Harms, G. (1995) Magnetic resonance imaging in brachial plexopathy of cancer. *Neurology* **45**, 421–427.

Tingle, A.J., Chantler, J.K., Pot, K.H., Paty, D.W. and Ford, D.K. (1985) Postpartum rubella immunization: association with development of prolonged arthritis, neurological sequelae, and chronic rubella viremia. *J. Infect. Dis.* **152**, 606–612.

Tobin, S.M. (1967) Carpal tunnel syndrome in pregnancy. *Am. J. Obstet. Gynecol.* **97**, 493–498.

Tola, M.R., Granieri, E., Caniatti, L., Paolino, E., Monetti, C., Dovigo, L., Scolozzi, R., De Bastiani, P. and Carreras, M. (1992) Systemic lupus erythematosus presenting with neurological disorders. *J. Neurol.* **239**, 61–64.

Töllner, U., Bechinger, D. and Pohlandt, F. (1980) Radial nerve palsy in a premature infant following long-term measurement of blood pressure. *J. Pediatr.* **96**, 921–922.

Toranto, I.R. (1989) Aneurysm of the median artery causing recurrent carpal tunnel syndrome and anatomic review. *Plast. Reconstr. Surg.* **84**, 510–512.

Touzard, R.C., Maigne, J.Y., Maigne, R. and Doursounian, L. (1989) Douleur de la region trochanterienne par striction canalaire de la branche perforante laterale cutanee du nerf iliohypogastrique. Indications de la neurolyse. [Pain in the trochanteric region caused by tunnel compression of the lateral cutaneous perforating branch of the ilio-hypogastric nerve. Indications for neurolysis.] *Chirurgie* **115**, 287–290.

Tranier, S., Durey, A., Chevallier, B. and Liot, F. (1992) Value of somatosensory evoked potentials in saphenous entrapment neuropathy. *J. Neurol. Neurosurg. Psychiatry* **55**, 461–465.

Trockel, U., Schroder, J.M., Reiners, K.H., Toyka, K.V., Goerz, G. and Freund, H.J. (1983) Multiple exercise-related mononeuropathy with abdominal colic. *J. Neurol. Sci.* **60**, 431–442.

Trojaborg, W. (1970) Rate of recovery in motor and sensory fibres of the radial nerve: clinical and electrophysiological aspects. *J. Neurol. Neurosurg. Psychiatry* **33**, 625–638.

Trojaborg, W. (1976) Motor and sensory conduction in the musculocutaneous nerve. *J. Neurol. Neurosurg. Psychiatry* **39**, 890–899.

Trojaborg, W. and Sindrup, E.H. (1969) Motor and sensory conduction in different segments of the radial nerve in normal subjects. *J. Neurol. Neurosurg. Psychiatry* **32**, 345–359.

Tsai, C.Y., Yu, C.L. and Tsai, S.T. (1996) Bilateral carpal tunnel syndrome secondary to tophaceous compression of the median nerves. *Scand. J. Rheumatol.* **25**, 107–108.

Tsairis, P., Dyck, P.J. and Mulder, D.W. (1972) Natural history of brachial plexus neuropathy. Report on 99 patients. *Arch. Neurol.* **27**, 109–117.

Tulwa, N., Limb, D. and Brown, R.F. (1994) Median nerve compression within the humeral head of pronator teres. *J. Hand Surg. [Br.]* **19**, 709–710.

Turan, I., Lindgren, U. and Sahlstedt, T. (1991) Computed tomography for diagnosis of Morton's neuroma. *J. Foot. Surg.* **30**, 244–245.

Tyrrell, P.J., Feher, M.D., and Rossor, M.N. (1989) Sciatic nerve damage due to toilet seat entrapment: another Saturday night palsy [letter]. *J. Neurol. Neurosurg. Psychiatry* **52**, 1113–1115.

Uchida, Y. and Sugioka, Y. (1990) Ulnar nerve palsy after supracondylar humerus fracture. *Acta Orthop. Scand.* **61**, 118–119.

Uncini, A., Lange, D.J., Solomon, M., Soliven, B., Meer, J. and Lovelace, R.E. (1989) Ring finger testing in carpal tunnel syndrome: a comparative study of diagnostic utility. *Muscle Nerve* **12**, 735–741.

Uncini, A., Di Muzio, A., Awad, J., Manente, G., Tafuro, M. and Gambi, D. (1993) Sensitivity of three median-to-ulnar comparative tests in diagnosis of mild carpal tunnel syndrome. *Muscle Nerve* **16**, 1366–1373.

Ungley, C.C., Channell, G.D. and Richards, R.L. (1945) The immersion foot syndrome. *Br. J. Surg.* **33**, 17–31.

Valer, A., Carrera, L. and Ramirez, G. (1993) Myxoma causing paralysis of the posterior interosseous nerve. *Acta Orthop. Belg.* **59**, 423–425.

van Alfen, N. and van Engelen, B.G.N. (1997) Lumbosacral plexus neuropathy. *Clin. Neurol. Neurosurg.* **99**, 138–141.

van Brakel, W.H. and Khawas, I.B. (1994) Nerve damage in leprosy: an epidemiological and clinical study of 396 patients in west Nepal. Part 1: Definitions, methods and frequencies. *Lepr. Rev.* **65**, 204–221.

van der Heijden, A., Spaans, F. and Reulen, J. (1994) Fasciculation potentials in foot and leg muscles of healthy young adults. *Electroencephalogr. Clin. Neurophysiol.* **93**, 163–168.

Vandertop, W.P. and Bosma, N.J. (1991) The piriformis syndrome. A case report. *J. Bone Joint Surg. [Am.]* **73**, 1095–1097.

Vandertop, W.P. and van't Verlaat, J.W. (1985) Neuropathy of the ulnar nerve caused by an aneurysm of the ulnar artery at the wrist. A case report and review of the literature. *Clin. Neurol. Neurosurg.* **87**, 139–142.

Van Diver, T. and Camann, W. (1995) Meralgia paresthetica in the parturient. *Int. J. Obstetr. Anesth.* **4**, 109–112.

van Eerten, P.V., Polder, T.W. and Broere, C.A. (1995) Operative treatment of meralgia paresthetica: transection versus neurolysis. *Neurosurgery* **37**, 63–65.

van Gijn, J. (1978) The Babinski sign and the pyramidal syndrome. *J. Neurol. Neurosurg. Psychiatry* **41**, 865–873.

van Horssen, N. (1995) Acetylsalicylzuur bij acute en postherpetische neuralgie niet oplossen in chloroform. [Acetylsalicylic acid for acute or post-herpetic neuralgia should not be dissolved in chlorophorm.] *Ned. Tijdschr. Geneeskd.* **139**, 1657.

Vanneste, J.A.L., Butzelaar, R.M.J.M. and Dicke, H.W. (1980) Ischiadic nerve entrapment by an extra- and intrapelvic lipoma: a rare case of sciatica. *Neurology* **30**, 532–534.

van Rossum, J., Buruma, O.J., Kamphuisen, H.A. and Onvlee, G.J. (1978) Tennis elbow – a radial tunnel syndrome? *J. Bone Joint Surg. [Br.]* **60**, 197–198.

van Rossum, J., Kamphuisen, H.A. and Wintzen, A.R. (1980) Management in the carpal tunnel syndrome: clinical and electromyographical follow-up in 62 patients. *Clin. Neurol. Neurosurg.* **82**, 169–176.

van Waalwijk van Doorn, E.S., Remmers, A. and Janknegt, R.A. (1992) Conventional and extramural ambulatory urodynamic testing of the lower urinary tract in female volunteers. *J. Urol.* **147**, 1319–1325.

Varghese, G., Williams, K., Desmet, A. and Redford, J.B. (1991) Nonarticular complication of heterotopic ossification: a clinical review. *Arch. Phys. Med. Rehabil.* **72**, 1009–1013.

Vargo, M.M., Robinson, L.R., Nicholas, J.J. and Rulin, M.C. (1990) Postpartum femoral neuropathy: relic of an earlier era? *Arch. Phys. Med. Rehabil.* **71**, 591–596.

Vastamäki, M. (1986) Decompression for peroneal nerve entrapment. *Acta Orthop. Scand.* **57**, 551–554.

Vastamäki, M. and Göransson, H. (1993) Suprascapular nerve entrapment. *Clin. Orthop.* 135–143.

Vaziri, N.D., Barton, C.H., Ravikumar, G.R., Martin, D.C., Ness, R. and Saiki, J. (1981) Femoral neuropathy: a complication of renal transplantation. *Nephron* **28**, 30–31.

Vecht, C.J., Van de Brand, H.J. and Wajer, O.J. (1989) Post-axillary dissection pain in breast cancer due to a lesion of the intercostobrachial nerve. *Pain* **38**, 171–176.

Venkatesh, S., Kothari, M.J. and Preston, D.C. (1995) The limitations of the dorsal ulnar cutaneous sensory response in patients with ulnar neuropathy at the elbow. *Muscle Nerve* **18**, 345–347.

Venna, N., Bielawski, M. and Spatz, E.M. (1991) Sciatic nerve entrapment in a child. Case report. *J. Neurosurg.* **75**, 652–654.

Verhaar, J. and Spaans, F. (1991) Radial tunnel syndrome. An investigation of compression neuropathy as a possible cause. *J. Bone Joint Surg. [Am.]* **73**, 539–544.

Verhaar, J., Walenkamp, G., Kester, A., van Mameren, H. and van der Linden, T. (1993) Lateral extensor release for tennis elbow. A prospective long-term follow-up study. *J. Bone Joint Surg. [Am.]* **75**, 1034–1043.

Verhagen, W.I., Gabreels-Festen, A.A., van Wensen, P.J., Joosten, E.M., Vingerhoets, H.M., Gabreels, F.J. and de Graaf, R. (1993) Hereditary neuropathy with liability to pressure palsies: a clinical, electroneurophysiological and morphological study. *J. Neurol. Sci.* **116**, 176–184.

Vincent, F.M. and Van, H.R. (1980) Trigeminal sensory neuropathy and bilateral carpal tunnel syndrome: the initial manifestation of mixed connective tissue disease. *J. Neurol. Neurosurg. Psychiatry* **43**, 458–460.

Vital, C., Aubertin, J., Ragnault, J.M., Amigues, H., Mouton, L. and Bellance, R. (1982) Sarcoidosis of the peripheral nerve: a histological and ultrastructural study of two cases. *Acta Neuropathol. Berl.* **58**, 111–114.

Vital, C., Deminiere, C., Lagueny, A., Bergouignan, F.X., Pellegrin, J.L., Doutre, M.S., Clement, A. and Beylot, J. (1988) Peripheral neuropathy with essential mixed cryoglobulinemia: biopsies from 5 cases. *Acta Neuropathol. (Berl.)* **75**, 605–610.

Vodusek, D.B., Janko, M. and Lokar, J. (1983) Direct and reflex responses in perineal muscles on electrical stimulation. *J. Neurol. Neurosurg. Psychiatry* **46**, 67–71.

Vogel, C.M., Albin, R. and Alberts, J.W. (1991) Lotus footdrop: sciatic neuropathy in the thigh. *Neurology* **41**, 605–606.

Vogel, P. and Vogel, H. (1982) Somatosensory cortical potentials evoked by stimulation of leg nerves: analysis of normal values and variability; diagnostic significance. *J. Neurol.* **228**, 97–111.

Vollertsen, R.S., Conn, D.L., Ballard, D.J., Ilstrup, D.M., Kazmar, R.E. and Silverfield, J.C. (1986) Rheumatoid vasculitis: survival and associated risk factors. *Medicine (Baltimore)* **65**, 365–375.

Vorenkamp, S.E. and Nelson, T.L. (1987) Ulnar nerve entrapment due to heterotopic bone formation after a severe burn. *J. Hand Surg. [Am.]* **12**, 378–380.

Vos, L.D., Bom, E.P., Vroegindeweij, D. and Tielbeek, A.V. (1995) Congenital pelvic arteriovenous malformation: a rare cause of sciatica. *Clin. Neurol. Neurosurg.* **97**, 229–232.

Vriesendorp, F.J., Dmytrenko, G.S., Dietrich, T. and Koski, C.L. (1993) Anti-peripheral nerve myelin antibodies and terminal activation products of complement in serum of patients with acute brachial plexus neuropathy. *Arch. Neurol.* **50**, 1301–1303.

Wadsworth, T.G. (1987) Tennis elbow: conservative, surgical, and manipulative treatment. *Br. Med. J. Clin. Res. Ed.* **294**, 621–624.

Wainapel, S.F., Kim, D.J. and Ebel, A. (1978) Conduction studies of the saphenous nerve in healthy subjects. *Arch. Phys. Med. Rehabil.* **59**, 316–319.

Walker, G.L. (1978) Neurological features of polyarteritis nodosa. *Clin. Exp. Neurol.* **15**, 237–247.

Wallach, H.W. and Oren, M.E. (1979) Sciatic nerve compression during anticoagulation therapy. Computerized tomography aids in diagnosis. *Arch. Neurol.* **36**, 448.

Walsh, C. and Walsh, A. (1992) Postoperative femoral neuropathy. *Surg. Gynecol. Obstet.* **174**, 255–263.

Wand, J.S. (1990) Carpal tunnel syndrome in pregnancy and lactation. *J. Hand Surg. [Br.]* **15**, 93–95.

Warndorff, D.K., Glynn, J.R., Fine, P.E., Jamil, S., de Wit, M.Y., Munthali, M.M., Stoker, N.G. and Klatser, P.R. (1996) Polymerase chain reaction of nasal swabs from tuberculosis patients and their contacts. *Int. J. Lepr. Other Mycobact. Dis.* **64**, 404–408.

Warner, M.A., Warner, M.E. and Martin, J.T. (1994) Ulnar neuropathy. Incidence, outcome, and risk factors in sedated or anesthetized patients. *Anesthesiology* **81**, 1332–1340.

Wartenberg, R. (1932) Cheiralgia paraesthetica. *Zentralbl. ges. Neur. Psychiat.* **141**, 145–155.

Waters, M.F. and Jacobs, J.M. (1996) Leprous neuropathies. *Baillière's Clin. Neurol.* **5**, 171–197.

Watson-Jones, R. (1949) Léri's pleonostosis, carpal tunnel compression of the median nerve and Morton's metatarsalgia. *J. Bone Joint Surg. [Br.]* **31**, 560–571.

Weber, E.R., Daube, J.R. and Coventry, M.B. (1976) Peripheral neuropathies associated with total hip arthroplasty. *J. Bone Joint Surg. [Am.]* **58**, 66–69.

Wehnert, M., Timmerman, V., Spoelders, P., Meuleman, J., Nelis, E. and Van Broeckhoven, C. (1997) Further evidence supporting linkage of hereditary neuralgic amyotrophy to chromosome 17q. *Neurology* **48**, 1719–1721.

Weikel, A.M. and Habal, M.B. (1977) Meralgia paresthetica: a complication of iliac bone procurement. *Plast. Reconstr. Surg.* **60**, 572–574.

Weintraub, M.I. (1997) Noninvasive laser neurolysis in carpal tunnel syndrome. *Muscle Nerve* **20**, 1029–1031.

Weinzweig, N. and Browne, E.Z., Jr. (1988) Infraclavicular median nerve compression caused by a lipoma. *Orthopedics* **11**, 1077–1078.

Weiss, A.P., Schenck, R.C., Jr, Sponseller, P.D. and Thompson, J.D. (1992) Peroneal nerve palsy after early cast application for femoral fractures in children. *J. Pediatr. Orthop.* **12**, 25–28.

Weiss, B.D. (1985) Nontraumatic injuries in amateur long distance bicyclists. *Am. J. Sports Med.* **13**, 187–192.

Welti, J.-J., Melekian, B. and Reveillaud, M. (1961) Paralysies périphériques ischémiques (paralysies périphériques provoquées par une embolie artérielle des membres). [Ischaemic peripheral palsies (peripheral palsies resulting from arterial embolism of limbs).] *Presse Méd.* **69**, 333–334.

Werner, C.O. (1979) Lateral elbow pain and posterior interosseous nerve entrapment. *Acta Orthop. Scand.* **174**(Suppl.), 1–62.

Wertsch, J.J. (1985) Pricer palsy [letter]. *N. Engl. J. Med.* **312**, 1645.

Wertsch, J.J. (1992) Anterior interosseous nerve syndrome (AAEM Case Report No. 25). *Muscle Nerve* **15**, 977–983.

White, S.M. and Witten, C.M. (1993) Long thoracic nerve palsy in a professional ballet dancer. *Am. J. Sports Med.* **21**, 626–628.

Widder, S. and Shons, A.R. (1988) Carpal tunnel syndrome associated with extra tunnel vascular compression of the median nerve motor branch. *J. Hand Surg. [Am.]* **13**, 926–927.

Wiederholt, W.C. (1992) Neurologic sequelae of thinking: compression neuropathies caused by a specific posture. *Neurology* **42**, 2223–2224.

Wiezer, M.J., Franssen, H., Rinkel, G.J.E. and Wokke, J.H.J. (1996) Meralgia paraesthetica: differential diagnosis and follow-up. *Muscle Nerve* **19**, 522–524.

Wilberger, J.E., Jr (1983) Lumbosacral radiculopathy secondary to abdominal aortic aneurysms. Report of three cases. *J. Neurosurg.* **58**, 965–967.

Wilbourn, A.J. (1986) AAEE case report No.12: common peroneal mononeuropathy at the fibular head. *Muscle Nerve* **9**, 825–836.

Wilbourn, A.J. and Aminoff, M.J. (1988) The electrophysiologic examination in patients with radiculopathies. *Muscle Nerve* **11**, 1099–1114.

Wilbourn, A.J., Furlan, A.J., Hulley, W. and Ruschhaupt, W. (1983) Ischemic monomelic neuropathy. *Neurology* **33**, 447–451.

Williams, P.H. and Trzil, K.P. (1991) Management of meralgia paresthetica. *J. Neurosurg.* **74**, 76–80.

Winkelmann, R.K., Connolly, S.M. and Doyle, J.A. (1982) Carpal tunnel syndrome in cutaneous connective tissue disease: generalized morphea, lichen sclerosus, fasciitis, discoid lupus erythematosus, and lupus panniculitis. *J. Am. Acad. Dermatol.* **7**, 94–99.

Witt, T.N. and Oberlander, D. (1981) Angeborene beidseitige Hypoplasie der Thenarmuskulatur. [Congenital bilateral hypoplasia of the thenar muscles.] *Nervenarzt* **52**, 484–487.

Witthaut, J., Steffens, K. and Koob, E. (1994) Ungewohnlicher Fall einer Metastase in die Weichteile der Hohlhand mit Kompression des N. medianus und N. ulnaris in Folge eines Nierenkarzinoms. Fallbericht. [An unusual case of metastasis to the soft tissues of the palm of the hand with compression of the median and ulnar nerve by kidney cancer. Case report.] *Handchir. Mikrochir. Plast. Chir.* **26**, 137–140.

Wolf, E., Shochina, M., Fidel, Y. and Gonen, B. (1983) Phrenic neuropathy in patients with diabetes mellitus. *Electromyogr. Clin. Neurophysiol.* **23**, 523–530.

Wolf, S.M., Schotland, D.L. and Phillips, L.L. (1965) Involvement of the nervous system in Behçet's disease. *Arch. Neurol.* **12**, 315–325.

Wolock, B.S., Baugher, W.H. and McCarthy, E.J. (1989) Neurilemoma of the sciatic nerve mimicking tarsal tunnel syndrome – report of a case. *J. Bone Joint Surg. [Am.]* **71**, 932–934.

Woltmann, H.W. and Learmonth, J.R. (1934) Progressive paralysis of the nervus interosseous dorsalis. *Brain* **57**, 25–31.

Wong, K.L., Woo, E.K., Yu, Y.L. and Wong, R.W. (1991) Neurological manifestations of systemic lupus erythematosus: a prospective study. *Q. J. Med.* **81**, 857–870.

Wood, M.J. (1994) Current experience with antiviral therapy for acute herpes zoster. *Ann. Neurol.* **35**(Suppl.), S65–S68.

Wooten, S.L. and McLaughlin, R.E. (1984) Iliacus hematoma and subsequent femoral nerve palsy after penetration of the medical acetabular wall during total hip arthroplasty. Report of a case. *Clin. Orthop.* 221–223.

Worth, R.M., Kettelkamp, D.B., Defalque, R.J. and Duane, K.U. (1984) Saphenous nerve entrapment. A cause of medial knee pain. *Am. J. Sports Med.* **12**, 80–81.

Wouda, E.J. and Vanneste, J.A.L. (1993) Leg pain associated with subgluteal lipoma. *Neurology* **43**, 2149–2150.

Yamout, B., Tayyim, A. and Farhat, W. (1994) Meralgia paresthetica as a complication of laparoscopic cholecystectomy. *Clin. Neurol. Neurosurg.* **96**, 143–144.

Yassini, P.R., Sauter, K., Schochet, S.S., Kaufman, H.H. and Bloomfield, S.M. (1993) Localized hypertrophic mononeuropathy involving spinal roots and associated with sacral meningocele. Case report. *J. Neurosurg.* **79**, 774–778.

Yasuoka, T., Yokota, T. and Tsukagoshi, H. (1993) [Deep peroneal nerve palsy associated with hypothyroidism]. *No. To. Shinkei.* **45**, 563–566.

Yee, W.C., Hahn, A.F., Hearn, S.A. and Rupar, A.R. (1989) Neuropathy in IgM lambda paraproteinemia. Immunoreactivity to neural proteins and chondroitin sulfate. *Acta Neuropathol. Berl.* **78**, 57–64.

Yip, K.M.H., Yurianto, H. and Lin, J. (1997) False aneurysm with median nerve palsy after iatrogenic brachial artery puncture. *Postgrad. Med. J.* **73**, 43–44.

Yoshikawa, H. and Dyck, P.J. (1991) Uncompacted inner myelin lamellae in inherited tendency to pressure palsy. *J. Neuropathol. Exp. Neurol.* **50**, 649–657.

Yoshioka, S., Okuda, Y., Tamai, K., Hirasawa, Y. and Koda, Y. (1993) Changes in carpal tunnel shape during wrist joint motion. MRI evaluation of normal volunteers. *J. Hand Surg. Br.* **18**, 620–623.

Young, A.W., Redmond, M.D. and Belandres, P.V. (1990) Isolated lesion of the lateral cutaneous nerve of the forearm. *Arch. Phys. Med. Rehabil.* **71**, 251–252.

Young, J.N., Friedman, A.H., Harrelson, J.M., Rossitch, E., Jr, Alston, S. and Rozear, M. (1991) Hemangiopericytoma of the sciatic nerve – case report. *J. Neurosurg.* **74**, 512–515.

Young, M.R. and Norris, J.W. (1976) Femoral neuropathy during anticoagulant therapy. *Neurology* **26**, 1173–1175.

Yuan, R.T. and Cohen, M.J. (1985) Lateral antebrachial cutaneous nerve injury as a complication of phlebotomy. *Plast. Reconstr. Surg.* **76**, 299–300.

Yuen, E.C., Olney, R.K. and So, Y.T. (1994) Sciatic neuropathy: clinical and prognostic features in 73 patients. *Neurology* **44**, 1669–1674.

Yuen, E.C., Yuen, T. and Olney, R.K. (1995) The electrophysiologic features of sciatic neuropathy in 100 patients. *Muscle Nerve* **18**, 414–420.

Zahrawi, F. (1984) Acute compression ulnar neuropathy at Guyon's canal resulting from lipoma. *J. Hand Surg. [Am.]* **9**, 238–239.

Zamora, J.L., Rose, J.E., Rosario, V. and Noon, G.P. (1986) Double entrapment of the median nerve in association with PTFE hemodialysis loop grafts. *South. Med. J.* **79**, 638–640.

Zeharia, A., Mukamel, M., Frishberg, Y., Weitz, R. and Mimouni, M. (1990) Benign plexus neuropathy in children. *J. Pediatr.* **116**, 276–278.

Zeuke, W. and Heidrich, R. (1974) Zur Pathogenese der isolierten, postoperativen Lahmung des Nervus musculocutaneus. [Pathogenesis of isolated postoperative paralysis of the musculocutaneous nerve.] *Schweiz. Arch. Neurol. Neurochir. Psychiatr.* **114**, 289–294.

Zingale, A., Consoli, V., Tigano, G., Pero, G. and Albanese, V. (1993) CT morphology of a median nerve neurilemmoma at the arm. Case report and review. *J. Neurosurg. Sci.* **37**, 57–59.

Zook, E.G., Kucan, J.O. and Guy, R.J. (1988) Palmar wrist pain caused by ulnar nerve entrapment in the flexor carpi ulnaris tendon. *J. Hand Surg. Am.* **13**, 732–735.

Zuniga, G., Ropper, A.H. and Frank, J. (1991) Sarcoid peripheral neuropathy. *Neurology* **41**, 1558–1561.

Index

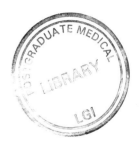